Innovative Therapeutics

Guest Editor

TED ROSEN, MD

DERMATOLOGIC CLINICS

www.derm.theclinics.com

Consulting Editor
BRUCE H. THIERS, MD

July 2010 • Volume 28 • Number 3

SAUNDERS an imprint of ELSEVIER, Inc.

W.B. SAUNDERS COMPANY
A Division of Elsevier Inc.

1600 John F. Kennedy Boulevard • Suite 1800 • Philadelphia, PA 19103-2899

http://www.theclinics.com

DERMATOLOGIC CLINICS Volume 28, Number 3
July 2010 ISSN 0733-8635, ISBN-13: 978-1-4377-2442-4

Editor: Carla Holloway

© **2010 Elsevier Inc. All rights reserved.**

This journal and the individual contributions contained in it are protected under copyright by Elsevier, and the following terms and conditions apply to their use:

Photocopying
Single photocopies of single articles may be made for personal use as allowed by national copyright laws. Permission of the Publisher and payment of a fee is required for all other photocopying, including multiple or systematic copying, copying for advertising or promotional purposes, resale, and all forms of document delivery. Special rates are available for educational institutions that wish to make photocopies for non-profit educational classroom use. For information on how to seek permission visit www.elsevier.com/permissions or call: (+44) 1865 843830 (UK)/(+1) 215 239 3804 (USA).

Derivative Works
Subscribers may reproduce tables of contents or prepare lists of articles including abstracts for internal circulation within their institutions. Permission of the Publisher is required for resale or distribution outside the institution. Permission of the Publisher is required for all other derivative works, including compilations and translations (please consult www.elsevier.com/permissions).

Electronic Storage or Usage
Permission of the Publisher is required to store or use electronically any material contained in this journal, including any article or part of an article (please consult www.elsevier.com/permissions). Except as outlined above, no part of this publication may be reproduced, stored in a retrieval system or transmitted in any form or by any means, electronic, mechanical, photocopying, recording or otherwise, without prior written permission of the Publisher.

Notice
No responsibility is assumed by the Publisher for any injury and/or damage to persons or property as a matter of products liability, negligence or otherwise, or from any use or operation of any methods, products, instructions or ideas contained in the material herein. Because of rapid advances in the medical sciences, in particular, independent verification of diagnoses and drug dosages should be made.

Although all advertising material is expected to conform to ethical (medical) standards, inclusion in this publication does not constitute a guarantee or endorsement of the quality or value of such product or of the claims made of it by its manufacturer.

Dermatologic Clinics (ISSN 0733-8635) is published quarterly by Elsevier Inc., 360 Park Avenue South, New York, NY 10010-1710. Months of publication are January, April, July, and October. Business and editorial offices: 1600 John F. Kennedy Blvd., Suite 1800, Philadelphia, PA 19103-2899. Customer service office: 11830 Westline Drive, St. Louis, MO 63146. Periodicals postage paid at New York, NY, and additional mailing offices. Subscription prices are USD 296.00 per year for US individuals, USD 431.00 per year for US institutions, USD 347.00 per year for Canadian individuals, USD 516.00 per year for Canadian institutions, USD 406.00 per year for international individuals, USD 516.00 per year for international institutions, USD 141.00 per year for US students/residents, and USD 204.00 per year for Canadian and international students/residents. International air speed delivery is included in all *Clinics* subscription prices. All prices are subject to change without notice. **POSTMASTER:** Send address changes to *Dermatologic Clinics*, Elsevier Health Sciences Division, Subscription Customer Service, 3251 Riverport Lane, Maryland Heights, MO 63043. **Customer Service: 1-800-654-2452 (U.S. and Canada); 314-447-8871 (outside U.S. and Canada). Fax: 314-447-8029. E-mail: journalscustomerservice-usa@elsevier.com (for print support); journalsonlinesupport-usa@elsevier.com (for online support).**

Reprints. For copies of 100 or more, of articles in this publication, please contact the Commercial Reprints Department, Elsevier Inc., 360 Park Avenue South, New York, New York 10010-1710. Tel.: (212) 633-3813; Fax: (212) 462-1935; Email: repritns@elsevier.com.

The *Dermatologic Clinics* is covered in *MEDLINE/PubMed (Index Medicus), Current Contents/Clinical Medicine, Excerpta Medica, Chemical Abstracts,* and *ISI/BIOMED*.

Printed and bound by CPI Group (UK) Ltd, Croydon, CR0 4YY
Transferred to Digital Print 2011

Contributors

CONSULTING EDITOR

BRUCE H. THIERS, MD
Professor and Chairman, Department of Dermatology and Dermatologic Surgery, Medical University of South Carolina, Charleston, South Carolina

GUEST EDITOR

TED ROSEN, MD
Professor, Department of Dermatology, Baylor College of Medicine; Chief, Dermatology Services, Michael E. DeBakey VA Medical Center, Houston, Texas

AUTHORS

WILLIAM ABRAMOVITS, MD
Professor of Dermatology, Department of Medicine, Baylor University Medical Center; Assistant Clinical Professor of Dermatology and Family Practice, The University of Texas Southwestern Medical School, Dallas, Texas

NATASHA ATANASKOVA, MD, PhD
Department of Dermatology, Cleveland Clinic Foundation, Cleveland, Ohio

YOON SOO BAE, MD
Department of Dermatology, Boston University School of Medicine, Boston, Massachusetts

TIMOTHY G. BERGER, MD
Department of Dermatology, University of California at San Francisco, San Francisco, California

YUVAL BIBI, MD, PhD
Department of Dermatology, Boston University School of Medicine, Boston, Massachusetts

DAVID R. CARR, MD
Department of Dermatology, Wright State University, Dayton, Ohio

C. STANLEY CHAN, MD
Department of Dermatology, Baylor College of Medicine, Houston, Texas

MENG CHEN, BA
Department of Dermatology, Baylor College of Medicine, Houston, Texas

ARNON D. COHEN, MD, MPH, PhD
Clalit Health Services; Siaal Research Center for Family Medicine and Primary Care, Faculty of Health Sciences, Ben-Gurion University, Beer-Sheva, Israel

SEAN D. DOHERTY, MD
Department of Dermatology, Baylor College of Medicine, Houston, Texas

JACOB DREIHER, MD, MPH
Clalit Health Services; Siaal Research Center for Family Medicine and Primary Care, Faculty of Health Sciences, Ben-Gurion University, Beer-Sheva, Israel

JAMISON D. FERAMISCO, MD, PhD
Department of Dermatology, University of California at San Francisco, San Francisco, California

ADINA FRASIN, MD
Unit of Dermatology, Ospedale A. Manzoni of Lecco, Italy

CARLO GELMETTI, MD
Full Professor, Department of Anesthesia, Intensive Care and Dermatologic Sciences, Università degli Studi di Milano; Head, Unit of Pediatric Dermatology, Fondazione IRCCS Ca' Granda "Ospedale Maggiore Policlinico," Mangiagalli eRegina Elena; Clinica Dermatologica, Milan, Italy

PATRICIA GRANOWSKI, BS
Research Assistant, Dermatology Treatment and Research Center; Neuroscience/BBS/ Pre-Medical; Department of Chemistry, The Research Group of Dr Mihaela Stefan, University of Texas at Dallas, Dallas, Texas

PETER HEALD, MD
Professor Emeritus of Dermatology, Department of Dermatology, Yale University School of Medicine, New Haven, Connecticut

MICHAEL P. HEFFERNAN, MD
Central Dermatology, St Louis, Missouri

NIKKI D. HILL, BSc
Department of Dermatology, Boston University School of Medicine, Boston, Massachusetts

SYLVIA HSU, MD
Professor, Department of Dermatology, Baylor College of Medicine, Houston, Texas

HAYDEE M. KNOTT, MD
Resident Physician, Cleveland Clinic, Department of Dermatology, Cleveland, Ohio

ANDREW N. LIN, MD, FRCPC
Associate Professor, Division of Dermatology and Cutaneous Sciences, University of Alberta, Edmonton, Alberta, Canada

JOSÉ DARÍO MARTÍNEZ, MD, IFAAD
Chief, Internal Medicine and Dermatology, Internal Medicine Clinic, University Hospital, University Autonomus of Nuevo León, Colonia Mitras Centro, Monterrey, Nuevo León, Mexico

JONI MAZZA, MA
Department of Dermatology, St Luke's-Roosevelt Hospital Center and Beth Israel Medical Center; Medical Student, Weill Cornell Medical College, New York, New York

BRIAN POLIGONE, MD, PhD
Assistant Professor of Dermatology and Oncology, Department of Dermatology; James P. Wilmot Cancer Center, University of Rochester School of Medicine, Rochester, New York

DEEPANI RATHNAYAKE, MD
Fellow, Department of Dermatology, St Vincent's Hospital Melbourne, Fitzroy, Melbourne, Victoria, Australia

LUCIA RESTANO, MD
Unit of Pediatric Dermatology, Fondazione IRCCS Ca' Granda "Ospedale Maggiore Policlinico," Mangiagalli eRegina Elena, Milan, Italy

TED ROSEN, MD
Professor, Department of Dermatology; Chief, Dermatology Services, Michael E. DeBakey VA Medical Center, Baylor College of Medicine, Houston, Texas

ANTHONY ROSSI, MD
Dermatology Resident, Department of Dermatology, St Luke's-Roosevelt Hospital Center and Beth Israel Medical Center, New York, New York

FAREESA SHUJA, MD
Department of Dermatology, Baylor College of Medicine, Houston, Texas

RODNEY SINCLAIR, MBBS, MD, FACD
Director, Dermatology Research, St Vincent's Hospital Melbourne; Professor, Department of Medicine, University of Melbourne; Skin and Cancer Foundation, Victoria, Australia

MARTIN STEINHOFF, MD, PhD
Department of Dermatology, University of California at San Francisco, San Francisco, California

KENNETH J. TOMECKI, MD
Department of Dermatology, Cleveland Clinic Foundation, Cleveland, Ohio

JEFFREY M. WEINBERG, MD
Director, Clinical Research Center, Department of Dermatology, St Luke's-Roosevelt Hospital Center and Beth Israel Medical Center; Associate Clinical Professor of Dermatology, Columbia University, New York, New York

V.E. GOTTFRIED WOZEL, MD
Professor, Department of Dermatology, University Hospital Carl Gustav Carus, Technical University of Dresden, Dresden, Germany

CATHERINE M. ZIP, MD
Clinical Associate Professor, Division of Dermatology, University of Calgary, Calgary, Alberta, Canada

Contents

Dermatologic Clinics

FORTHCOMING ISSUES

October 2010

Vulvar Dermatologic Disease
Libby Edwards, MD,
Guest Editor

January 2011

Tropical Dermatology
Scott Norton, MD and
Aisha Sethi, MD,
Guest Editors

April 2011

Oncologic Surgery in Dermatology
Allison Vidimos,
Guest Editor

RECENT ISSUES

April 2010

Epidermolysis Bullosa: Part II – Diagnosis and Management
Dédée F. Murrell, MA, BMBCh, FAAD, MD,
Guest Editor

January 2010

Epidermolysis Bullosa: Part I – Pathogenesis and Clinical Features
Dédée F. Murrell, MA, BMBCh, FAAD, MD,
Guest Editor

October 2009

Cosmetic Dermatology
Vic A. Narurkar, MD, FAAD,
Guest Editor

RELATED INTEREST

Dermatologic Clinics April 2007 (Vol. 25, Issue 2)
Drug Actions, Reactions, and Interactions
James Q. Del Rosso, DO, FAOCD, *Guest Editor*
www.derm.theclinics.com

THE CLINICS ARE NOW AVAILABLE ONLINE!

Access your subscription at:
www.theclinics.com

Preface
Innovative Therapeutics

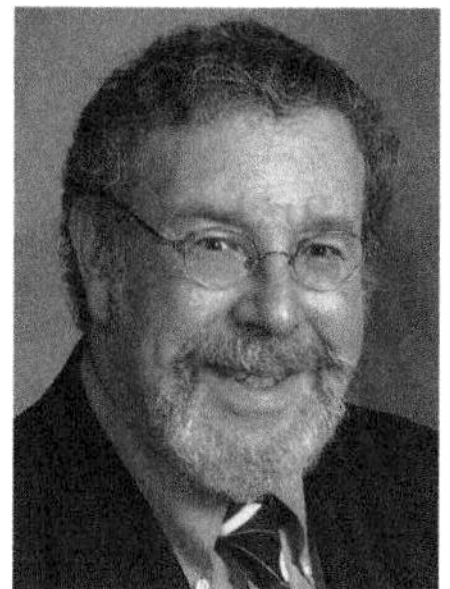

Ted Rosen, MD
Guest Editor

Many disorders presenting to the dermatologist are generally well managed, using widely accepted therapeutic regimens and employing one or more of sundry medications or devices that are approved by the US Food and Drug Administration for the indication at hand. Conversely, we are often presented with exceptions to this rule. Some common diseases may prove frustratingly refractory to first- or second-line interventions. Pruritus and furunculosis are good examples of this phenomenon. Other maladies are routinely difficult to control under the best of circumstances. Hidradenitis suppprativa and severe hand eczema exemplify the latter situation. Still other problems are considered to be quite manageable but require, with some degree of regularity, a modicum of out-of-the-box thinking; for example, lupus erythematosus. For this issue, I have invited well-known expert clinicians to offer pragmatic approaches to these varying situations.

Dermatological treatment is also constantly evolving, both with the steady advent of newly approved agents (ie, topical calcineurin inhibitors, rituximab, and TNF-alpha blockers) and via the incessant "reinvention" of older drugs. The latter involves discovery of novel uses for seemingly antique agents, largely facilitated by a better understanding of known and theoretical mechanisms of action. So it is that dapsone, thalidomide, spironolactone, and pharmacologic doses of zinc continue to find ever-expanding roles in our armamentarium. I have invited another set of authors to address selected therapeutic agents, both old and new. Hopefully, their articles will reveal ways to help you utilize these drugs more effectively.

Finally, I have requested a distinguished clinician-investigator to provide an update on new ways to manage cases in pediatric-aged individuals—our most vulnerable patients, often with vexing disorders.

You will notice that the titles of most of the articles included herein contain the word "innovative." That is neither an accident nor a coincidence. The purpose of this issue is to emphasize the inventive, and frequently creative, ways in which dermatologists provide highly cost-effective treatment for those who entrust their cutaneous health to us. Dermatology has a long and storied history of combining solid basic research, translational trials, and common sense ingenuity to enhance our collective ability to alleviate suffering. This is true globally, as attested to by the many scholarly manuscripts prepared by the international authors included in this issue of the *Dermatologic Clinics*. If nothing else, this issue is a vivid reminder of the ongoing, positive contributions a relatively small specialty can make to health care.

I would like to thank you for reading some, or all, of this volume. I would also like to express my appreciation to the authors and coauthors whose selfless dedication to education and to patient care made this issue possible. Without their expertise and skill, the pages that follow would never have happened!

Ted Rosen, MD
Department of Dermatology
Baylor College of Medicine
6620 Main Street, Suite 1425
Houston, TX 77030, USA

E-mail address:
vampireted@aol.com

Dermatol Clin 28 (2010) xiii
doi:10.1016/j.det.2010.03.016
0733-8635/10/$ – see front matter © 2010 Elsevier Inc. All rights reserved.

Innovative Management of Severe Hand Dermatitis

William Abramovits, MD[a,b,*], Patricia Granowski, BS[c,d]

KEYWORDS

• Evaluation • Management • Quality of life • Hand dermatitis

Severe HD is pragmatically defined as that which does not respond to simple preventive measures, barrier repair and protection, topical steroids, or brief courses of systemic steroids, or that which recurs rapidly after the foregoing measures are tapered or discontinued, having protracted episodes and a chronic, relapsing course. Intuitively, severe hand dermatitis (HD) also has lesion-related symptoms that limit function and adversely affect the quality of life (QoL).

HD is a comprehensive term that, for the purpose of this review, encompasses all skin inflammatory disorders involving the hands. It includes hand eczema (HE) and a long list of inflammatory dermatoses ranging from atopic dermatitis (AD) and psoriasis to other reactions, many of external causation, such as allergic and irritant contact dermatitis (ICD), infections, and reactions of internal etiology such as drug eruptions, auto and heteroimmunity conditions.

In this article, the term HE is reserved for the clinical syndrome characterized by pruritus, pale erythematous to violaceous hues, scaling, vesiculation or bulla formation, erosion, exudation and crusting, lichenification, fissuring, and excoriation, that typically results in a genetically determined faulty barrier function plus a dysregulated response of the immune system to common antigens, often involving immunoglobin E (IgE), predominantly affecting the hands. A connection between the filaggrin gene and HE is questionable.[1,2]

There are several ways to classify HD, most reflect the pathogenesis or the clinical pattern. Classification schemes address extrinsic aspects of contact dermatitis (CD) such as nonallergic, irritant, nutritional, physical or chemical burns, and allergic CD (ACD) to intrinsic factors (genetic or inherited, metabolic, age related, neoplastic, dyskeratotic or acantholytic, autoimmune), and infectious causes as well as multifactorial conditions such as psoriasis, pityriasis rubra pilaris, AD, PsEmA (psoriasis/eczema overlap syndrome), lichen planus, and reactive arthritis.[3–9]

Patterns involving specific selected areas of the hands, such as dorsal, ventral (palmar or volar), junctional (webs, finger sides, and canthal), and miscellaneous (ring, pulpitic, apron, lenticular, unilateral, and onychial), may be sufficiently characteristic as to suggest a diagnosis. Allergic reactions to ingredients in protective gloves are often limited to the back of the hands and wrists; isolated lesions localized to the fingertips of the dominant hand suggest acrylate allergy (particularly in dental personnel), plant or vegetable dermatitis, or chromate allergy.[10–14] Changing patterns, such as webs to fingertips or volar to dorsal, should alert the physician to consider patch testing.

Other classifications use signs that best correlate with the natural history of HD, dividing it into

[a] Department of Medicine, Baylor University Medical Center, Dallas, TX, USA
[b] The University of Texas Southwestern Medical School, Dallas, TX, USA
[c] Dermatology Treatment & Research Center, 5310 Harvest Hill Road, Suite 160, Dallas, TX 75230-5808, USA
[d] Neuroscience/BBS/Pre-Medical and Department of Chemistry, The Research Group of Dr Mihaela Stefan, University of Texas at Dallas, Dallas, TX, USA
* Corresponding author. Dermatology Treatment & Research Center, 5310 Harvest Hill Road, Suite 160, Dallas, TX 75230.
E-mail address: dra@dermcenter.us

Dermatol Clin 28 (2010) 453–465
doi:10.1016/j.det.2010.03.001
0733-8635/10/$ – see front matter © 2010 Elsevier Inc. All rights reserved.

acute, subacute, or chronic. These may be differentiated into wet, intermediate, dry, and less common/harder to categorize. Wet typically corresponds with acute, oozing, macerated, ulcerated, excoriated, pompholyx (dishydrotic), or relapsing forms. Dry typically corresponds to scaly, hyperkeratotic, or lichenified, usually chronic forms. Less common/harder to categorize may correspond with follicular, pustular, bullous, ulcerative, purpuric, lichenoid, dyspigmented, and erythema exsudativum multiforme-like, eruptions.[11,14–20]

Dyshidrotic eczema (DE) or pompholyx merits separate attention. DE is a chronic, recurrent HD characterized by flares that start as tiny, tense, pruritic vesicles that may coalesce into large blisters and evolve into pustular lesions usually affecting the palms and volar and lateral aspects of the fingers. Although DE may be totally idiopathic, it may be associated with underlying atopy, contactants, and fungal or bacterial infection with hypersensitivity.[21,22]

EPIDEMIOLOGY

The most frequent causes of HD include soap, plain water, detergents, solvents, acidic and alkaline agents, repeated friction, mechanical abrasion, thermal trauma, exposure to metals, fragrances, preservatives, food proteins, animal dander, rubber, and latex proteins. Less common/unusual causes recently reported include white-stemmed gum moth, cercaria, shiitake mushroom, hydrangea, aspen bark, henna, hop, phytophotodermatitis, pierced ears and tongue, radiation, photoallergic eczema, posttraumatic eczema, drugs, topical steroid allergy and dependence, quaternium-15, newer biocides used as preservatives, parvovirus, and Papillon-Lefevre syndrome.[8,13,23–44] Additional rare factors include asparagus, artichokes, *Paeonia* (peony), melamide formaldehyde resins (in a plywood worker), and a case of contact uticaria from raw potatoes.[45–49] Although often implicated as causing or aggravating factor, smoking was recently found to be not clearly associated in a study involving 13,452 individuals.[50]

In a retrospective study of 714 consecutive individuals with HD, the precise etiologic diagnosis of HE was not distinguishable by clinical pattern, prevalence of personal atopy, or nickel sensitivity.[51]

During systemic treatment of cancer, methotrexate, 6-mercaptopurine, carbamazepine, multikinase inhibitors like sorafenib and sunitinib, and inhibitors of vascular endothelium growth factor signal transduction (eg, monoclonal antibodies bevacizumab and ranibizumab) may all produce a painful hand-foot syndrome requiring awareness by physicians caring for patients at risk.[52,53]

HD represents 20% to 25% of all cases of eczematous dermatitis seen by dermatologists[54] and 20% to 35% of all dermatitis affects the hands.[55]

QOL

Effective therapy is needed because HD significantly affects QoL. Pertinent issues include occupational, domestic, social, psychological, and economic factors. Major livelihood changes, like job transfers, may not lead to QoL improvements, and substantially increase cost of care. One study found that medical costs translated to $70 per patient per month; a burden that may be an underestimation when adjusted for inflation and the omission of over-the-counter drugs and indirect expenses.[56] In another study, the highest number of claims due to HD from latex gloves came from nurses (30.8%), nursing aides and orderlies (24.6%), dental assistants (13.8%), clinical laboratory technicians (9.2%), and institutional maids/housemen (4.6%). By contrast, food preparers, laundry workers, therapists, general office clerks, private household cleaners, cooks, and personal service occupations filed the fewest claims. The average claim cost was $8309.48.[57] Preventing exposure to noxious chemicals is recommended to reduce claims and facilitate healing from occupation-related skin diseases of the hands.[58]

Patients from the Danish National Board of Industrial Injuries Registry with newly recognized occupational HE (OHE) were assessed with 1-year follow-ups. Underlying AD, age greater than 40 years and a low socioeconomic status at baseline were predictors of severe OHE, prolonged sick leave, and job loss.[59] Substantially greater severity was observed among those with irritant occupational CD and AD. Prolonged sick leave because of OHE was reported by 19.9% of patients and was associated with AD. Severe OHE occurred more often among those in food-related occupations (27.2%) compared with those in wet (20.1%) and other occupations (16.5%).[60] Persons with childhood AD had a significantly increased risk for job change (9% of the cases vs 2% of controls) and sick leave (10% vs 2%), both being related to HD.[61]

CD has a significant effect on emotional well-being when it affects the hands or face, or interferes with normal occupation. Itching, irritation, and chronicity are most bothersome. Patients who elect to change jobs because of their skin condition report significantly worse QoL than those who do not.[62] CD and HE are associated with impaired health-related QoL. Early diagnosis and intervention are associated with QoL improvements. Contradicting reports exist where disease duration, AD, age, and gender do not seem to have significant effects.[63]

Among hospital employees self-reporting HD, 75% observed symptom worsening in direct relation to work, 79% improved during leisure time, and 48% declared psychological distress from their lesions.[64]

High subjective reactions (high-SR) to stress correlated with high HD severity and depression scores, more itching, and life events. High-SR subgroups were younger and had earlier onset of HD. Those with high-SR but negative patch-test results recorded significantly higher values for itching, helplessness, and search for information, suggesting a greater need for adjunctive mental health intervention and psychological care.[65] Chronicity in ICD is an initiator of emotional, physical, and financial stress. The hardening phenomenon is a questionable and poorly understood part of the healing process in HD; elucidating it should lead to better treatments.[66]

DIAGNOSTIC TECHNIQUES

Diagnostic methods include appropriate direct examinations and cultures to exclude bacterial, fungal, and viral causes. Biopsies for routine histology or immunofluorescence and special stains, confocal microscopy, and other imaging techniques, when necessary, may help characterize HD. Extensive or focused patch testing remains the gold standard to identify responsible antigens. A comprehensive occupational and recreational history may identify irritant exposures.

SEVERITY ASSESSMENTS

The Hand Eczema Severity Index (HECSI) was developed in response to a need for a standardized clinical grading system, mostly for research purposes. Agreement for inter- and intraobserver reliability was achieved, but the inclusion of patient-rated symptoms is suggested to add value to this tool.[67] A severity assessment tool developed for palmar eczema collated 3 standardized tools (the global assessment of severity, a standard eczema severity scale (grading erythema, edema/induration/papulation, excoriation, oozing/weeping, scaling, and lichenification), and a scale that integrates body surface area, course, and itch) and gave a near-linear score distribution without end clustering, suggesting that it is accurate.[68]

Differences between self-rated severity (visual analog scale [VAS], 0–10) and The Danish National Board of Industrial Injury severity rating based on morphology, extent of eczema, and frequency of eruptions, suggest that researchers should include ratings from patients and physicians.[69] A guide composed of 5 severity levels, with 4 photographs per level, showed high interrater reliability and test-retest reproducibility.[70] Asking "Do you have hand eczema?" had a higher sensitivity and specificity than grading erythema, papules or vesicles, scaling, and fissuring/lichenification.[71]

Patients with HE were followed for 6 months from their first visit to identify factors associated with severe initial disease and poor prognosis using the HECSI and a self-administered photographic guide; overall improvement occurred by 6 months, but many symptoms remained noteworthy. Older age, AD, frequent flares, and being an unskilled worker (presumably exposed to sundry irritants or allergens) were predictors of a poor prognosis.[72]

PATCH TESTING

Patch testing is an effective and relevant method for determining the cause of allergic reactions. Patch testing with ammonia-preserved natural rubber latex (NRL) identifies patients in whom delayed-type hypersensitivity needs to be differentiated from IgE type 1 response.[73] The addition of methyldibromo glutaronitrile, a preservative in liquid soaps and cosmetics, to the European standard patch test resulted in its ban after many cases of HD attributable to it were detected.[74]

A study that patch tested 644 patients with suspected textile-induced ACD identified a typical distribution pattern that included areas of friction on the trunk and extremities, with the hands being affected less frequently. Allergic reactions to dye or resin were experienced by 12.9% of those patients. The highest incidence of sensitization was from disperse blue (DB) (30.6%), DB 106 (27%), DB 85 (8.1%), and melamine formaldehyde (20.7%). In the resin group, ethyleneurea melamine formaldehyde (20.7%) and urea formaldehyde (18.3%) caused the most reactions.[16]

A patch-tested population that included students, farmers, housewives engaged in farming, laborers, paramedical workers, salesmen, teachers, and photographers, with pompholyx, revealed 40% of subjects reacting to 1 or more allergens; nickel sulfate was the most common (14%), followed by potassium dichromate, phenylenediamine and dinitrofurazone (8%), fragrance mix (FM; 6%), and cobalt chloride (4%).[75]

Among patch-test–positive gold allergic individuals, total avoidance of gold jewelry on hands and wrists benefited a subgroup with facial and eyelid dermatitis who wore powder, eye shadow, or foundation on those areas. Titanium dioxide may adsorb gold particles from jewelry.[76]

Patch testing patients with discoid eczema found hands and feet (44%), hands and forearms (30%), legs and feet (12%), and trunk and limbs (12%) to be the most common distribution patterns. Potassium dichromate, (20%) was followed by nickel, (16%) cobalt chloride, and fragrances (12%) as the most common allergens.[77]

Comparing the FM in the European standard series with a novel selection of 14 fragrance allergens to which hand exposure would likely occur, 10.2% of 658 consecutive HD patients reacted to at least 1 allergen; the most common reactions to fragrances not in the FM series were to citral, hydroxyisohexyl-3-cyclohexene carboxaldehyde, and 1-limonene; more than half would have been missed by the FM.[78]

Compositae dermatitis is 1 of the top 10 contact sensitivities in Europe with a prevalence of 0.7% to 1.4% in the general population. Patch testing with sesquiterpene lactone mix, Compositae extracts screening mix, and Compositae plant extract is recommended.[79] Because of the frequency of positive responses and an annual increase in propolis allergy, it is recommended that it be excluded from topical products used by children.[80]

The hands were the most frequently affected area in 82% of 281 packing station and field workers evaluated by physical examination, standard patch tests, and pesticide patch tests. Reactions to chlorothalonil (51.4%), thiabendazole (12.8%), imazalil (10.2%), and aluminum hydroxide (10.2%) were the most common.[81]

Contact hypersensitivity was less common in patients with HD than in those without (46.7% vs 63.2% respectively) among 105 consecutive adult HD patients (vs 361 suspected nonhand ACD) patch tested. Irritant factors may explain these results.[82]

In summary, several common allergens have been identified and should be sought as a cause of HD in patients who have an occupation or lifestyle that could conceivably place them at high risk for ACD. Randomly chosen patients with HD who undergo extensive patch testing may occasionally be found to have a reversible exposure to an unsuspected allergen.

OCCUPATION

Professions reported to have an increased risk of developing HD include hairdressers; musicians; food industry, agricultural, factory, and electronics workers; cleaners/washers and housekeepers; printers; builders; and medical and dental personnel. Estimates of HD in individuals with work-related skin diseases ranged from 80% to 88% in the 1980s, although recent figures suggest a decrease to 10% to 15%.[83–86] Biocides are frequent hand irritants in medicine, agriculture and forestry, and industry.[24]

The hands were the primary body part affected in 64% of ACD cases and 80% of ICD among 5839 patients who were patch tested. Frequently encountered allergens include carba mix, thiuram mix, epoxy resin, formaldehyde, and nickel.[87] ACD and ICD of the hands were work related in 16.5% and 44.4% of 360 consecutive health care workers with HCD.[88] Among 59 workers with HE, 72.8% had positive patch tests, 30.5% of which had a strong relationship to occupation; significantly less than was observed with other types of eczema (55% of 160 patients). The rate of atopic history did not differ.[21] Among electronic workers, HD was found most frequently with wafer bonding, cutting, printing/photomasking, softening/degluing, impregnation, and tin plating; 35.5% had ICD and 3.8% ACD.[89]

HD was associated with contact allergy to epoxy resin among 325 patch-tested workers in the wind turbine industry. Although women washed their hands more often and used more moisturizers/protection creams at work than men, no gender differences were found.[27] This suggests that some common-sense maneuvers may not be effective at preventing HD or HE, even when clear-cut exposures are identified. Among 1355 metal workers, of whom 96.7% were men, implementation and acceptance of recommended skin protection at a German factory was shown to be low, even though barrier creams and moisturizers were highly recommended as a potentially effective means to prevent dermatitis.[90]

Prolonged or repeated contact with gasoline caused hyperkeratosis, dryness, onychosis, fissuring, and dermatitis among 52 exposed workers in a matched epidemiologic study in the solvent industry.[91] Prevalence of nickel allergy among older female hairdressers, who use scissors and crochet hooks, was higher than among younger individuals, probably as result of regulations to exclude nickel from such instruments.[92] In large cohort studies that included a clinical examination, the prevalence of HD among hairdressers was 16.4%, compared with 80% in smaller questionnaire-based studies.[93] Among 209 hairdressers, paraphenylenediamine caused the greatest number of positive patch tests, followed by paratoluenediamine sulfate, monthioglycolate, and ammonium persulphate.[94] Total avoidance of these materials is difficult because they are essential to the hairdressing trade.

HD was more prevalent in intensive care unit (ICU) nurses (65%) than among in-patient clinic nurses (50%) at a hospital in the United States.[95] Twelve-month prevalence data (from a self-reporting questionnaire) showed a correlation between history of allergic rash, increased hand washing, and HD, in a cohort of 148 Australian hospital nurses. The period prevalence was higher than in other reports.[96] The rate of HD among Chinese nursing students was similar to that of their Japanese counterparts, but higher than that of nursing students from Germany, Holland, and Australia.[97]

In the dental vocation, among 107 nurses examined, 29 cases of ACD, 15 of contact urticaria, and 12 of ICD, were found. Rubber chemicals, NRL in protective gloves, and methacrylates (dental-restorative materials) were the most common causes of allergy.[98] In a recent questionnaire-based investigation, 17.4% of Norwegian orthodontists reported occupational dermatoses of the hands and fingers (vs 40% in 1987), a reduction explained by changes in hygiene factors such as soaps and detergents, as biomaterial-related reactions persisted unchanged.[99] Prospective data from the National Board of Industrial Industry Registry and a self-administered questionnaire found OHE as a result of ICD to be the most frequent work-related disease in Denmark. The prevalence of AD was low (16.4%) and men had a greater rate of ACD. OHE occurred frequently among bakers, hairdressers, and dental surgery assistants.[100]

Hand and mouth dermatitis among musicians was most frequent in string and wind instrument players; colophony, exotic woods, nickel sulfate, varnishes, and propolis (bee glue) were the most common allergens.[101] As with hairdressers, total avoidance of true allergens might be difficult for those who must come in contact with these materials to play their instruments.

CD is common among beekeepers, due to allergy to propolis, an ingredient in some toothpastes, ointments, and cosmetics.[102] The most frequent hand problems in paddy field workers were nail dystrophy, paronychia, and hyperkeratosis, 73% reporting work-related itch.[103] Repetitive trauma to the hands caused nodules and plaques in 150 carpet weavers.[104]

RISK FACTORS

Of 50 consecutive patients with HE, most had a personal history of atopy; 58% had known contact allergy, 67.4% hay fever, 25.6% asthma, 82% other eczema/dermatitis, 44% fungal infection, and 52% familial atopy.[68] AD and contact allergy were confirmed as important risk factors for HE but did not adequately account for the aggregation. HE in a population-based study involving 1076 individual twins suggests an unrecognized independent genetic risk factor.[105] Skin atopy, previous HD, and flexural dermatitis were predictive for the development of HD. By contrast, there was no association with respiratory atopy among food industry apprentices suffering HD.[106] Among 59 workers with DE, 72.8% had positive patch tests and 30.5% a strong relationship to occupation, much less than with other types of eczema (55% of 160 patients); the rate of atopic history did not differ.[21] A perplexing relapsing case of HD after connubial contact between husband and wife with the same occupation (gardening) is described.[33]

In a retrospective study of 3000 individuals from the general Swedish population, there was no gender difference in the incidence rates of HE in those older than 30 years. Female sex, childhood eczema, and asthma/hay fever were associated with HE in those less than 30 years.[107] HD in psoriasis occurred with similar frequency in men and women, and a higher number of female patients had HE in an analysis of treatment practices in a dermatology outpatient clinic. More frequent and intense therapy was provided to men; women used more topical preparations.[108]

The retrospective analysis of a patch-tested population at a dermatologic referral clinic found that 32% had HD, 56% of it was occupational, 54.4% allergic, and 27.4% irritant. Among women, the prevalence of ACD remained constant between the ages of 21 and 60 years, whereas ICD peaked in the third decade; the prevalence of ICD and ACD peaked in the fifth decade for men.[109] Among 502 (458 men, 44 women) patch-test–negative subjects, analyzed retrospectively, 8.8% had adult-onset AD, and the hands were the most frequently affected area; 5.6% were pure adult-onset, whereas 3.2% had prior contact sensitization.[110]

LABORATORY

Laboratory evaluations may be used to measure the effect of various media that can cause sensitization of hand skin. The release of cobalt, nickel, and chromium from hard metal alloys was tested in cobalt-sensitized patients; cobalt concentration was high enough to generate ACD in sensitized patients. Because the materials in the discs are used in wear parts of hard metal tools, individuals with contact allergy to cobalt can develop HE when handling them.[111]

Manipulation tests simulating everyday coin handling provide a reliable means to evaluate contamination. The introduction of the Euro has led to a decrease in nickel exposure; coins are now an unlikely cause of nickel allergy, unless a simultaneous increase in copper exposure causes synergistic sensitization.[112] A newly designed, more reliable method of quantifying nickel on the skin in occupationally exposed individuals consists in immersing thumbs and indexes into tubes containing ultrapure water.[113] In 15 patients with patch-test–positive eczema to a given fragrance, there was no concordance between immersion in a solution containing the fragrance and patch-test results.[114]

African American skin proved superior to White skin in terms of barrier function, stratum corneum disruption, and presence of parakeratosis and spongiosis in a study of ICD on hands evaluated by confocal microscopy, fluorescence, and transepidermal water loss.[115]

THERAPY

In all cases, a thorough exploration of environmental factors, many of which were discussed earlier, is appropriate. The trigger of HD, when known from a carefully obtained history and dermatologic examination, should be addressed first, be it by discontinuing a drug or contactant, or by treating a specific cause. When the trigger is not known, or the condition does not respond to conventional therapy, a series of steps must be considered.

Prevention

Regardless of HD type, education and lifestyle modification are essential. Measures contributing to a successful treatment include avoidance of irritants, use of protective gloves, application of protective creams and foams, appropriate moisturization, and use of barrier-restorative materials. Some oil-containing lotions or barrier creams help to protect the hands against dryness, chemical irritation, and skin breakdown.[116–118]

Through the implementation of an evidence-based prevention program that included frequent use of protective gloves, cotton gloves worn underneath rubber or plastic gloves, and increased discussion of skin problems, the frequency of HE at a European factory was significantly reduced from 56.2% at baseline to 41.0% at the 1-year follow up.[119] HD symptoms can be diminished by reducing the exposure to irritants through training, frequent but short-duration hypoallergenic glove use, and limited hand washing with soap.[120]

A guideline from the Centers for Disease Control and Prevention promotes alcohol-based hand rubs containing emollients instead of irritating soaps and detergents to reduce skin damage, dryness, and irritation. Frequency of ICD was highest with preparations containing 4% chlorhexidine gluconate, less with nonantimicrobial soaps, and least with alcohol-based hand rubs containing emollients. Washing after application of an alcohol-based hand rub is not recommended.[121] A summary of the evidence justifying recommendations of glove occlusion during wet activities and of alcohol rub as the preferred hand disinfectant is available.[122] Another article reviews hand-hygiene practices emphasizing promotion programs and provides guidelines for hand antisepsis for health care workers.[123]

Hand contact dermatitis (HCD) usually results from exposures to monomers and additives in the occupational setting. Resin- and additive-induced direct CD usually affects the hands, fingers, and forearms, whereas indirect exposure affects the face and neck. Industrial hygiene prevention techniques are essential when handling resin systems.[124]

The low irritation index (IrIn) of some soaps and cleansers was established for White Dove, Dove Baby, Dove liquid cleanser for hands, Dove Pink (Lever Pond's, Toronto, Ontario, Canada), Cetaphil bar (Galderma Laboratory, Forth Worth, TX, USA), and Aderma (Pierre Fabre, Dermo-Cosmetique, Boulagne, France). Camay Classic (Procter & Gamble, Cincinnati, OH, USA) had the lowest IrIn.[125] Prevention of HD with general skin protective measures seems to be more effective than UV light hardening.[126]

Topical Agents

Corticosteroids remain first-line agents for HD. Topical calcineurin inhibitors have been studied for chronic eczematous skin diseases, and are particularly favored to treat the dorsal aspect of the hands, and as steroid-sparing agents. Recently introduced device creams for eczema, containing glycyrrhetinic acid and telmesteine or palmitoylethanolamide, alginate, and trolamine, await testing to prove their value in HD. Refractory chronic pruritic eruptions hydrated for 20 minutes before bedtime followed by the application of mid- to high-strength corticosteroids led to clearing or dramatic symptom improvement in a retrospective study of 28 patients.[127]

Statistically significant improvement is obtained in mild to moderate and moderate to severe chronic HD with pimecrolimus 1% cream applied twice daily under occlusion. Pimecrolimus blood concentrations remain below the limit of quantitation.[128] Most patients with hand and foot dermatitis improved significantly in erythema, scaling, induration, fissuring, and pruritus with tacrolimus 0.1% ointment applied to affected areas 3 times daily for 8 weeks.[129–131]

Bexarotene gel was well tolerated and showed a good clinical effect in an open-label randomized study of 55 patients comparing its use alone versus in combination with low- and midpotency corticosteroids.[132] Alitretinoin also seems promising for refractory HD.[133]

Botulinum toxin may be an alternative or an adjunctive therapy for vesicular eczema. In 39% of patients with pompholyx, itch improvement occurred on the treated side (compared with a 52% increase in symptoms on the untreated side). A mean decrease in Dyshidrotic Eczema Area and Severity Index (DASI) from 36 to 3 on the hand treated with topical corticosteroids plus intradermal botulinum (compared with a mean decrease from 28 to17 with topical therapy alone) was reported in another study.[134,135]

Ionizing Radiation

Radiation therapy is often mentioned as useful in reviews on HE treatment.[136] A comprehensive review of past studies using superficial x-rays and grenz rays, revealed contradictory findings.[137] Of a subgroup of patients treated with grenz rays for CD (94% of them with HD), 64% stated that such radiation was worthwhile and 77% would choose it again if needed.[138] Megavoltage equipment producing low-dose external beam radiation was used to induce long-term remission in a patient for whom conventional treatments, including systemic steroids, failed.[139] Although few dermatologists still offer ionizing radiation therapy in the ambulatory setting, this modality is available in hospitals or medical centers.

Nonionizing Radiation

Topical and systemic psoralen combined with ultraviolet A irradiation (PUVA) has been used to treat patients with different forms of HD. UVA-psoralen gel is a potentially less expensive alternative to PUVA bath therapy in severe recalcitrant palmar-plantar dermatoses.[140]

Preliminary results using 308-nm excimer laser light suggests its efficacy and safety in the treatment of HD. The palmar-plantar pustular form did better than plaque-type, chronic atopic, and non-AD.[141]

A prospective open study of 30 patients with chronic hand dermatoses treated with hand UVB-TL01 found that psoriatics responded best; 9 of 11 patients improved after 20 to 38 treatments (compared with 11 of 16 patients with eczema who improved after 11–31 treatments).[142]

UVA-1 irradiation for DE was superior to placebo, assessed by DASI and VAS, after 2 and 3 weeks in a randomized, double-blind, placebo-controlled study of 28 patients receiving irradiation 5 times per week for 3 weeks. There was no difference in response between individuals with increased and normal IgE levels.[143,144]

Systemic Treatment

Antihistamines, leukotriene antagonists, corticosteroids, cyclosporine, methotrexate, mycophenolate mofetil, azathioprine, hydroxyurea, thalidomide, botulinum toxin, several retinoids, and biologics have all been used to treat HD. Nonetheless, a systematic review of 100 studies, including 31 randomized clinical trials, concluded that this body of evidence constituted an inadequate guide to proper clinical practice.[142] Paradoxically, topical exposure to azathioprine and mycophenolate mofetil have been reported to induce HD.[145,146]

Cyclosporine has been repeatedly found, in isolated case reports and in small series, to be effective.[147–150] Acrodermatitis continua–type pustular psoriasis has also been reported to respond to low-dose cyclosporine.[151] The theoretical risk of superinfection during cyclosporine therapy has also been confirmed.[152]

Recent reports on retinoids suggest that oral alitretinoin, a panagonist of retinoid receptors, works well on chronic, severe HE unresponsive to potent topical corticosteroids. In a double-blind placebo-controlled study involving more than 1000 patients, 80% cleared or almost cleared on drug (compared with 8% on placebo).[153]

The use of biologics has been successful in HD, particularly if related to psoriasis. Etanercept has been found to bring long-term control to acrodermatitis continua–type pustular psoriasis. A good response occurred in a patient previously refractory to infliximab, another anti-TNF-α agent.[154] Inconsistent responses to etanercept are reported for pompholyx-type HD.[155] A psoriasiform dermatitis to infliximab involving the hands has been reported.[41] The successful use of adalimumab treating acrodermatitis continua of Hallopeau, and its use with acitretin in a patient who failed to respond to cyclosporine, acitretin, and infliximab, was recently reported. A literature search crossing HD and adalimumab failed to bring up any other reports of success or failure.[156] Alefacept may be a treatment option for refractory chronic HD as suggested by a dramatic and lasting improvement in a patient who failed to respond to class I topical corticosteroids, topical calcineurin inhibitors, intralesional triamcinolone, and phototherapy. The benefit was noted 30 weeks after therapy was initiated, and was sustained for at least 28 weeks with the aid of a mild topical corticosteroid.[157] Efalizumab, once considered to be a usable drug in palmoplantar pustular forms of dermatitis, particularly if associated with psoriasis, was involved in a serious adverse infectious event, requiring its withdrawal from the market.

Tetracycline, along with betamethasone valerate under occlusion, produced a dramatic improvement within a week in a patient with acrodermatitis continua.[158]

Thalidomide combined with UVB therapy succeeded for an infant with acrodermatitis continua of Hallopeau.[159]

Iatrogenic phytophotodermatitis occurred in a 56-year-old farmer after ingesting a herbal decoction prescribed for his chronic HD.[34]

SUMMARY

The treatment of severe HD varies by cause. After that is established, if trigger avoidance or a specific treatment is available that is clearly successful (based on evidence-based medicine), that should be tried first. For recalcitrant forms, a more advanced search for the cause may be needed and, again, if it explains the condition, a tailored approach should work. An array of modalities including education, prevention, QoL interventions, topical medication, phototherapy or ionizing radiation, and systemic medications are available to bring gratifying results to those with the most complicated forms of HD.

REFERENCES

1. Molin S, Vollmer S, Weiss EH, et al. Filaggrin mutations may confer susceptibility to chronic hand eczema characterized by combined allergic and irritant contact dermatitis. Br J Dermatol 2009; 161(4):801–7.
2. Brown SJ, Cordell HJ. Are filaggrin mutations associated with hand eczema or contact allergy?—We do not know. Br J Dermatol 2008;158(6):1383–4.
3. Tamiya Y. Hand eczema. The clinical classification of the roles of endogenous and exogenous factors in each type. Nippon Ika Daigaku Zasshi 1994; 61(4):286–94.
4. Hornstein OP. Remarks and recommendations on the definition and classification of eczematous diseases. Z Hautkr 1986;61(18):1281–96.
5. Abramovits W, Cockerell C, Stevenson L, et al. PsEma - a hitherto unnamed dermatologic entity with clinical features of both psoriasis and eczema. Skinmed 2005;4(5):275–81.
6. McMullen E, Gawkrodger DJ. Physical friction is under-recognized as an irritant that can cause or contribute to contact dermatitis. Br J Dermatol 2006;154(1):154–6.
7. Kaukiainen A, Riala R, Martikainen R, et al. Chemical exposure and symptoms of hand dermatitis in construction painters. Contact Dermatitis 2005; 53(1):14–21.
8. Tan C, Zhu WY. Furazolidone induced nonpigmenting fixed drug eruptions affecting the palms and soles. Allergy 2005;60(7):972–4.
9. Korinth G, Goen T, Koch HM, et al. Visible and subclinical skin changes in male and female dispatch department workers of newspaper printing plants. Skin Res Technol 2005;11(2): 132–9.
10. Rycroft RJG. Occupational contact dermatitis. In: Rycroft RJG, Menne T, Frosch PJ, editors. Textbook of contact dermatitis. Heidelberg: Springer Verlag; 1995. p. 341.
11. Avnstorp C, Rastogi SC, Menne T. Acute fingertip dermatitis from temporary tattoo and quantitative chemical analysis of the product. Contact Dermatitis 2002;47(2):119–20.
12. Ortiz de Frutos FI, Vergara A, Isarria MI, et al. Occupational allergic contact eczema in a dental assistant. Actas Dermosifiliogr 2005;96(1):56–8.
13. Rademaker M. Occupational contact dermatitis to hydrangea. Australas J Dermatol 2003;44(3): 220–1.
14. Saeki H, Watanabe R, Tsunemi Y, et al. Severe hyperkeratotic palmoplantar eczema (eczema tyloticum). J Dermatol 2009;36(6):362–3.
15. Fox G, Harrell C, Mehregan D. Extensive lichenoid drug eruption due to glyburide: a case report and review of the literature. Cutis 2005;76:41–5.
16. Lazarov A. Textile dermatitis in patients with contact sensitization in Israel: a 4-year prospective study. J Eur Acad Dermatol Venereol 2004;18(5): 531–7.
17. Sugimura C, Katsuura J, Moriue T, et al. Dyshidrosiform pemphigoid: report of a case. J Dermatol 2003;30(7):525–9.
18. Canonne-Courivaud D, Carpentier O, Dejobert Y, et al. Lichenoid drug reaction to leflunomide. Ann Dermatol Venereol 2003;130(4):435–7.
19. Bryld LE, Agner T, Menne T. Relation between vesicular eruptions on the hands and tinea pedis, atopic dermatitis and nickel allergy. Acta Derm Venereol 2003;83(3):186–8.
20. Bukhari IA. Successful treatment of chronic persistent vesicular hand dermatitis with topical pimecrolimus. Saudi Med J 2005;26(12):1989–91.
21. Lehucher-Michel MP, Koeppel MC, Lanteaume A, et al. Dyshidrotic eczema (DE) and occupation: a

descriptive study. Contact Dermatitis 2000;43(4): 200–5.
22. Wolff HH, Kutzner H. How do I treat dyshidrosiform eruptions? Z Hautkr 1986;61(11):815–8.
23. Kabigting FD, Kempiak SJ, Alexandrescu DT, et al. Sea urchin granuloma secondary to *Strongylocentrotus purpuratus* and *S. franciscanus*. Sea urchin induced granuloma. Dermatol Online J 2009;15(5):9.
24. Maier LE, Lampel HP, Bhutani T, et al. Hand dermatitis: a focus on allergic contact dermatitis to biocides. Dermatol Clin 2009;27(3):251–64, v–vi.
25. Murphy R, Gawkrodger DJ. Contact allergens in 200 patients with hand dermatitis. Contact Dermatitis 2003;48(4):227–8.
26. Bauer A. Hand dermatitis: uncommon presentations. Clin Dermatol 2005;23:465–9.
27. Ponten A, Carstensen O, Rasmussen K, et al. Epoxy-based production of wind turbine rotor blades: occupational dermatoses. Contact Dermatitis 2004;50(6):329–38.
28. Balit CR, Geary MJ, Russell RC, et al. Clinical effects of exposure to the white-stemmed gum moth (*Chelepteryx collesi*). Emerg Med Australas 2004;16(1):74–81.
29. Farahanak A, Essalat M. A study on cercarial dermatitis in Khuzestan province, south western Iran. BMC Public Health 2003;3:35.
30. Aolto-Korte K, Susitaival P, Kaminska R, et al. Occupational protein contact dermatitis from shiitake mushroom and demonstration of shiitake-specific immunoglobulin E. Contact Dermatitis 2005;53(4):211–3.
31. Aolto-Korte K, Valimaa J, Henriks-Eckerman ML, et al. Allergic contact dermatitis from salicyl alcohol and salicylaldehyde in aspen bark. Contact Dermatitis 2005;52(2):93–5.
32. Nawaf AM, Joshi A, Nour-Eldin O. Acute allergic contact dermatitis due to para-phenylenediamine after temporary henna painting. J Dermatol 2003; 30(11):797–800.
33. Spiewak R, Dutkiewicz J. Occupational airborne and hand dermatitis to hop with non-occupational relapses. Ann Agric Environ Med 2002;9(2):249–52.
34. Moloney FJ, Parnell J, Buckley CC. Iatrogenic phytophotodermatitis resulting from herbal treatment of an allergic contact dermatitis. Clin Exp Dermatol 2006;31(1):39–41.
35. Abramovits W, Stevenson LC. Hand eczema in a 22 year-old woman with piercings. Proc (Bayl Univ Med Cent) 2004;17(2):211–3.
36. Artignan S, Conso F, Hazebroucq V. Radiodermatitis in interventional radiology (hand dose measurement, screening and compensation). J Radiol 2003;84(3):317–9.
37. Lasa Elgezua O, Gorrotxategi PE, Gardeazabal Garcia J, et al. Photoallergic hand eczema due to benzydamine. Eur J Dermatol 2004;14(1):69–70.
38. Markman M, Kulp B, Peterson G. Grade 3 liposomal-doxorubicin-induced skin toxicity in a patient following complete resolution of moderately severe sunburn. Gynecol Oncol 2004;94(2): 578–80.
39. Ozkaya-Bayazit E. Independent lesions of fixed drug eruption caused by trimethoprim-sulfamethoxazole and tenoxicam in the same patient: a rare case of polysensitivity. J Am Acad Dermatol 2004;51(2 Suppl):S102–4.
40. Kastalli S, El Aidli S, Daghfous R, et al. Fixed drug eruption induced by sulfaguanidine. Ann Dermatol Venereol 2004;131(4):382–4.
41. Verea MM, Del Pozo J, Yebra-Pimentel MT, et al. Psoriasiform eruption induced by infliximab. Ann Pharmacother 2004;38(1):54–7.
42. Cahill J, Nixon R. Allergic contact dermatitis to quaternium 15 in a moisturizing lotion. Australas J Dermatol 2005;46(4):2284–5.
43. Pavlovic MD. Papular-purpuric "gloves and socks" syndrome caused by parvovirus B19. Vojnosanit Pregl 2003;60(2):223–5.
44. Patel S, Davidson LE. Papillon-Lefevre syndrome: a report of two cases. Int J Paediatr Dent 2004; 14(4):288–94.
45. Rademaker M, Yung A. Contact dermatitis to *Asparagus officinalis*. Australas J Dermatol 2000; 41(4):262–3.
46. Pipili C, Cholongitas E, Ioannidou D. Phytocontact dermatitis caused by artichoke: an exceptionally rare case. Clin Exp Dermatol 2009;34(4):534–5.
47. Timmermans MW, Pentiga SE, Rustemeyer T, et al. Contact dermatitis due to *Paeonia* (peoney); a rare sensitizer? Contact Dermatitis 2009; 60(4):232–3.
48. Garcia GJ, Loureiro MM, Fernandez-Redondo V, et al. Contact dermatitis from melamine formaldehyde resins in a patient with a negative patch-test reaction to formaldehyde. Dermatitis 2008; 19(2):E5–6.
49. de Lagran ZM, de Frutos FJ, de Arribas MG, et al. Contact uticaria from raw potato. Dermatol Online J 2009;15(5):14.
50. Mending B, Alderling M, Albin M, et al. Does tobacco smoking influence the occurrence of hand eczema? Br J Dermatol 2009;160(3):514–8.
51. Magina S, Barros MA, Ferreira JA, et al. Atopy, nickel sensitivity, occupation, and clinical patterns in different types of hand dermatitis. Am J Contact Dermatitis 2003;14(2):63–8.
52. Anderson R, Jatoi A, Robert C, et al. Search for evidence-based approaches for the prevention and palliation of hand-foot skin reaction (HFSR) caused by the multikinase inhibitors (MKIs). Oncologist 2009;14(3):291–302.
53. Oh SH, Kim DS, Kwon YS, et al. Concurrence of palmoplantar psoriasiform eruptions and hair loss

during carbamazepine treatment. Acta Derm Venereol 2008;88(5):532–3.
54. Wilkinson DS. Introduction, definition and classification. In: Menne T, Maibach HI, editors. Hand eczema. Boca Raton (FL): CRC Press; 1994. p. 2–12.
55. Elston DM, Ahmed DDF, Watsky KL, et al. Hand dermatitis. J Am Acad Dermatol 2002;47:291–9.
56. Fowler JF, Ghosh A, Sung J, et al. Impact of chronic hand dermatitis on quality of life, work productivity, activity impairment, and medical costs. J Am Acad Dermatol 2006;54(3):448–57.
57. Horwitz LB, Kammeyer-Mueller J, McCall BP. Workers' compensation claims related to natural rubber latex gloves among Oregon healthcare employees from 1987–1998. BMC Public Health 2002;18(2):2l.
58. Neidner R. Occupational burden of the skin: the example of hands. Bundesgesundheitblatt Geshundheitsforschung Gesundheitsschutz 2008; 51(3):334–9.
59. Cvetkovski RS, Zachariae R, Jensen H, et al. Prognosis of occupational hand eczema (OHE): a follow-up study. Arch Dermatol 2006;142(3): 305–11.
60. Cvetkovski RS, Rothman KJ, Olsen J, et al. Relation between diagnoses on severity, sick leave and loss of job among patients with occupational hand eczema (OHE). Br J Dermatol 2005;152(1):93–8.
61. Nyren M, Lindberg M, Sternberg B, et al. Influence of childhood atopic dermatitis on future worklife. Scand J Work Environ Health 2005;31(6):474–8.
62. Kadyk DL, McCarter K, Achen F, et al. Quality of life (QoL) in patients with allergic contact dermatitis (ACD). J Am Acad Dermatol 2003;49(6):1037–48.
63. Skoet R, Zachariae R, Agner T. Contact dermatitis (CD) and quality of life (QoL): a structured review of the literature. Br J Dermatol 2003;149(3):452–6.
64. Szepietowski J, Salomon J. Hand dermatitis: a problem commonly affecting nurses. Rocz Akad Med Bialysmst 2005;50(Suppl 1):46–8.
65. Niemeier V, Nippesen M, Kupfer J, et al. Psychological factors associated with hand dermatoses: which subgroup needs additional psychological care? Br J Dermatol 2002;146(6):1031–7.
66. Watkins SA, Maibach HI. The hardening phenomenon in irritant contact dermatitis: an interpretive update. Contact Dermatitis 2009;60(3):123–30.
67. Held E, Skoet R, Johansen JD, et al. The hand eczema severity index (HECSI): a scoring system for clinical assessment of hand eczema. A study of inter- and intraobserver reliability. Br J Dermatol 2005;152(2):302–7.
68. Abramovits W, Stevenson L. Atopic profiles, familial histories, and coexisting conditions associated with hand eczema. Skinmed 2005;4(4):204–10.
69. Cvetkovski RS, Jensen H, Olsen J, et al. Relation between patients' and physicians' assessment of occupational hand eczema. Br J Dermatol 2005; 153(3):596–600.
70. Coenraads PJ, Van Der Walle H, Thestrup-Pedersen K, et al. Construction and validation of a photographic guide for assessing severity of chronic hand dermatitis. Br J Dermatol 2005; 152(2):199–201.
71. Svensson A, Lindberg M, Meding B, et al. Self-reported hand eczema: symptom-based reports do not increase the validity of diagnosis. Br J Dermatol 2002;147(2):281–4.
72. Hald M, Agner T, Blands J, et al. Allergens associated with severe symptoms of hand eczema and a poor prognosis. Contact Dermatitis 2009; 61(2):101–8.
73. Sommer S, Wilkinson SM, Beck MH, et al. Type IV hypersensitivity reactions to natural rubber latex: results of a multicenter study. Br J Dermatol 2002; 146(1):114–7.
74. Bruze M, Gruvberger B, Zimerson E. A clinically relevant contact allergy to methyldibromoglutaronitrile (MDBGN) at 1% (0.32 mg/cm) detected by a patch test. Contact Dermatitis 2006;54(1):14–7.
75. Jain VK, Aggarwal K, Passi S, et al. Role of contact allergens in pompholyx. J Dermatol 2004;31(3): 188–93.
76. Nedorost S, Wagman A. Positive patch-test reactions to gold: patients' perception of relevance and the role of titanium dioxide in cosmetics. Dermatitis 2005;16(2):67–70.
77. Khurana S, Jain VK, Aggarwal K, et al. Patch testing in discoid eczema. J Dermatol 2002;29(12):763–7.
78. Heydorn S, Johansen JD, Andersen KE, et al. Fragrance allergy in patients with hand eczema – a clinical study. Contact Dermatitis 2003;48(6): 317–23.
79. Jovanovic M, Poljacki M. Compositae dermatitis. Med Pregl 2003;56(1–2):43–9.
80. Giusti F, Miglietta R, Pepe P, et al. Sensitization to propolis in 1255 children undergoing patch testing. Contact Dermatitis 2004;51(5–6):255–8.
81. Penagos HG. Contact dermatitis caused by pesticides among banana plantation workers in Panama. Int J Occup Environ Health 2002;8(1): 14–8.
82. Li WF, Wang J. Contact hypersensitivity in hand dermatitis. Contact Dermatitis 2002;47:206–9.
83. Emmett EA. Occupational contact dermatitis I. Incidence and return to work pressures. Am J Contact Dermatitis 2002;13:30–4.
84. Bureau of Labor Statistics. Occupational injuries and illnesses in the United States. [Bulletin 2512]. Washington (DC): US Department of Labor, Bureau of Labor Statistics; 1999.
85. Lushniak BD. The epidemiology of occupational contact dermatitis. Dermatol Clin 1995; 13:671–9.

86. Vestey JP, Gawkrodger DJ, Wong WK, et al. An analysis of 501 consecutive contact clinic consultations. Contact Dermatitis 1986;15:119–25.
87. Rietschel RL, Mathias CG, Fowler JF Jr, et al. North American Contact Dermatitis Group. Relationship of occupation to contact dermatitis (OCD): evaluation in patients tested from 1998 to 2000. Am J Contact Dermatitis 2002;13(4):170–6.
88. Nettis E, Colanardi MC, Soccio AL, et al. Occupational irritant and allergic contact dermatitis (ACD) among healthcare workers. Contact Dermatitis 2002;46(2):101–7.
89. Shiao JS, Sheu HM, Chen CJ, et al. Prevalence and risk factors of occupational hand dermatoses in electronics workers. Toxicol Ind Health 2004;20(1–5):1–7.
90. Kutting B, Weistenhofer W, Baumeister T, et al. Current acceptance and implementation of preventive strategies for occupational hand eczema in 1355 metal workers in Germany. Br J Dermatol 2009;161(2):390–6.
91. Jia X, Xiao P, Jin X, et al. Adverse effects of gasoline on the skin of exposed workers. Contact Dermatitis 2002;46(1):44–7.
92. Thyssen JP, Milting K, Bregnhoj A, et al. Nickel allergy in patch-tested female hairdressers and assessment of nickel release from hairdressers' scissors and crochet hooks. Contact Dermatitis 2009;61(5):281–6.
93. Khumalo NP, Jessop S, Ehrlich R. Prevalence of cutaneous adverse effects of hairdressing: a systemic review. Arch Dermatol 2006;142(3):377–83.
94. Iorizzo M, Parente G, Vincenzi C, et al. Allergic contact dermatitis in hairdressers: frequency and source of sensitization. Eur J Dermatol 2002;12(2):179–82.
95. Lampel HP, Patel N, Boyse K, et al. Prevalence of hand dermatitis in inpatient nurses at a United States hospital. Dermatitis 2007;18(3):140–2.
96. Smith DR, Smyth W, Leggat PA, et al. Prevalence of hand dermatitis among hospital nurses working in a tropical environment. Aust J Adv Nurs 2005;22(3):28–32.
97. Smith DR, Wei N, Zhang RX, et al. Epidemiology of hand dermatitis among rural nursing students in mainland China: results from a preliminary study. Rural Remote Health 2004;4(2):270.
98. Alanko K, Susitaival P, Jolanki R, et al. Occupational skin diseases among dental nurses. Contact Dermatitis 2004;50(2):77–82.
99. Jacobsen N, Hensten-Pettersen A. Changes in occupational health problems and adverse patient reactions in orthodontics from 1987 to 2000. Eur J Orthod 2003;25(6):591–8.
100. Skoet R, Olsen J, Mathiesen B, et al. A survey of occupational hand eczema in Denmark. Contact Dermatitis 2004;51(4):159–66.
101. Lombardi C, Bottello M, Caruso A, et al. Allergy and skin diseases in musicians. Allerg Immunol 2003;35(2):52–5.
102. Munsted K, Hellener M, Hackenthal A, et al. Contact allergy to propolis in beekeepers. Allergol Immunopathol (Madr) 2007;35(3):95–100.
103. Shenoi SD, Davis SV, Rao S, et al. Dermatoses among paddy field workers-a descriptive, cross-sectional pilot study. Indian J Dermatol Venereol Leprol 2005;71(4):254–8.
104. Noorbala MT. Skin lesions in carpet hand-weavers. Dermatol Online 2008;14(3):5.
105. Bryld LE, Hindsberger C, Kyvik KO, et al. Risk factors influencing the development of hand eczema in a population-based twin sample. Br J Dermatol 2003;149(6):1214–20.
106. Bauer A, Bartsch R, Hersmann C, et al. Occupational hand dermatitis in food industry apprentices: results of a 3-year follow-up cohort study. Int Arch Occup Environ Health 2001;74(6):437–42.
107. Meding B, Jarvholm B. Incidence of hand eczema (HE) - a population based retrospective study. J Invest Dermatol 2004;122(40):873–7.
108. Osika I, Evengard B, Waernulf L, et al. The laundry-basket project–gender differences to the very skin. Different treatment of some common skin diseases in men and women. Lakartidningen 2005;102(40):2846–8, 2850–1.
109. Templet JT, Hall S, Belsito DV. Etiology of hand dermatitis among patients referred for patch testing. Dermatitis 2004;15(1):25–32.
110. Ingordo V, D'Andria G, D'Angria C. Adult-onset atopic dermatitis in a patch test population. Dermatology 2003;206(3):197–203.
111. Julander A, Hindsén M, Skare L, et al. Cobalt-containing alloys and their ability to release cobalt and cause dermatitis. Contact Dermatitis 2009;60(3):165–70.
112. Fournier PG, Govers TR. Contamination by nickel, copper and zinc during the handling of euro coins. Contact Dermatitis 2003;48(4):181–8.
113. Staton I, Ma R, Evans N, et al. Dermal nickel exposure associated with coin handling and in various occupational settings: assessment using a newly developed finger immersion method. Br J Dermatol 2006;154(4):658–64.
114. Heydorn S, Menne T, Andersen KE, et al. The fragrance hand immersion study – an experimental model simulating real-life exposure for allergic contact dermatitis of the hands. Contact Dermatitis 2003;48(6):324–30.
115. Astner S, Burnett N, Rius-Diaz F, et al. Irritant contact dermatitis induced by a common household irritant: a noninvasive evaluation of ethnic variability in skin response. J Am Acad Dermatol 2006;54(3):458–65.

116. McCormick RD, Buchman TL, Maki DG. Double-blind, randomized trial of scheduled use of a novel barrier cream and an oil-containing lotion for protecting the hands of health care workers. Am J Infect Control 2000;28(4):302–10.
117. Fowler JF. Efficacy of a skin-protective foam in the treatment of chronic hand dermatitis. Am J Contact Dermatitis 2000;11(3):165–9.
118. Slade HB, Fowler J, Draelos ZD, et al. Clinical efficacy evaluation of a novel barrier protection cream. Cutis 2008;82(Suppl 4):21–8.
119. Flyvholm MA, Mygind K, Sell L, et al. A randomized controlled intervention study on prevention of work related skin problems among gut cleaners in swine slaughterhouses. Occup Environ Med 2005;62(9): 642–9.
120. Jungbauer FH, Van der Harst JJ, Schuttelaar ML, et al. Characteristics of wet work in the cleaning industry. Contact Dermatitis 2004;51(3):131–4.
121. Kampf G, Kramer A. Epidemiologic background of hand hygiene and evaluation of the most important agents for scrubs and rubs. Clin Microbiol Rev 2004;17(4):863–93, table of contents.
122. Jungbauer FH, Van Der Harst JJ, Groothoff JW, et al. Skin protection in nursing work: promoting the use of gloves and hand alcohol. Contact Dermatitis 2004;51(3):135–40.
123. Boyce JM, Pittet D, Healthcare Infection Control Practices Advisory Committee, et al. Guideline for hand hygiene in health-care settings. Recommendations of the Healthcare Infection Control Practices Advisory Committee and the HICPAC/SHEA/APIC/IDSA Hand Hygiene Task Force. Society for Healthcare Epidemiology of America/Association for Professionals in Infection Control/Infectious Diseases Society of America. MMWR Recomm Rep 2002;51(RR-16):1–45 [quiz: CE 1–4].
124. Cao LY, Sood A, Taylor JS. Hand/face/neck localized pattern: sticky problems—resins. Dermatol Clin 2009;27(3):227–49, v.
125. Baranda L, Gonzalez-Amaro R, Torres-Alvarez B, et al. Correlation between pH and irritant effect of cleansers marketed for dry skin. Int J Dermatol 2002;41(8):494–9.
126. Bauer A, Kelterer D, Bartsch R, et al. Prevention of hand dermatitis in bakers' apprentices: different efficacy of skin protection measures and UVB hardening. Int Arch Occup Environ Health 2002; 75(7):491–9.
127. Gutman AB, Kligman AM, Sciacca J, et al. Soak and smear: a standard technique revisited. Arch Dermatol 2005;141(12):1556–9.
128. Andersen KE, Broesby-Olsen S. A case of allergic contact dermatitis from oleyl alcohol in a pimecrolimus cream has been reported. Contact Dermatitis 2006; 55(6):354–6.
129. Belsito DV, Fowler JF Jr, Marks JG Jr, et al. Multicenter investigator group. Pimecrolimus cream 1%: a potential new treatment for chronic hand dermatitis. Cutis 2004;73(1):31–8.
130. Thaçi D, Steinmeyer K, Ebelin ME, et al. Occlusive treatment of chronic hand dermatitis with pimecrolimus cream 1% results in low systemic exposure, is well tolerated, safe, and effective. An open study. Dermatology 2003;207(1):37–42.
131. Thelmo MC, Lang W, Brooke E, et al. An open-label pilot study to evaluate the safety and efficacy of topically applied tacrolimus ointment for the treatment of hand and/or foot eczema. J Dermatolog Treat 2003;14(3):136–40.
132. Hanifin JM, Stevens V, Sheth P, et al. Novel treatment of chronic severe hand dermatitis with bexarotene gel. Br J Dermatol 2004; 150(3):545–53.
133. Molin S, Ruzicka T. Alitretinoin: a new treatment option for chronic refractory hand eczema. Hautarzt 2008;59(9):703–4 706–9.
134. Wollina U, Karamfilov T. Adjuvant botulinum toxin A in dyshydrotic hand eczema: a controlled prospective pilot study with left-right comparison. J Eur Acad Dermatol Venereol 2002;16(1):40–2.
135. Swartling C, Naver H, Lindberg M, et al. Treatment of hand dermatitis with intradermal botulinum toxin. J Am Acad Dermatol 2002;47(5):667–71.
136. Veien NK, Menne T. Treatment of hand eczema. Skin Therapy Lett 2003;8(5):4–7.
137. Warshaw E. Therapeutic options for chronic hand dermatitis. Dermatol Ther 2004;4:17240–50.
138. Schalock PC, Zug KA, Carter JC, et al. Efficacy and patient perception of Grenz ray therapy in the treatment of dermatoses refractory to other medical therapy. Dermatitis 2008;19(2):90–4.
139. Stembaugh MD, DeNittis AS, Wallner PE, et al. Complete remission of refractory dyshidrotic eczema with the use of radiation therapy. Cutis 2000;65(4):211–4.
140. Schiener R, Gottlober P, Muller B, et al. PUVA-gel vs PUVA-bath therapy for severe recalcitrant palmoplantar dermatoses. A randomized, single-blinded prospective study. Photodermatol Photoimmunol Photomed 2005;21(2):62–7.
141. Aubin F, Vigan M, Puzenat E, et al. Evaluation of a novel 308-nm monochromatic excimer light delivery system in dermatology: a pilot study in different chronic localized dermatoses. Br J Dermatol 2005;152(1):99–103.
142. Nordal EJ, Christensen OB. Treatment of chronic hand dermatoses with UVB-TL01. Acta Derm Venereol 2004;84(4):302–4.
143. Polderman MC, Govaert JC, le Cessie S, et al. A double-blind placebo-controlled trial of UVA-1 in the treatment of dyshidrotic eczema. Clin Exp Dermatol 2003;28(6):584–7.

144. Diepgen TL, Svensson A, Coenraads PJ. Therapy of hand eczema. What can we learn from the published clinical studies? Hautarzt 2005;56(3): 224–31.
145. Soni BP, Sherertz EF. Allergic contact dermatitis from azathioprine. Am J Contact Dermatitis 1996; 7(2):116–7.
146. Semhoun-Ducloux D, Miguel JP. Mycophenolate mofetil-induced dyshidrotic eczema. Ann Intern Med 2000;132(5):417.
147. Bowers PW, Julian CG. Dogger Bank Itch and cyclosporine. J Dermatolog Treat 2001;12(1): 23–4.
148. Granlund H, Erkko P, Reitamo S. Long-term follow-up of eczema patients treated with cyclosporine. Acta Derm Venereol (Stockh) 1998;78(1):40–3.
149. Granlund H, Erkko P, Reitamo S. Comparison of the influence of cyclosporine and topical betamethasone-17,21-dipropionate treatment on quality of life in chronic hand eczema. Acta Derm Venereol 1997;77(1):54–8.
150. Petersen CS, Menné T. Cyclosporin A responsive chronic severe vesicular hand eczema. Acta Derm Venereol 1992;72(6):436–7.
151. Peter RU, Ruzicka T, Donhauser G, et al. Acrodermatitis continua-type of pustular psoriasis responds to low-dose cyclosporine. AM Acad Dermatol 1990;23(3 Pt 1):515–6.
152. Monari P, Sala R, Calzavara-Pinton P. Norwegian scabies in a healthy woman during oral cyclosporine therapy. Eur J Dermatol 2007;17(2):173.
153. Garnock-Jones KP, Perry CM. Alitretinoin: in severe chronic hand eczema. Am J Clin Dermatol 2009; 10(6):421–2.
154. Thielen AM, Barde C, Marazza G, et al. Long-term control with etanercept of a severe acrodermatitis continua of Hallopeau refractory to infliximab. Dermatology 2008;217(2):137–9.
155. Ogden S, Clayton TH, Goodfield MJ. Recalcitrant hand pompholyx: variable response to etanercept. Clin Exp Dermatol 2006;31(1):145–6.
156. Tobin AM, Kirby B. Successful treatment of recalcitrant acrodermatitis continua of Hallopeau (ACH) with adalimumab and acitretin. Br J Dermatol 2005;153(2):445–6.
157. Aronson PJ, Yeung-Yue KA. Treatment of hand dermatitis with alefacept. Dermatitis 2008;19(3): 161–2.
158. Piquero-Casals J, Fonseca de Mello AP, Dal Coleto C, et al. Using oral tetracycline and topical betamethasone valerate to treat acrodermatitis continua of Hallopeau. Cutis 2002;70(2):106–8.
159. Kiszewski AE, De Villa D, Scheibel I, et al. An infant with acrodermatitis continua of Hallopeau: successful treatment with thalidomide and UVB therapy. Pediatr Dermatol 2009;26(1):105–6.

Innovative Management of Pruritus

Jamison D. Feramisco, MD, PhD, Timothy G. Berger, MD,
Martin Steinhoff, MD, PhD*

KEYWORDS

- Pruritus • Itch • Uremia • Renal • Cholestasis
- Neuropathy • Treatment

Itch is defined as the unpleasant sensation of the skin resulting in a desire to scratch[1] and is often classified as acute and chronic. Pruritus can be an extremely distressing symptom that dramatically affects the quality of life. Other classifications of itch are based on where the sensation is located (generalized versus localized or shifting): specifically, as pruritus on diseased or inflamed skin; as pruritus on nondiseased or noninflamed skin; or as pruritus presenting with severe, chronic secondary lesions related to scratching.[2] The incidence of pruritus in the general population is poorly documented. However, chronic renal failure and liver failure are associated with pruritus in up to 75% of patients. In this article the authors focus on pruritus affecting noninflamed or nondiseased skin. Processes in this category include cholestasis, uremia, neuropathic derangement, thyroid disorders, iron deficiency, polycythemia vera, essential thrombocytosis, malignancy, human immunodeficiency virus (HIV)/AIDS, and medication-induced itch. In many of these conditions, the pruritus is best resolved by treatment of the underlying condition; however, this treatment may not always be possible or sufficient. Thus, the authors review current mechanisms and new innovative therapies to treat intractable pruritus of selected systemic diseases.

PRURITUS WORKUP

Itch can be caused by inflammatory skin diseases, exogenous trigger factors (eg, mites, virus), endogenous trigger factors (eg, systemic drugs), or systemic diseases (eg, chronic renal insufficiency). To properly treat a patient with pruritus, an effort must be made to determine the precise cause of the itch. The authors recommend that when a patient presents to the dermatologist with a chronic itch (lasting longer than 6 weeks), a detailed history and full skin examination should be performed. Of note, the skin of a patient with pruritus may seem normal. It may alternatively reveal an underlying disease, show specific features of a dermatosis (eg, hives in urticaria), or may only show unspecific scratching "artifacts" (ie, pruritus on primary nondiseased skin). If a primary dermatologic or systemic process is identified, then appropriate disease-specific workup and treatment is indicated. If the patient has pruritus without inflamed or diseased skin, the authors suggest that, in addition to the full skin examination and detailed medical and medication history, a set of general laboratory studies be obtained, including a complete blood count with differential, sedimentation rate, levels of creatinine and glucose, liver function tests (aspartate aminotransferase, alanine aminotransferase, alkaline phosphatase, total bilirubin), thyroid function tests (thyroid stimulating hormone, free T4); iron studies (transferrin saturation, ferritin, iron), rapid plasma reagin for syphilis, HIV antibody test, and a chest radiograph. More specialized tests may be indicated based on medical history (eg, antinuclear antibody, hepatitis serology, antimitochondrial antibody, antigliadin antibody,

Funding and conflicts of interest: None.
Department of Dermatology, University of California at San Francisco, 1701 Divisadero Street, 3rd floor, San Francisco, CA 94115, USA
* Corresponding author.
E-mail address: SteinhoffM@derm.ucsf.edu

Dermatol Clin 28 (2010) 467–478
doi:10.1016/j.det.2010.03.004
0733-8635/10/$ – see front matter © 2010 Elsevier Inc. All rights reserved.

antitransglutaminase antibody, parathyroid hormone, calcium, phosphate, specific immunoglobulin (Ig) E, functional anti-IgE Fc receptor antibody, serum tryptase, serotonin and its metabolites, stool for ova and parasites or stool occult blood examination). Sometimes, allergy testing (prick or patch testing), histologic examination of affected skin, and direct immunofluorescence and internal evaluations such as ultrasound or radiologic imaging (magnetic resonance imaging [MRI], computed tomography [CT]) may also be beneficial. An age-appropriate malignancy workup is warranted if these initial studies are unremarkable or if the history and review of systems suggest a possible malignancy. Thus, the approach to identify the origin of pruritus may be complex and multidisciplinary.

CHOLESTATIC ITCH

Cholestasis refers to conditions whereby the flow of bile is reduced from its pathway to the intestine from the liver. In some forms of liver disease, pruritus is often an early finding. It can be associated with a variety of liver and biliary diseases, including hepatitis, primary sclerosing cholangitis, primary biliary cirrhosis (PBC), tumors, gallstones, congenital malformations, and medications.[3] Pruritus is a common symptom in cholestatic disease and is more often seen in the context of intrahepatic rather than extrahepatic obstruction.[4–6] In one study, 69% of patients with PBC reported itch. This result is consistent with prior estimates of prevalence as well as associated depression and reduced quality of life in such patients.[7–9] The mechanism of itch in cholestasis remains largely unknown. Some hypotheses include derangements in bile salt production and excretion, alterations in progesterone metabolites, histamine imbalance, substance P dysregulation, and alterations of endogenous opioids.[6,10]

There have been few randomized controlled trials (RCTs) evaluating treatment modalities in cholestatic itch. Of these, even fewer have included controls for individual disease processes. As such, recent attempts to provide guidelines for the treatment of cholestasis-associated pruritus are based mostly on descriptive studies and case series.[9] Studies evaluating the efficacy of topical therapies in cholestatic itch have demonstrated equivocal results at best. Antihistamines are traditionally given to treat pruritus, but remain largely ineffective in cholestatic itch, and medication side effects often worsen symptoms.[10] An observation that pruritus can be relieved in patients with partial biliary obstruction by intermittent external biliary drainage motivated Datta and Sherlock[11,12] to treat 10 patients with oral cholestyramine, relieving itch in 8 participants. Since then, cholestyramine and other nonabsorbable anion exchange resins have become a mainstay for the treatment of cholestatic pruritus.[13] But cholestyramine is not very palatable and must be taken on an empty stomach and not within 4 hours of other oral medications, all these features making it inconvenient for patients. Dosing regimens start at 4 g daily and increase to a maximum dose of 16 g/d.[6,9] Rifampicin (or rifampin) has been studied at total daily doses of 300 to 600 mg divided twice daily and has been shown to be effective in RCTs and in a meta-analysis.[13–15] As with other treatments, the mechanism of action of rifampicin as an antipruritic is unknown, but an older report indicates that it may alter intracellular bile acid composition.[16]

Higher levels of endogenous opioids are present in animal and human models of cholestasis; however, it is unclear whether they correlate with prurtius.[17–20] After an original report in 1979 describing the relief of pruritus with naloxone administration,[21] μ-opioid antagonists have been shown in several clinical trials as an effective treatment of cholestatic pruritus.[13,16,22–24] Dosing schedules vary, but common regimens include oral naltrexone (25–150 mg/d), oral nalmefene (40–120 mg/d), and intravenous (IV) naloxone (IV bolus of 0.4 mg followed by 0.2 μg/kg/min). To decrease the opiate withdrawal-like symptoms that commonly occur in the first days of treatment, one can give IV naloxone (at 0.002 μg/kg/min) increasing gradually or oral clonidine (100 mg 3 times daily) before switching to oral naltrexone (titrating slowly by 25 mg by mouth daily every 3 days).[25,26] In preliminary studies, κ-opioid receptor agonists, such as butorphanol (1 mg intranasally) and nalfurafine (5 μg IV following dialysis 3 times weekly) have been shown to be effective for the treatment of uremic and cholestatic pruritus.[27,28]

Psychotropic medications have also been used in patients with cholestatic pruritus, including both the serotonin 5-HT_3 antagonist ondansetron and the selective serotonin reuptake inhibitors (SSRIs) sertraline and paroxetine. Although the SSRIs have been shown to relieve pruritus of cholestasis (oral sertraline at 75–100 mg/d and oral paroxetine at 20 mg/d) in controlled trials,[29–31] ondansetron has demonstrated mixed efficacy (at oral doses of 4–24 mg/d).[6] As with many treatments for intractable pruritus, a known mechanism of action is lacking for this class of drug.

Ursodeoxycholic acid (UDCA) is a small component of the bile acid pool in humans and is used as an anticholestatic agent in PBC. Although UDCA was initially thought to decrease morbidity and mortality in PBC and to improve pruritus (doses of 10–15 mg/kg/d), a recent Cochrane Review of the literature did not support these initial findings.[32,33]

Other oral and IV medications that have shown efficacy in treating pruritus of cholestasis in small case series or case reports include phenobarbital (2–5 mg/kg/d orally), the cannabinoid receptor ligand dronabinol (5 mg 3 times daily by mouth), thalidomide (50–100 mg/d orally), propofol (10–15 mg IV bolus and 1 mg/kg/h), and lidocaine (100 mg/d IV).[6] Unfortunately, gabapentin was no better than placebo in a well-conducted, double-blind RCT for the treatment of cholestatic itch.[34]

Nonmedical therapies have also been studied. Cholestatic pruritus is intermittent and cyclical in nature, and in mouse models, disruption of the circadian clock results in dysregulation of bile acid homeostasis that mimics cholestatic disease. As such, bright-light therapy was tested and facilitated a modest decrease of hourly scratching assay score in 7 of 8 patients.[35] The use of phototherapy with either UV-A or UV-B rays has proven effective in case series but has not yet been tested in an RCT.[36,37] Alternative approaches to the management of cholestatic itch, including plasma separation and anion absorption, plasmapheresis, ileal diversion, and molecular adsorbent recirculating system therapy, have also been successful in case reports.[6] Finally, liver transplant is a consideration for the treatment of intractable pruritus of cholestasis, even without evidence of objective cellular hepatobiliary derangement (**Fig. 1**).[9]

RENAL PRURITUS

Pruritus is a common symptom in patients with end-stage renal disease (ESRD), affecting between 22% and 90% of these patients (with most estimates centered on 40%–50%); the variation is based on some studies measuring lifetime prevalence and some measuring snapshot prevalence.[38–44] As technology in dialysis has improved during the past decade, the incidence of renal-associated pruritus has also decreased.[45] Often, the pruritus of renal disease is severe and refractory to treatment. In such cases, this condition (1) has been shown to decrease the quality of life, (2) contributes to insomnia, (3) leads to other poor patient outcomes, and (4) is an independent factor predictive of increased mortality.[46–50] Surprisingly, the prevalence of uremic pruritus may also be underestimated by nephrologists.[47]

The mechanism of renal pruritus is most likely multifactorial and has been postulated to be caused by 1 or more of the following derangements present in uremia: uremic xerosis, secondary hyperparathyroidism and an abnormal calcium-phosphorus product, changes in κ- and μ-opioid receptors, altered signaling in epidermal and dermal nerve fibers, hypervitaminosis A, peripheral neuropathy, iron deficiency anemia, and altered levels of serum inflammatory markers.[49,51–55] Thus, the term renal pruritus is superior to uremic pruritus because the correlation between blood urea nitrogen levels and occurrence of itch is poor. Currently, there is much debate as to the relative contributions of each of these processes to uremia-associated itch. Although some have postulated simply that the severity of uremic xerosis correlates with degree of pruritus symptoms,[54,56–58] experimental data are lacking to support this assertion.[59,60] The relationship between uremic itch and serum markers also remains controversial. Some reports implicate lower transferrin saturation levels, higher C-reactive protein levels, and increased alpha-1 glycoprotein in hemodialysis (HD) patients with pruritus as compared with HD patients without itch.[39] Recently, there has been discussion of mid- and macrosized molecule toxins and cytokines contributing to renal itch, akin to a chronic inflammatory state with increased proinflammatory cytokine activation.[61–64]

During the past few decades, numerous treatment approaches have been used to alleviate uremic pruritus. Similar to other subclasses of pruritus, there is no magic bullet that can uniformly and reliably treat this difficult medical problem. Because the cause of uremic pruritus is likely multifactorial, as described earlier, the treatment plan often incorporates multiple modalities and is often patient specific. Treatment options can be separated fundamentally by method of delivery.

Topical medications address xerosis and alterations in the stratum corneum barrier function (with increased transepidermal water loss), which likely contribute to itching in end-stage renal disease.[53,58,65–67] Emollients have been used for many years, with a paucity of evidence-based trials. This paucity may be because of the variability in the composition of emollients. In an open uncontrolled trial using aqueous cream applied twice daily, there was a significant improvement of pruritus in 9 of 21 patients.[58] Capsaicin has been reported to deplete substance P in neurons and has been effective in treating uremic pruritus in many trials. For example, in a double-blind, controlled, crossover study, relief of itch was seen in 14 of 17 patients using 0.025% capsaicin cream 4 times a day.[68] One percent pramoxine lotion showed good efficacy when used twice daily for 4 weeks in a randomized,

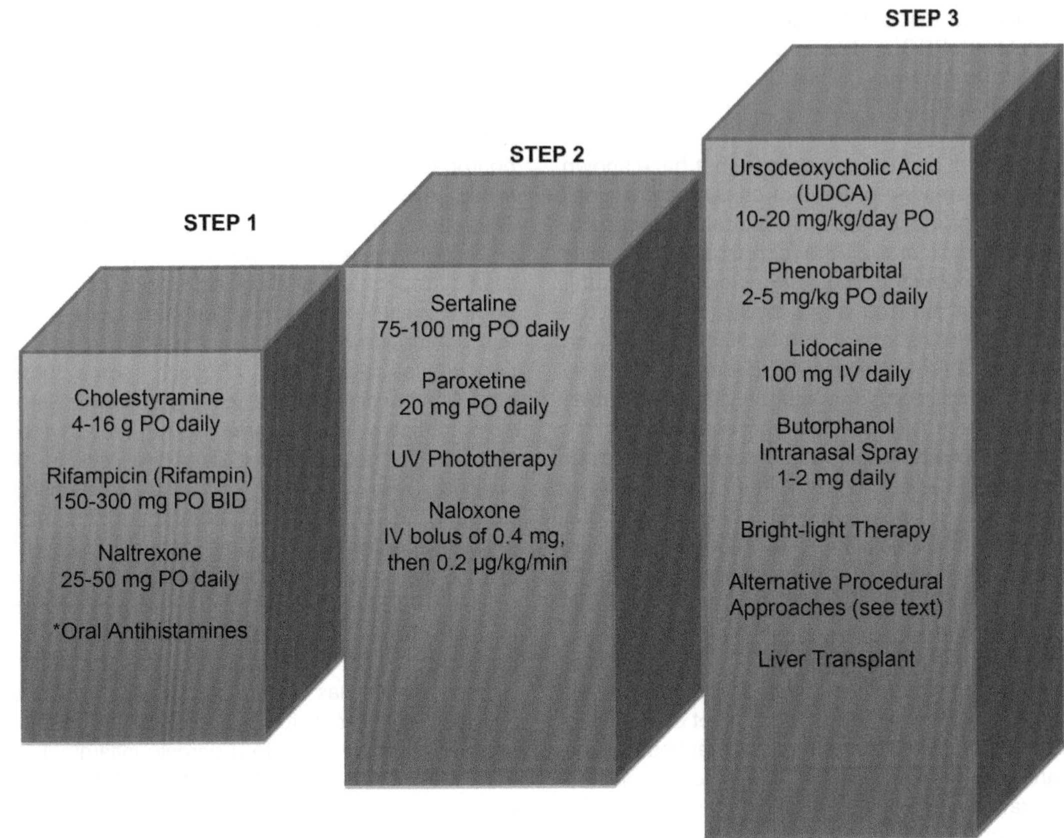

Fig. 1. Stepwise approach to treatment of cholestatic pruritus. * Antihistamines may be effective in treating pruritus and have a benign side-effect profile. However, there are no RCTs to support their use.

double-blind controlled study, revealing a 61% decrease in itch intensity in the treatment group compared with a 12% reduction in the control group.[48] In another controlled, double-blind, crossover study, gamma-linolenic acid (2.2% cream applied once daily to entire body and 3 times daily to itchy areas) decreased the average traditional visual analog scale and pruritus questionnaire scores in 17 dialysis patients.[69] Although an initial case series demonstrated that topical tacrolimus 0.03% cream improved refractory uremic pruritus,[70] a recent RCT did not support these findings.[71] Topical steroids have been used anecdotally and in case reports, but there have not been any controlled studies showing their efficacy.

Although numerous systemic medications have been prescribed to attempt to treat uremic pruritus, the authors have consolidated the literature to focus on the small subset of medications that have either shown efficacy or represented pertinent negatives. Oral antihistamines are frequently used for the treatment of many types of itch, but they are strikingly ineffective in the treatment of uremic pruritus.[72–74] There are a few notable exceptions. Ketotifen, the antihistamine and mast cell stabilizer, produced a decrease in pruritus (without altering the plasma histamine levels) in all 5 patients taking the medication for 8 weeks in 1 report.[75] Similarly, the antihistamine prodrug of fexofenadine, terfenidine, which was banned by the Food and Drug Administration in 1997, was also effective.[76] Gabapentin, classically thought of as an anticonvulsant, has been used in the treatment of neuropathic pain and pruritus syndromes, such as postherpetic neuralgia, diabetic neuropathy, HIV neuropathy, and brachioradial pruritus.[77–86] In 2004, a randomized, double-blind, controlled study showed that with the use of 300 mg gabapentin given after dialysis 3 times a week, patients' had a significant decrease in pruritus over 4 weeks of use, with many patients experiencing complete remission of itch.[87] Subsequent RCTs have substantiated these findings and suggest that a dose of 100 mg orally after each dialysis session is adequate to control symptoms and may reduce the risk of developing neurotoxicity.[88–91] The tricyclic antidepressant and anti-H_1 histaminic receptor, doxepin, produced a complete resolution of pruritus in approximately 50% of patients (vs 10% in placebo group) and an improvement in an additional 30% when used at 10 mg orally twice daily for 1 week in a randomized, double-blind, crossover study.[92] Doxepin can also be considered a good choice in patients with ESRD as it may concurrently alleviate other common symptoms of depression and anxiety in this group.[93,94] Doxepin blood levels can be monitored adding a level of safety.

As in cholestatic pruritus, psychotropic medications have been tested to treat uremic itch. Initial studies indicate inconsistency in the reported plasma blood levels of serotonin in dialysis patients,[95–97] and to that end, serotonin receptor antagonists have had varied success in treating uremic pruritus. Ondansetron (a serotonin type 3 receptor [5-HT$_3$] antagonist) given orally at 8 mg 3 times a day for 2 weeks in an RCT was no better than placebo in controlling HD-associated itch,[98] but another highly selective 5-HT$_3$ blocker, granisetron (given orally at 1 mg twice a day for 1 month), showed a significant decrease in mean pruritus scores.[99] The observation in Brazil that thalidomide administered for the treatment of leprosy improved itch in a dialysis patient sparked a randomized, double-blind, controlled, crossover study to formally evaluate thalidomide as a treatment of uremic itch. This study by Silva and colleagues[100] showed that more than half of patients taking 100 mg thalidomide each night for 1 week greatly reduced their pruritus score (by approximately 75%–80%). In 2 independent RCTs, activated charcoal given at 6 g daily showed either a complete or a partial reduction in itch symptoms in most patients.[101,102] Primrose oil also generated a decrease in subjective itch questionnaire score after 6 weeks of 2 g/d orally.[103]

A French study from 1989 performed a papaverine skin test on dialysis patients with and without itch, and those patients with itch had a significantly smaller wheal response, suggesting an altered vascular tone. Accordingly, the same group tested nicergoline therapy (an ergoline, both a dopamine-receptor agonist and a partial α-adrenergic blocker) in a double-blind crossover study to evaluate its use in the treatment of uremic pruritus. They found that nicergoline was effective in ameliorating itch in 13 of 15 patients when 5 mg was given intravenously during dialysis. When IV treatment was stopped, all patients' itch relapsed, but half of them again found their symptoms in remission when given 30 mg of oral nicergoline daily.[104] Additional systemic medications that have efficacy in the treatment of uremic pruritus in case reports or case series include mirtazapine (15 mg orally each night)[105] and cromolyn sodium (100 mg orally 4 times a day).[106] Recently, 1 group hypothesized that oral nicotinamide could represent a novel potential therapy.[107]

Although the oral μ-receptor antagonist naltrexone (25–100 mg/d) did not show efficacy in reducing renal-induced itch,[108] the κ-opioid receptor antagonist nalfurafine (5 μg 3 times weekly after dialysis) produced a marked reduction in itching intensity, sleep disturbance, and excoriations in a multicenter RCT.[27] Additional IV or subcutaneous agents have been tried with varied success and include IV lidocaine (200 mg/d), heparin (75–100 mg twice daily), and erythropoietin (36 units/kg 3 times a week).[109]

In 1977, Gilchrest and colleagues[110] suggested that ultraviolet phototherapy (using conventional sunburn-spectrum wavelengths) is an effective and safe modality to treat uremic pruritus. Since then, there have been several studies and many more case reports and case series supporting this finding and clarifying that it is specifically broadband UV-B and not UV-A irradiation that is valuable in treating uremic pruritus.[111–114] Of note, there have been varied results with the use of narrowband UV-B on the treatment of uremic pruritus.[115,116]

Alternative methods including dry sauna bath, acupuncture, and homeopathic medications have also been found to improve the symptoms of pruritus in renal failure.[53,117–121] Finally, renal transplant may be the ultimate intervention to cease debilitating pruritus in these patients (**Fig. 2**).[51,122]

NEUROPATHIC ITCH

Patients can also present with complaints of pruritus, paresthesias, or pain related to underlying neuropathies. The differentiation of these symptoms by patients is often difficult, and treatment often needs to address more than 1 sensation. Neuropathic pruritus manifests from a dysfunction of signaling, sensation, or synthesis at any level of the afferent pathway from the skin (eg, herpes zoster) to the brain (eg, central nervous system tumor).[123,124] Specific conditions affecting either the peripheral nervous system or the central nervous system (brachioradial pruritus, notalgia paresthetica, gonyalgia paresthetica, postherpetic neuropathy, small fiber neuropathy, anogenital pruritus, vulvodynia, burning mouth syndrome, erythromelalgia, neuropathic rosacea, diabetes mellitus–associated neuropathy, idiopathic sudomotor failure, multiple sclerosis, brain tumors, abscesses, aneurysms and others) are collectively referred to as neurocutaneous dermatoses. Not surprisingly, the mechanisms underlying

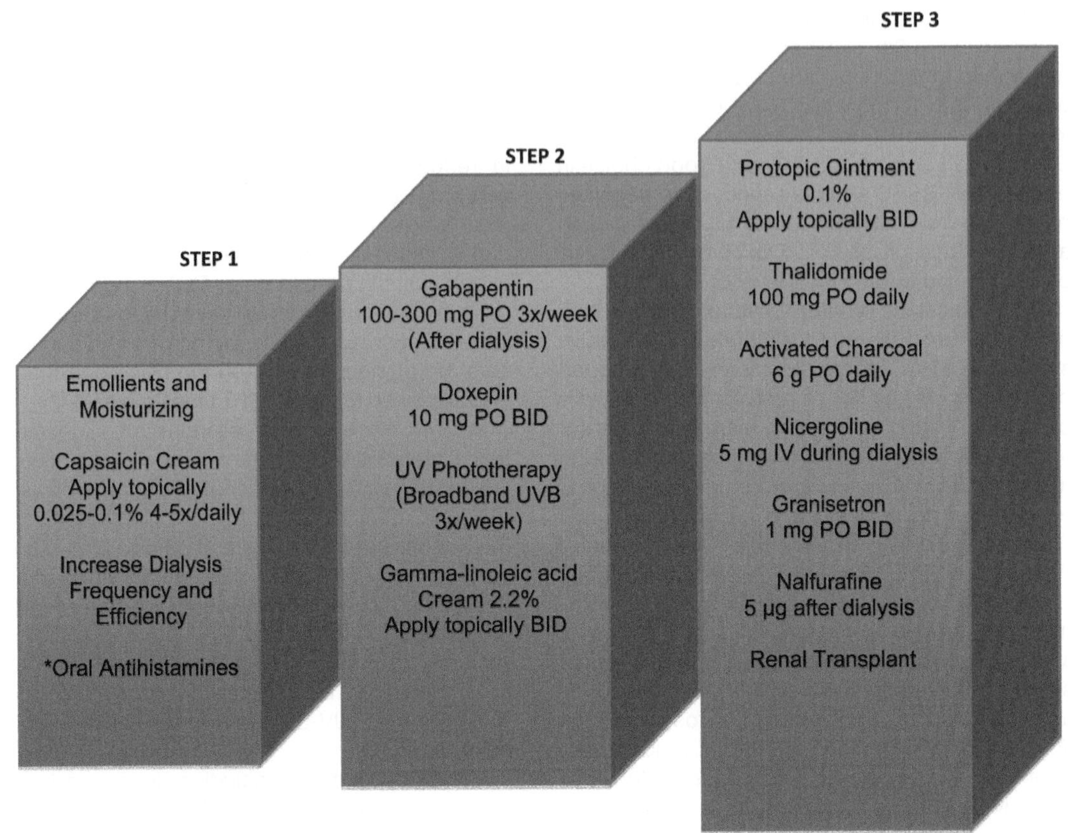

Fig. 2. Stepwise approach to treatment of renal pruritus. * Antihistamines may be effective in treating pruritus and have a benign side-effect profile. However, there are no RCTs to support their use.

neuropathic pruritus remain mysterious and are the focus of much basic and translational research. Recent evidence suggests that there are distinct subsets of small C-nerve fibers with differential sensitivity to histamine and cowhage, and it is these fibers that participate in itch transmission across the circuitry of the nervous system.[125–127] The evaluation and workup of a patient with neuropathic itch is similar to that outlined earlier. However, a visit to a neurologist with clinical workup as well as diagnostic procedures including MRI, CT, electromyography, and nerve conduction studies are also indicated when nerve root impingement is suspected as in brachioradial pruritus or severe notalgia paresthetica.

Brachioradial pruritus was first described by Waisman in 1968 (affecting a patient in Florida) as a neurocutaneous dermatosis localized to the dorsolateral forearm overlying the proximal head of the brachioradialis muscle. Involvement of the upper arms and shoulders is also common in this disease.[128–130] Brachioradial pruritus can be unilateral or bilateral scratching, and sun exposure often worsen the sensation, and the condition is often associated with cervical nerve (C5–C8) injury or nerve compression. Patients report that the application of cold packs frequently provides symptomatic relief.[131] The most effective treatments, however, are those directed at the neurologic cause of the disease. The application of topical capsaicin, oral amitriptyline, oral gabapentin, oral carbamazepine, cervical spine manipulation, and even surgical resection of a cervical rib or spinal fusion have been reported to alleviate brachioradial pruritus in case series or reports.[82,132–137,138]

Herpes zoster is common and so thus is postherpetic neuralgia. There have been various RCTs evaluating treatment modalities for this condition. But most other subsets of neuropathic itch have only been evaluated via case reports and case series. Although the later discussion outlines tested treatments for postherpetic neuralgia with pruritus, identical approaches can be used in treating neuropathic itch from various impingements and neurodegenerative processes. In postherpetic zoster, pain is the classic

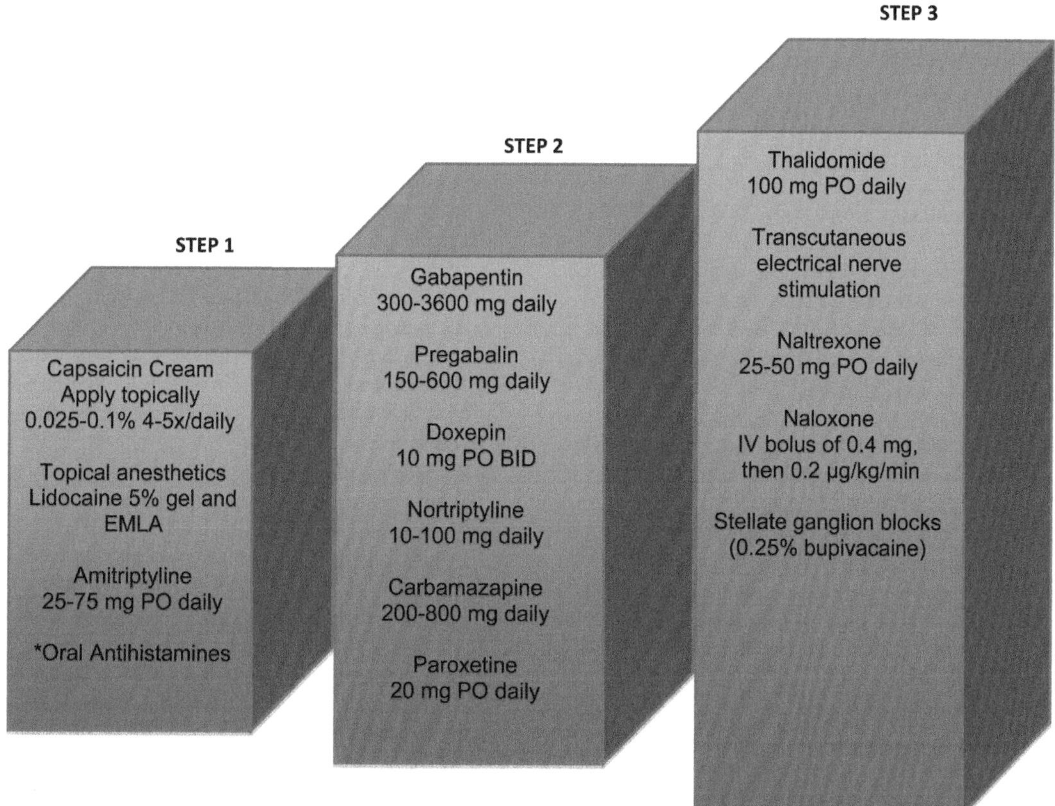

Fig. 3. Stepwise approach to treatment of neuropathic pruritus. * Antihistamines may be effective in treating pruritus and have a benign side-effect profile. However, there are no RCTs to support their use.

associated symptom, but pruritus is also common, affecting approximately 50% of individuals.[139,140] Treatments with proved efficacy include topical and oral agents. Topical capsaicin is used to treat both pain and pruritus (doses ranging from 0.025%–0.075% 4 times a day).[141,142] Topical anesthetics such as 5% lidocaine gel and plaster and eutectic mixture of local anesthetics (EMLA) (2.5% lidocaine and 2.5% prilocaine)[143] and oral tricyclic and other antidepressants have been used with good success in treating postzoster neuralgia. For severe pain, antidepressants can be even combined with weak opioids such as oxycodone. Oral gabapentin (300–3600 mg daily, divided 3 times a day), nortriptyline (10–100 mg daily), pregabalin (150–450 mg/day, divided 2–3 times a day), and carbamazepine (400–800 mg/day) have been shown in cases and RCTs to treat both pain and pruritus of postherpetic neuralgia.[83,144–150] Recently, a case report highlighted the effective treatment of postherpetic itch with serial stellate ganglion blocks with 0.25% bupivacaine.[151]

The treatment of many other forms of neuropathic itch has not been evaluated using RCTs and we are limited to reviewing case reports, case series, and personal experience to suggest therapeutic options (**Fig. 3**).

SUMMARY

Pruritus can be associated with either cutaneous or systemic disease and can be extremely difficult to treat effectively. To do so, it is essential to first establish its cause and address the underlying condition if possible. For pruritus without clinically obvious dermatoses, controlled therapeutic ladders can be used to find the appropriate and effective treatment for each individual. To this end, more basic research investigating the pathogenesis of pruritus and many more RCTs are necessary to help the patients get rid of pruritus. In this article, the authors review current available therapeutics.

REFERENCES

1. Savin JA. How should we define itching? J Am Acad Dermatol 1998;39(2 Pt 1):268–9.

2. Ständer S, Weisshaar E, Mettang T, et al. Clinical classification of itch: a position paper of the International Forum for the Study of Itch. Acta Derm Venereol 2007;87:291–4.
3. Zollner G, Trauner M. Mechanisms of cholestasis. Clin Liver Dis 2008;12:1–26, vii.
4. Lindor KD, Gershwin ME, Poupon R, et al. Primary biliary cirrhosis. Hepatology 2009;50:291–308.
5. Talwalkar JA, Souto E, Jorgensen RA, et al. Natural history of pruritus in primary biliary cirrhosis. Clin Gastroenterol Hepatol 2003;1:297–302.
6. Kremer AE, Beuers U, Oude-Elferink RPJ, et al. Pathogenesis and treatment of pruritus in cholestasis. Drugs 2008;68:2163–82.
7. Bergasa NV, Mehlman JK, Jones EA. Pruritus and fatigue in primary biliary cirrhosis. Baillieres Best Pract Res Clin Gastroenterol 2000;14:643–55.
8. Rishe E, Azarm A, Bergasa NV. Itch in primary biliary cirrhosis: a patients' perspective. Acta Derm Venereol 2008;88:34–7.
9. Heathcote EJ. Management of primary biliary cirrhosis. The American Association for the Study of Liver Diseases practice guidelines. Hepatology 2000;31:1005–13.
10. Bergasa NV. Pruritus in primary biliary cirrhosis: pathogenesis and therapy. Clin Liver Dis 2008;12: 385–406.
11. Datta DV, Sherlock S. Cholestyramine for long term relief of the pruritus complicating intrahepatic cholestasis. Gastroenterology 1966;50:323–32.
12. Datta DV, Sherlock S. Treatment of pruritus of obstructive jaundice with cholestyramine. Br Med J 1963;1:216–9.
13. Tandon P, Rowe BH, Vandermeer B, et al. The efficacy and safety of bile acid binding agents, opioid antagonists, or rifampin in the treatment of cholestasis-associated pruritus. Am J Gastroenterol 2007;102:1528–36.
14. Ghent CN, Carruthers SG. Treatment of pruritus in primary biliary cirrhosis with rifampin. Results of a double-blind, crossover, randomized trial. Gastroenterology 1988;94:488–93.
15. Khurana S, Singh P. Rifampin is safe for treatment of pruritus due to chronic cholestasis: a meta-analysis of prospective randomized-controlled trials. Liver Int 2006;26:943–8.
16. Ghent CN. Pruritus of cholestasis is related to effects of bile salts on the liver, not the skin. Am J Gastroenterol 1987;82:117–8.
17. Terg R, Coronel E, Sordá J, et al. Efficacy and safety of oral naltrexone treatment for pruritus of cholestasis, a crossover, double blind, placebo-controlled study. J Hepatol 2002;37:717–22.
18. Kaplan MM. Primary biliary cirrhosis. N Engl J Med 1996;335:1570–80.
19. Spivey JR, Jorgensen RA, Gores GJ, et al. Methionine-enkephalin concentrations correlate with stage of disease but not pruritus in patients with primary biliary cirrhosis. Am J Gastroenterol 1994;89:2028–32.
20. Thornton JR, Losowsky MS. Plasma leucine enkephalin is increased in liver disease. Gut 1989;30:1392–5.
21. Bernstein JE, Swift R. Relief of intractable pruritus with naloxone. Arch Dermatol 1979;115:1366–7.
22. Wolfhagen FH, Sternieri E, Hop WC, et al. Oral naltrexone treatment for cholestatic pruritus: a double-blind, placebo-controlled study. Gastroenterology 1997;113:1264–9.
23. Bergasa NV, Alling DW, Talbot TL, et al. Effects of naloxone infusions in patients with the pruritus of cholestasis. A double-blind, randomized, controlled trial. Ann Intern Med 1995;123:161–7.
24. Carson KL, Tran TT, Cotton P, et al. Pilot study of the use of naltrexone to treat the severe pruritus of cholestatic liver disease. Am J Gastroenterol 1996;91:1022–3.
25. Thornton JR, Losowsky MS. Opioid peptides and primary biliary cirrhosis. BMJ 1988;297:1501–4.
26. Jones EA, Neuberger J, Bergasa NV. Opiate antagonist therapy for the pruritus of cholestasis: the avoidance of opioid withdrawal-like reactions. QJM 2002;95:547–52.
27. Wikström B, Gellert R, Ladefoged SD, et al. Kappa-opioid system in uremic pruritus: multicenter, randomized, double-blind, placebo-controlled clinical studies. J Am Soc Nephrol 2005;16:3742–7.
28. Bergasa NV. Medical palliation of the jaundiced patient with pruritus. Gastroenterol Clin North Am 2006;35:113–23.
29. Mayo MJ, Handem I, Saldana S, et al. Sertraline as a first-line treatment for cholestatic pruritus. Hepatology 2007;45:666–74.
30. Browning J, Combes B, Mayo MJ. Long-term efficacy of sertraline as a treatment for cholestatic pruritus in patients with primary biliary cirrhosis. Am J Gastroenterol 2003;98:2736–41.
31. Zylicz Z, Krajnik M, Sorge AA, et al. Paroxetine in the treatment of severe non-dermatological pruritus: a randomized, controlled trial. J Pain Symptom Manage 2003;26:1105–12.
32. Gong Y, Huang ZB, Christensen E, et al. Ursodeoxycholic acid for primary biliary cirrhosis. Cochrane Database Syst Rev 2008;3:CD000551. DOI: 10.1002/14651858. CD000551.pub2.
33. Poupon RE, Lindor KD, Cauch-Dudek K, et al. Combined analysis of randomized controlled trials of ursodeoxycholic acid in primary biliary cirrhosis. Gastroenterology 1997;113:884–90.
34. Bergasa NV, McGee M, Ginsburg IH, et al. Gabapentin in patients with the pruritus of cholestasis: a double-blind, randomized, placebo-controlled trial. Hepatology 2006;44:1317–23.

35. Bergasa NV, Link MJ, Keogh M, et al. Pilot study of bright-light therapy reflected toward the eyes for the pruritus of chronic liver disease. Am J Gastroenterol 2001;96:1563–70.
36. Hanid MA, Levi AJ. Phototherapy for pruritus in primary biliary cirrhosis. Lancet 1980;2:530.
37. Cerio R, Murphy GM, Sladen GE, et al. A combination of phototherapy and cholestyramine for the relief of pruritus in primary biliary cirrhosis. Br J Dermatol 1987;116:265–7.
38. Hajheydari Z, Makhlough A. Cutaneous and mucosal manifestations in patients on maintenance hemodialysis: a study of 101 patients in Sari, Iran. Iran J Kidney Dis 2008;2:86–90.
39. Melo NC, Elias RM, Castro MC, et al. Pruritus in hemodialysis patients: the problem remains. Hemodial Int 2009;13:38–42.
40. Udayakumar P, Balasubramanian S, Ramalingam KS, et al. Cutaneous manifestations in patients with chronic renal failure on hemodialysis. Indian J Dermatol Venereol Leprol 2006;72:119–25.
41. Picó MR, Lugo-Somolinos A, Sánchez JL, et al. Cutaneous alterations in patients with chronic renal failure. Int J Dermatol 1992;31:860–3.
42. Robinson-Bostom L, DiGiovanna JJ. Cutaneous manifestations of end-stage renal disease. J Am Acad Dermatol 2000;43:975–86 [quiz: 987–90].
43. Zucker I, Yosipovitch G, David M, et al. Prevalence and characterization of uremic pruritus in patients undergoing hemodialysis: uremic pruritus is still a major problem for patients with end-stage renal disease. J Am Acad Dermatol 2003;49:842–6.
44. Kuypers DR. Skin problems in chronic kidney disease. Nat Clin Pract Nephrol 2009;5:157–70.
45. Patel TS, Freedman BI, Yosipovitch G. An update on pruritus associated with CKD. Am J Kidney Dis 2007;50:11–20.
46. Tessari G, Dalle Vedove C, Loschiavo C, et al. The impact of pruritus on the quality of life of patients undergoing dialysis: a single centre cohort study. J Nephrol 2009;22:241–8.
47. Weisshaar E, Matterne U, Mettang T. How do nephrologists in haemodialysis units consider the symptom of itch? Results of a survey in Germany. Nephrol Dial Transplant 2009;24:1328–30.
48. Young TA, Patel TS, Camacho F, et al. A pramoxine-based anti-itch lotion is more effective than a control lotion for the treatment of uremic pruritus in adult hemodialysis patients. J Dermatolog Treat 2009;20:76–81.
49. Narita I, Alchi B, Omori K, et al. Etiology and prognostic significance of severe uremic pruritus in chronic hemodialysis patients. Kidney Int 2006;69:1626–32.
50. Kurban MS, Boueiz A, Kibbi A. Cutaneous manifestations of chronic kidney disease. Clin Dermatol 2008;26:255–64.
51. Chou FF, Ho JC, Huang SC, et al. A study on pruritus after parathyroidectomy for secondary hyperparathyroidism. J Am Coll Surg 2000;190:65–70.
52. Keithi-Reddy SR, Patel TV, Armstrong AW, et al. Uremic pruritus. Kidney Int 2007;72:373–7.
53. Lugon JR. Uremic pruritus: a review. Hemodial Int 2005;9:180–8.
54. Khopkar U, Pande S. Etiopathogenesis of pruritus due to systemic causes: implications for treatment. Indian J Dermatol Venereol Leprol 2007;73:215–7.
55. Hampers CL, Katz AI, Wilson RE, et al. Disappearance of "uremic" itching after subtotal parathyroidectomy. N Engl J Med 1968;279:695–7.
56. Szepietowski JC, Sikora M, Kusztal M, et al. Uremic pruritus: a clinical study of maintenance hemodialysis patients. J Dermatol 2002;29:621–7.
57. Balaskas EV, Chu M, Uldall RP, et al. Pruritus in continuous ambulatory peritoneal dialysis and hemodialysis patients. Perit Dial Int 1993;13(Suppl 2):S527–32.
58. Morton CA, Lafferty M, Hau C, et al. Pruritus and skin hydration during dialysis. Nephrol Dial Transplant 1996;11:2031–6.
59. Yosipovitch G, Reis J, Tur E, et al. Sweat secretion, stratum corneum hydration, small nerve function and pruritus in patients with advanced chronic renal failure. Br J Dermatol 1995;133:561–4.
60. Kato A, Hamada M, Maruyama T, et al. Pruritus and hydration state of stratum corneum in hemodialysis patients. Am J Nephrol 2000;20:437–42.
61. Chen ZJ, Cao G, Tang WX, et al. A randomized controlled trial of high-permeability haemodialysis against conventional haemodialysis in the treatment of uraemic pruritus. Clin Exp Dermatol 2009;34:679–83.
62. Stam F, van Guldener C, Schalkwijk CG, et al. Impaired renal function is associated with markers of endothelial dysfunction and increased inflammatory activity. Nephrol Dial Transplant 2003;18:892–8.
63. Stenvinkel P, Pecoits-Filho R, Lindholm B. Coronary artery disease in end-stage renal disease: no longer a simple plumbing problem. J Am Soc Nephrol 2003;14:1927–39.
64. Kimmel M, Alscher DM, Dunst R, et al. The role of micro-inflammation in the pathogenesis of uraemic pruritus in haemodialysis patients. Nephrol Dial Transplant 2006;21:749–55.
65. Szepietowski JC, Reich A, Schwartz RA. Uraemic xerosis. Nephrol Dial Transplant 2004;19:2709–12.
66. Ståhle-Bäckdahl M. Uremic pruritus. Semin Dermatol 1995;14:297–301.
67. Nielsen T, Andersen KE, Kristiansen J. Pruritus and xerosis in patients with chronic renal failure. Dan Med Bull 1980;27:269–71.

68. Tarng DC, Cho YL, Liu HN, et al. Hemodialysis-related pruritus: a double-blind, placebo-controlled, crossover study of capsaicin 0.025% cream. Nephron 1996;72:617–22.
69. Chen Y, Chiu W, Wu M. Therapeutic effect of topical gamma-linolenic acid on refractory uremic pruritus. Am J Kidney Dis 2006;48:69–76.
70. Pauli-Magnus C, Klumpp S, Alscher DM, et al. Short-term efficacy of tacrolimus ointment in severe uremic pruritus. Perit Dial Int 2000;20:802–3.
71. Duque MI, Yosipovitch G, Fleischer AB, et al. Lack of efficacy of tacrolimus ointment 0.1% for treatment of hemodialysis-related pruritus: a randomized, double-blind, vehicle-controlled study. J Am Acad Dermatol 2005;52(3 Pt 1):519–21.
72. Schwartz IF, Iaina A. Uraemic pruritus. Nephrol Dial Transplant 1999;14:834–9.
73. Narita I, Iguchi S, Omori K, et al. Uremic pruritus in chronic hemodialysis patients. J Nephrol 2008;21: 161–5.
74. Manenti L, Tansinda P, Vaglio A. Uraemic pruritus: clinical characteristics, pathophysiology and treatment. Drugs 2009;69:251–63.
75. Francos GC, Kauh YC, Gittlen SD, et al. Elevated plasma histamine in chronic uremia. Effects of ketotifen on pruritus. Int J Dermatol 1991;30:884–9.
76. Russo GE, Spaziani M, Guidotti C, et al. [Pruritus in chronic uremic patients in periodic hemodialysis. Treatment with terfenadine (an antagonist of histamine H1 receptors)]. Minerva Urol Nefrol 1986;38: 443–7 [in Italian].
77. Mizoguchi H, Watanabe C, Yonezawa A, et al. New therapy for neuropathic pain. Int Rev Neurobiol 2009;85:249–60.
78. Quilici S, Chancellor J, Löthgren M, et al. Meta-analysis of duloxetine vs. pregabalin and gabapentin in the treatment of diabetic peripheral neuropathic pain. BMC Neurol 2009;9:6.
79. Sandercock D, Cramer M, Wu J, et al. Gabapentin extended release for the treatment of painful diabetic peripheral neuropathy: efficacy and tolerability in a double-blind, randomized, controlled clinical trial. Diabetes Care 2009;32:e20.
80. Hahn K, Arendt G, Braun JS, et al. A placebo-controlled trial of gabapentin for painful HIV-associated sensory neuropathies. J Neurol 2004;251: 1260–6.
81. Bueller HA, Bernhard JD, Dubroff LM. Gabapentin treatment for brachioradial pruritus. J Eur Acad Dermatol Venereol 1999;13:227–8.
82. Winhoven SM, Coulson IH, Bottomley WW. Brachioradial pruritus: response to treatment with gabapentin. Br J Dermatol 2004;150:786–7.
83. Gilron I, Bailey JM, Tu D, et al. Nortriptyline and gabapentin, alone and in combination for neuropathic pain: a double-blind, randomised controlled crossover trial. Lancet 2009;374:1252–61.
84. Irving G, Jensen M, Cramer M, et al. Efficacy and tolerability of gastric-retentive gabapentin for the treatment of postherpetic neuralgia: results of a double-blind, randomized, placebo-controlled clinical trial. Clin J Pain 2009;25:185–92.
85. Zin CS, Nissen LM, Smith MT, et al. An update on the pharmacological management of post-herpetic neuralgia and painful diabetic neuropathy. CNS Drugs 2008;22:417–42.
86. Rowbotham M, Harden N, Stacey B, et al. Gabapentin for the treatment of postherpetic neuralgia: a randomized controlled trial. JAMA 1998;280: 1837–42.
87. Gunal AI, Ozalp G, Yoldas TK, et al. Gabapentin therapy for pruritus in haemodialysis patients: a randomized, placebo-controlled, double-blind trial. Nephrol Dial Transplant 2004;19:3137–9.
88. Manenti L, Vaglio A, Borgatti PP. Gabapentin as a therapeutic option in uremic pruritus. Kidney Int 2008;73:512 [author reply: 512–3].
89. Naini AE, Harandi AA, Khanbabapour S, et al. Gabapentin: a promising drug for the treatment of uremic pruritus. Saudi J Kidney Dis Transpl 2007; 18:378–81.
90. Manenti L, Vaglio A, Costantino E, et al. Gabapentin in the treatment of uremic itch: an index case and a pilot evaluation. J Nephrol 2005;18:86–91.
91. Razeghi E, Eskandari D, Ganji MR, et al. Gabapentin and uremic pruritus in hemodialysis patients. Ren Fail 2009;31:85–90.
92. Pour-Reza-Gholi F, Nasrollahi A, Firouzan A, et al. Low-dose doxepin for treatment of pruritus in patients on hemodialysis. Iran J Kidney Dis 2007;1:34–7.
93. Feighner J, Hendrickson G, Miller L, et al. Double-blind comparison of doxepin versus bupropion in outpatients with a major depressive disorder. J Clin Psychopharmacol 1986;6:27–32.
94. Rickels K, Feighner JP, Smith WT. Alprazolam, amitriptyline, doxepin, and placebo in the treatment of depression. Arch Gen Psychiatry 1985; 42:134–41.
95. Weisshaar E, Dunker N, Röhl F, et al. Antipruritic effects of two different 5-HT3 receptor antagonists and an antihistamine in haemodialysis patients. Exp Dermatol 2004;13:298–304.
96. Weisshaar E, Dunker N, Domröse U, et al. Plasma serotonin and histamine levels in hemodialysis-related pruritus are not significantly influenced by 5-HT3 receptor blocker and antihistaminic therapy. Clin Nephrol 2003;59:124–9.
97. Balaskas EV, Bamihas GI, Karamouzis M, et al. Histamine and serotonin in uremic pruritus: effect of ondansetron in CAPD-pruritic patients. Nephron 1998;78:395–402.
98. Murphy M, Reaich D, Pai P, et al. A randomized, placebo-controlled, double-blind trial of ondansetron in renal itch. Br J Dermatol 2003;148:314–7.

99. Layegh P, Mojahedi MJ, Malekshah PE, et al. Effect of oral granisetron in uremic pruritus. Indian J Dermatol Venereol Leprol 2007;73:231–4.
100. Silva SR, Viana PC, Lugon NV, et al. Thalidomide for the treatment of uremic pruritus: a crossover randomized double-blind trial. Nephron 1994;67:270–3.
101. Pederson JA, Matter BJ, Czerwinski AW, et al. Relief of idiopathic generalized pruritus in dialysis patients treated with activated oral charcoal. Ann Intern Med 1980;93:446–8.
102. Giovannetti S, Barsotti G, Cupisti A, et al. Oral activated charcoal in patients with uremic pruritus. Nephron 1995;70:193–6.
103. Yoshimoto-Furuie K, Yoshimoto K, Tanaka T, et al. Effects of oral supplementation with evening primrose oil for six weeks on plasma essential fatty acids and uremic skin symptoms in hemodialysis patients. Nephron 1999;81:151–9.
104. Bousquet J, Rivory JP, Maheut M, et al. Double-blind, placebo-controlled study of nicergoline in the treatment of pruritus in patients receiving maintenance hemodialysis. J Allergy Clin Immunol 1989;83:825–8.
105. Davis MP, Frandsen JL, Walsh D, et al. Mirtazapine for pruritus. J Pain Symptom Manage 2003;25:288–91.
106. Rosner MH. Cromolyn sodium: a potential therapy for uremic pruritus? Hemodial Int 2006;10:189–92.
107. Namazi MR, Fallahzadeh MK, Roozbeh J. Nicotinamide as a potential novel addition to the anti-uremic pruritus weaponry. Saudi J Kidney Dis Transpl 2009;20:291–2.
108. Pauli-Magnus C, Mikus G, Alscher DM, et al. Naltrexone does not relieve uremic pruritus: results of a randomized, double-blind, placebo-controlled crossover study. J Am Soc Nephrol 2000;11:514–9.
109. De Marchi S, Cecchin E, Villalta D, et al. Relief of pruritus and decreases in plasma histamine concentrations during erythropoietin therapy in patients with uremia. N Engl J Med 1992;326:969–74.
110. Gilchrest BA, Rowe JW, Brown RS, et al. Relief of uremic pruritus with ultraviolet phototherapy. N Engl J Med 1977;297:136–8.
111. Rivard J, Lim HW. Ultraviolet phototherapy for pruritus. Dermatol Ther 2005;18:344–54.
112. Gilchrest BA, Rowe JW, Brown RS, et al. Ultraviolet phototherapy of uremic pruritus. Long-term results and possible mechanism of action. Ann Intern Med 1979;91:17–21.
113. Blachley JD, Blankenship DM, Menter A, et al. Uremic pruritus: skin divalent ion content and response to ultraviolet phototherapy. Am J Kidney Dis 1985;5:237–41.
114. Lazrak S, Skali H, Benchikhi H, et al. [Phototherapy and hemodialysis pruritus]. Nephrologie 2004;25:293–5 [in French].
115. Ada S, Seçkin D, Budakoğlu I, et al. Treatment of uremic pruritus with narrowband ultraviolet B phototherapy: an open pilot study. J Am Acad Dermatol 2005;53:149–51.
116. Hsu MM, Yang CC. Uraemic pruritus responsive to broadband ultraviolet (UV) B therapy does not readily respond to narrowband UVB therapy. Br J Dermatol 2003;149:888–9.
117. Gao H, Zhang W, Wang Y. Acupuncture treatment for 34 cases of uremic cutaneous pruritus. J Tradit Chin Med 2002;22:29–30.
118. Che-Yi C, Wen CY, Min-Tsung K, et al. Acupuncture in haemodialysis patients at the Quchi (LI11) acupoint for refractory uraemic pruritus. Nephrol Dial Transplant 2005;20:1912–5.
119. Duo LJ. Electrical needle therapy of uremic pruritus. Nephron 1987;47:179–83.
120. Cavalcanti AM, Rocha LM, Carillo R, et al. Effects of homeopathic treatment on pruritus of haemodialysis patients: a randomised placebo-controlled double-blind trial. Homeopathy 2003;92:177–81.
121. Snyder D, Merrill JP. Sauna baths in the treatment of chronic renal failure. Trans Am Soc Artif Intern Organs 1966;12:188–92.
122. Altmeyer P, Kachel HG, Schäfer G, et al. [Normalization of uremic skin changes following kidney transplantation]. Hautarzt 1986;37:217–21 [in German].
123. Ikoma A, Steinhoff M, Ständer S, et al. The neurobiology of itch. Nat Rev Neurosci 2006;7:535–47.
124. Steinhoff M, Bienenstock J, Schmelz M, et al. Neurophysiological, neuroimmunological, and neuroendocrine basis of pruritus. J Invest Dermatol 2006;126:1705–18.
125. Schmelz M, Schimdt R, Bickel A, et al. Specific C-receptors for itch in human skin. J Neurosci 1997;17:8003–8.
126. Ikoma A, Rukwied R, Ständer S, et al. Neurophysiology of pruritus: interaction of itch and pain. Arch Dermatol 2003;139:1475–8.
127. Yosipovitch G, Greaves MW, Schmelz M. Itch. Lancet 2003;361:690–4.
128. Heyl T. Brachioradial pruritus. Arch Dermatol 1983;119:115–6.
129. Veien NK, Hattel T, Laurberg G, et al. Brachioradial pruritus. J Am Acad Dermatol 2001;44:704–5.
130. Waisman M. Solar pruritus of the elbows (brachioradial summer pruritus). Arch Dermatol 1968;98:481–5.
131. Bernhard JD, Bordeaux JS. Medical pearl: the ice-pack sign in brachioradial pruritus. J Am Acad Dermatol 2005;52:1073.

132. Knight TE, Hayashi T. Solar (brachioradial) pruritus–response to capsaicin cream. Int J Dermatol 1994;33:206–9.
133. Barry R, Rogers S. Brachioradial pruritus–an enigmatic entity. Clin Exp Dermatol 2004;29:637–8.
134. Kanitakis J. Brachioradial pruritus: report of a new case responding to gabapentin. Eur J Dermatol 2006;16:311–2.
135. Tait CP, Grigg E, Quirk CJ. Brachioradial pruritus and cervical spine manipulation. Australas J Dermatol 1998;39:168–70.
136. Rongioletti F. Pruritus as presenting sign of cervical rib. Lancet 1992;339:55.
137. Binder A, Fölster-Holst R, Sahan G, et al. A case of neuropathic brachioradial pruritus caused by cervical disc herniation. Nat Clin Pract Neurol 2008;4:338–42.
138. Wang KC, Berger TG. Dermatological-neurological interactions. In: Aminoff MJ, editor. Neurology and general medicine. 4th edition. Philadelphia (PA): Churchill Livingstone; 2008. p. 217–25.
139. Oaklander AL, Cohen SP, Raju SV. Intractable postherpetic itch and cutaneous deafferentation after facial shingles. Pain 2002;96:9–12.
140. Oaklander AL, Bowsher D, Galer B, et al. Herpes zoster itch: preliminary epidemiologic data. J Pain 2003;4:338–43.
141. Summey BT, Yosipovitch G. Pharmacologic advances in the systemic treatment of itch. Dermatol Ther 2005;18:328–32.
142. Garroway N, Chhabra S, Landis S, et al. Clinical inquiries: what measures relieve postherpetic neuralgia? J Fam Pract 2009;58:384d–f.
143. Binder A, Bruxelle J, Rogers P, et al. Topical 5% lidocaine (lignocaine) medicated plaster treatment for post-herpetic neuralgia: results of a double-blind, placebo-controlled, multinational efficacy and safety trial. Clin Drug Investig 2009;29:393–408.
144. Semionov V, Shvartzman P. Post herpetic itching–a treatment dilemma. Clin J Pain 2008;24:366–8.
145. Ehrchen J, Ständer S. Pregabalin in the treatment of chronic pruritus. J Am Acad Dermatol 2008;58:S36–7.
146. Porzio G, Aielli F, Verna L, et al. Efficacy of pregabalin in the management of cetuximab-related itch. J Pain Symptom Manage 2006;32:397–8.
147. Tassone DM, Boyce E, Guyer J, et al. Pregabalin: a novel gamma-aminobutyric acid analogue in the treatment of neuropathic pain, partial-onset seizures, and anxiety disorders. Clin Ther 2007;29:26–48.
148. Yesudian PD, Wilson NJE. Efficacy of gabapentin in the management of pruritus of unknown origin. Arch Dermatol 2005;141:1507–9.
149. Gore M, Sadosky A, Tai K, et al. A retrospective evaluation of the use of gabapentin and pregabalin in patients with postherpetic neuralgia in usual-care settings. Clin Ther 2007;29:1655–70.
150. McKeage K, Keam SJ. Pregabalin: in the treatment of postherpetic neuralgia. Drugs Aging 2009;26:883–92.
151. Peterson RC, Patel L, Cubert K, et al. Serial stellate ganglion blocks for intractable postherpetic itching in a pediatric patient: a case report. Pain Physician 2009;12:629–32.

Innovative Management of Recurrent Furunculosis

Natasha Atanaskova, MD, PhD, Kenneth J. Tomecki, MD*

KEYWORDS

- Furunculosis • *Staphylococcus aureus* • MRSA
- Colonization • Management

Dermatologists confront a variety of cutaneous infections in an era when infections are becoming more prevalent and also more aggressive. For example, the emergence of organisms with rapidly expanding resistance leads to common skin commensals causing life-threatening conditions. Such skin and soft tissue infections (SSTIs) are frequent causes of emergency room visits and hospitalizations. Most of the treatment of SSTIs is based primarily on anecdotal evidence and addresses only acute management; thus, recommendations in this body of evidence may be inadequate to suggest appropriate steps to prevent recurrent or relapsing cutaneous infection.

One of the most common bacterial infections of the skin and soft tissue is furunculosis (boil), an inflammatory nodule that involves the hair follicle, with small abscess formation extending through the dermis into the subcutaneous layers (**Fig. 1**). Etiologically, a furuncle is essentially the suppurative sequela of folliculitis.[1] When infection involves several adjacent follicles, producing a coalescent inflammatory mass with pus draining from multiple orifices, the larger nodule is then termed a carbuncle.

Patients with furunculosis present with a painful reddened nodule, sometimes with an overlying pustule, commonly at a site associated with trauma, and most frequently on the extremities.[2] Occasionally and usually mistakenly, furuncles are thought to follow a spider bite.[3] The duration and course of furunculosis are variable: some patients may experience only 1 episode whereas others develop recurrences for months or even years. Recurrence is generally defined as 3 or more attacks within 12 months.[4] When furunculosis is recurrent, infection often spreads to other family members. Familial occurrence is the sole independent factor associated with recurrent furunculosis, which raises concern that currently recommended routine therapy is inadequate and that affected family members should receive some type of concomitant treatment as well.[5]

BACTERIAL MILIEU

Effective therapy needs to target the infectious agent, usually *Staphylococcus aureus*—a gram-positive, coagulase-positive bacterium, which is a commensal on human skin and mucosa; 20% of the population harbors the organism chronically and 60% intermittently.[6] Although a colonizer, *S aureus* is the leading cause of SSTIs, lower respiratory infections, and bloodstream infections worldwide.[7] The primary human reservoir for *S aureus* is the anterior nares, and nasal carriage is a documented risk factor for staphylococcal infections. In recent years, carriage has also been noted to occur in other warm, moist skin folds, such as behind the ears, under pendulous breast, in the groin, and on perianal skin.

S aureus has the ability to adapt to antibiotics, especially penicillins, and to evolve to a more potent and penetrant organism. In response to

Department of Dermatology, Cleveland Clinic Foundation, A61, 9500 Euclid Avenue, Cleveland, OH 44195, USA
* Corresponding author.
E-mail address: tomeckk@ccf.org

Dermatol Clin 28 (2010) 479–487
doi:10.1016/j.det.2010.03.013
0733-8635/10/$ – see front matter © 2010 Elsevier Inc. All rights reserved.

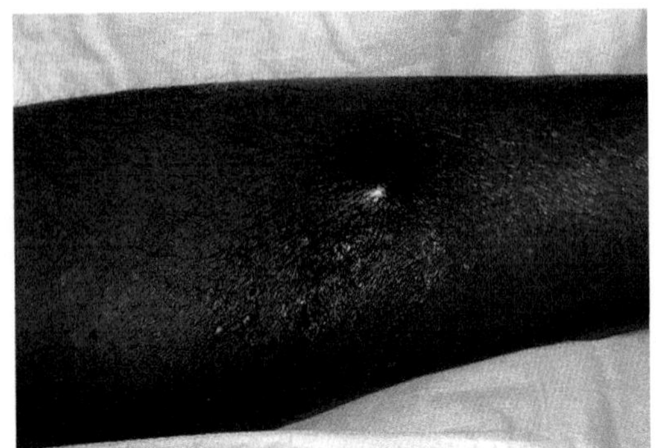

Fig. 1. Furunculosis of different stages on leg.

penicillin, *S aureus* produces β-lactamase and resistance develops rapidly. Methicillin, a penicillinase-resistant semisynthetic penicillin created in 1960, temporarily resolved this problem until the emergence of methicillin-resistant *S aureus* organisms (MRSA) 1 year later.[8] Initially, the methicillin-resistant species arose as hospital-acquired infections (HA-MRSA), associated with pneumonia, bacteremia, urinary tract infections, and surgical wound infections. HA-MRSA is primarily prevalent in the elderly, patients requiring frequent hospitalizations and invasive procedures, and residents of long-term facilities.[9]

When a similar MRSA variant appeared in healthy adults and children in the past 2 decades, the scope of this problem significantly expanded. This community-acquired MRSA variant (CA-MRSA) is a different entity in terms of history, epidemiology, and molecular characteristics.[10] The delineation between these 2 entities, HA-MRSA and CA-MRSA, is becoming less clear as newer variants, such as community-associated HA-MRSA, are described.[11]

MOLECULAR PATHOGENESIS

CA-MRSA infection typically affects young, healthy individuals (median age 23), producing SSTIs in 85% of cases; at present, MRSA infections are the leading cause of cutaneous abscesses in the United States.[12] Furunculosis is the main clinical presentation of CA-MRSA infections. Necrotizing pneumonia is an uncommon presentation that generally occurs after influenza in otherwise healthy adults and children. Pneumonia may occur with furunculosis, leucopenia, and hemoptysis, resulting in a fulminant course with 37% mortality.[13]

Rarely, CA-MRSA may produce musculoskeletal infections, endocarditis, bacteremia, brain abscesses, and sinusitis. Methicillin resistance of *S aureus* is mediated by alteration of genes on the staphylococcal cassette chromosome, also found in *S epidermidis* strains, which might explain MRSA's propensity for cutaneous colonization and infections.[14] Leukocidin toxins account for some of the distinctive clinical characteristics of CA-MRSA; the toxins cause pyogenic infections by irreversibly damaging the responding immune effector cells.[15] Panton-Valentine leukocidin (PVL) is a pore-forming toxin of staphylococci that causes cell lysis of neutrophils, monocytes, and macrophages. PVL may account for MRSA's ability to form abscesses by promoting inflammation, neutrophil infiltration, secretion of degenerative enzymes, and generation of superoxide species.[16] The PVL cascade produces tissue necrosis of the dermonecrotic centers of MRSA furuncles, which may mimic an insect assault.

RISK FACTORS

In the past decade, the incidence of CA-MRSA infections has increased to become the most common cause of SSTIs in the emergency room setting; prevalence now approaches 60%.[3] *S aureus* is the most common causative organism of recurrent furunculosis, isolated in approximately 90% of cases, but lacks any distinct virulent features to explain the recurrence.[10] Nasal carriage is common, but airborne spread is another, albeit uncommon, mode of *S aureus* transmission in SSTIs. The main risk factor for furunculosis is direct physical contact with infected individuals, primarily family members or health care personnel.[17]

Close contact within a household, living facility, or workplace has been associated with outbreaks of MRSA SSTIs. The ability of *S aureus* to survive on fomites creates a potential source of cross contamination: some species can survive for weeks on fabrics and plastics. This phenomenon tends to enhance the likelihood of recurrent furunculosis in crowded areas and in those with compromised hygiene.[18] Individuals who live in hot, humid climates are at a higher risk for developing skin lesions, and household pets may act as vectors for MRSA SSTIs in humans.[19]

An individual's overall health is another factor that may predispose to recurrent furunculosis (eg, obesity, anemia, diabetes mellitus, immunotherapy, HIV infection, and end-stage renal disease tend to predispose individuals to SSTIs).[4] Established skin diseases increase the susceptibility to bacterial colonization, and patients with atopic dermatitis, burn injuries, chronic wounds, or leg ulcers are more prone to developing refractory furunculosis.[20] Inherited immune-deficiency states, in particular those with impaired neutrophil function, also correlate with increased risk for recurrent furunculosis.[21]

DIAGNOSIS

Initial evaluation of affected patients requires a bacterial culture of the furuncle content to confirm the causative organism and to yield data on prevalence. Standard technique is a swab from the center of the furuncle or, with larger wounds, a rotating maneuver from the outer edges inward.[22] Molecular assays, such as polymerase chain reaction, allow amplification and rapid detection of organisms within hours, with minimal false-negative rates; however, this kind of testing is not standard due to cost concerns.[23] Skin biopsy for tissue culture is another diagnostic option but is only rarely necessary.

Although uncommon, some cutaneous lesions may mimic furunculosis (eg, an inflamed epidermal cyst or dermal myiasis). Thus, caution should be used in making the diagnosis of furunculosis if the situation seems at all uncertain.

TREATMENT

The mainstay of therapy for acute furunculosis is simple incision and drainage. Drainage alone without use of adjunctive antibiotic is usually sufficient to treat a single abscess smaller than 5 cm.[24] Systemic antibiotics should be reserved for abscesses larger than 5 cm or if cellulitis or fever is present. Other situations that warrant the use of antibiotics are central facial disease, extremes of age (very young or old patients), other comorbidities (ie, immunosupression), or previously failed treatment.[25,26] Patients with fever, cellulitis, or other comorbidities, usually require hospitalization and intravenous antibiotic (eg, vancomycin) with the goal of preventing bacteremia. Patients with MRSA bacteremia have a poor outcome compared with patients with methicillin-susceptible *S aureus* (MSSA) bacteremia.[27]

RECURRENT FURUNCULOSIS

Therapy becomes more complicated in patients with recurrent or multiple furunculosis. Incision and drainage of many nodules/abscesses is painful and impractical, necessitating treatment with an antibiotic. The greatest challenge in treating recurrent furunculosis is that most treatment recommendations rely on anecdotal evidence that predates the MRSA era.[28] Successful therapy consists of a therapeutic triad: antibiotics, decolonization, and decontamination.

Antibiotic Therapy in Recurrent Furunculosis

For recurrent furunculosis, bacterial culture and sensitivity ultimately dictate the antibiotic choice, and culture is warranted with each outbreak. Clindamycin, doxycycline, and trimethoprim-sulfamethoxazole (TMP-SMX) are the most commonly used antibiotics for outpatient treatment of MRSA-related SSTI in the United States.[29] TMP-SMX (Bactrim or Septra) is an effective and inexpensive drug for MRSA furunculosis, but empiric use is limited by its suboptimal efficacy against group A streptococcal organisms (**Table 1**). TMP-SMX is a good second-line treatment of severe MRSA infections when patients are unable to tolerate first-line drugs.[30,31] Side effects of TMP-SMX are infrequent but potentially serious (eg, toxic epidermal necrolysis and Stevens-Johnson syndrome) but benefits should outweigh this risk. Clindamycin, favored by pediatricians, can be used as first-line treatment of MRSA skin infections unless inducible resistance emerges. The latter varies by geographic region.[31] Bacterial sensitivity to clindamycin should be assessed before treatment, which is not always practical. An important advantage of clindamycin is its ability to suppress production of PVL and other virulence factors in MRSA.[32] The long-acting tetracyclines, specifically minocycline and doxycycline, are good drugs for MRSA furunculosis. They are well absorbed by the gastrointestinal tract and have good tissue penetration, with response rates against MRSA at 80% to 100%.[33] Minocycline and doxycycline have better documented efficacy against staphylococcal skin infections than tetracycline. In vitro data suggest that minocycline has better antistaphylococcal activity than doxycycline, but clinical superiority has not been demonstrated.[34] In children, doxycyline should

Table 1
Oral antibiotics for treatment of MRSA furunculosis

Agent	Dose
Clindamycin	300–600 mg every 6–8 hours Pediatric dosage: 2–8 mg/kg every 6–8 h
TMP-SMX	2 DS (160/800) tabs every 12 hours
Doxycyline	100 mg every 12 hours
Minocycline	100 mg every 12 hours
Fusidic acid	500 mg 2–3 times daily (usually with Rifampin 300 mg every 12 hours)

be reserved for those older than 8 years of age. Emergence of resistance to the tetracyclines in USA300 clones of MRSA has occurred.[35]

Rifampicin is an oral antimicrobial with excellent in vitro activity against MRSA, but it cannot be administered as monotherapy because of rapidly inducible resistance during therapy. If used, rifampin must be combined with another antibiotic, usually in combination with tetracyclines or TMP-SMX. Rifampicin and TMP-SMX exhibit in vitro antagonism when used together.[36] The combination of fusidic acid (500 mg 2–3 times daily) and rifampin (300 mg twice daily) is used widely in Europe, Canada, and Asia as effective treatment of skin infections due to MRSA.[37] This combinations helps prevent mutual emergence of resistance during therapy. Fusidic acid is a bacteriostatic agent, effective against gram-positive organisms, including MSSA and MRSA; when used alone, resistance develops quickly during the course of treatment.[38] Fusidic acid is not available in the United States.

For patients who require hospitalization, a variety of parenteral agents are available (eg, vancomycin, linezolid, daptomycin, quinupristin-dalfopristin, and tigecycline) (**Table 2**). Vancomycin is the gold standard of therapy for serious MRSA infections. Despite more than 50 years of use, vancomycin is still a safe and effective treatment. Vancomycin-resistant strains of *S aureus* (VRSA) are an anecdotal phenomenon, and the strains have not been associated with invasive disease.[39] Linezolid, an oxazolidinone, is a new antibiotic available intravenously and orally. It is the only oral antibiotic with proved efficacy against MRSA in controlled clinical trials.[40] Linezolid exhibits bacteriostatic activity against MRSA via binding to the 50S ribosomal subunit and preventing toxin formation. It also has excellent activity against group A streptococci and is efficacious in the treatment of necrotizing fasciitis. Its major advantage is low cross-resistance with other antimicrobial agents. The oral bioavailability is 100%, allowing sequential intravenous to oral use (600 mg twice daily) without changing the drug dose or regimen. Compared with vancomycin treatment, patients treated with linezolid spent 5 to 8 fewer days (median) hospitalized.[41] Linezolid is generally well tolerated, although some patients experience gastrointestinal distress. Serious adverse effects (eg, bone marrow suppression and peripheral and optic neuropathy) are uncommon and invariably associated with prolonged use (ie, more than 28 days). Linezolid is a weak monoamine oxidase inhibitor and should be avoided in patients receiving serotonin reuptake inhibitors due to the possibility of serotonin syndrome.[42] The high cost of linezolid limits its use as outpatient therapy.

Daptomycin is a bactericidal, cyclic lipoprotein that causes depolarization of bacterial cell membranes. Its clinical efficacy is comparable to vancomycin, and 97% of *S aureus* strains are susceptible to daptomycin, including some VRSA strains.[43] Its half-life is 8 hours, and most of the drug is excreted by the kidney, nonmetabolized.[44] Daptomycin is the drug of choice for patients with severe MRSA infections or bacteremia who are intolerant of vancomycin or for patients with VRSA infections, which are daptomycin susceptible. Resistance to daptomycin has been reported in *S aureus* species previously treated with vancomycin but not with other antimicrobials. Side effects are rare, mainly rhabdomyolysis with elevated serum creatinine phosphokinase, and are usually reversible with discontinuation of the drug. Other side effects are paresthesias, dysesthesias, and peripheral neuropathy.[45]

The streptogramin combination of quinupristin-dalfopristin (Synercid) has synergistic antibacterial activity in vitro against a wide array of gram-positive organisms, including most MRSA strains. The drug is bactericidal for resting and proliferating bacteria. Administration is intravenous, usually via central venous catheter to offset thrombophlebitis at infusion site. Other side effects include arthralgias, myalgias, hyperbilirubinemia, liver toxicity, and QT prolongation.[46]

Tigecycline, a glycycline, is a novel minocycline derivative whose large size allows it to avoid efflux from bacterial cells, thus preventing bacterial

Table 2
Intravenous antibiotics for treatment of MRSA furunculosis

Agent	Dose
Vancomycin	2–3 g daily divided into doses every 6–12 hours
Linezolid	600 mg every 12 hours (equivalent oral dosing)
Daptomycin	4 mg/kg every 24 hours
Quinupristin-dalfopristin	7.5 mg/kg every 12 hours
Tigecycline	Initial dose of 100 mg once, then 50 mg every 12 hours

resistance. Tigecycline is bacteriostatic against MRSA with documented in vitro activity against VRSA and vancomycin-insensitive *S aureus*.[47] The drug is administered twice daily via 1-hour infusions. Side effects are nausea, vomiting, and headaches.

Newer MRSA agents include the semisynthetic lipoglycopeptides, dalbavacin, telavancin, and oritavancin, all of which are bactericidal and inhibit cell wall synthesis. Dalbavacin has a long half-life, which allows a simple dosing schedule (100 mg on day 1 and 500 mg on day 8 of treatment).[48] Telavancin has rapid, concentration-dependent bactericidal effects against MRSA and gram-positive bacteria resistant to vancomycin.[49] Dose adjustments are required in patients with renal failure. Oritavancin is an efficient drug for complicated MRSA and VRSA SSTIs and is also active against *Clostridium difficile* and vancomycin-resistant enterococcus.[50]

Ceftobiprole and ceftaroline are novel cephalosporins that target aberrant bacterial penicillin-binding proteins involved with MRSA furunculosis.[51]

Colonization in Chronic Furunculosis

Eradication of *S aureus* carriage reduces the risk of recurrent infections in colonized patients and decolonization can prevent cross-transmission of organisms to others.[52] Routine decolonization of carriers probably contributes to the decreasing incidence of MRSA in some European countries.[30,53] Nonetheless, the comparative overall efficacy of various MRSA decolonization strategies remains controversial.

Several topical and systemic agents have been used for MRSA decolonization, all with limited success. The nares are commonly cultured for *S aureus* colonization but yield only 52% detection sensitivity. This raises the need to screen additional body sites for colonization; sampling the combination of nares and throat results in 88% sensitivity of *S aureus* detection.[54] In addition to colonization of the nasopharynx, it is increasingly recognized that pathogenic bacteria may also inhabit other warm, moist skin sites: under pendulous breasts, in the upper-inner thigh, and in the gluteal cleft. Topical attempts at decolonization with mupirocin and chlorhexidine can reduce the incidence of subsequent *S aureus* infections, albeit at different levels of efficacy.[55] Decolonization usually consists of a 5-day application of mupirocin ointment (Bactroban) twice daily to nares, and daily body washing with 4% chlorhexidine soap. Further improvement can be achieved with oral rinsing with 0.2% chlorhexidine solution 3 times daily for 5 days, which decreases pharyngeal flora.[55] The combination 3-pronged approach reduces colonization by 40% to 70% in sensitive patients.[56,57] Although low-level resistance to mupirocin has emerged, a direct link with MRSA recolonization has not been clearly established. Topical gentian violet 0.3% solution is an inexpensive antiseptic that can be applied to nares twice daily for 2–3 weeks to eradicate nasal MRSA carriage.[58]

When topical antimicrobial treatment is unsuccessful, the need for systemic therapy arises. Decolonization with a combination of topical and systemic antimicrobial agents is highly effective, yielding clearance rates of 87% in treated patients.[37,59,60] Most oral antibiotics do not reach nasal mucosa secretions, but parenteral clindamycin is effective in eradicating nasal colonization of *S aureus*.[61] If furunculosis recurs despite nasal clearance, affected patients should have rectal swab cultures to assess gastrointestinal colonization, a potentially important MRSA reservoir, which facilitates recolonization of other body sites when not treated.[62] Oral vancomycin (1 g twice daily for 5 days) can eradicate 80% to 100% of MRSA gut colonization and reduce SSTI rates.[63,64] The urogenital tract may also warrant decolonization. Cotrimoxazole (800/160 mg twice daily for 5 days) is effective against urinary MRSA. *S aureus* vaginal colonization is related to recurrent furunculosis of the genitals and buttocks in women and their sexual partners.[65,66] Vaginal cultures should be obtained from such women; if colonized, treatment with povidone-iodine ovule (Betadine) should be administered once daily for 5 days.[66]

Most patients can be successfully decolonized with 2 or 3 combination courses of the above measures **(Table 3)**.[66] If initial attempts of

Table 3
Therapy for *S aureus* colonization

Site	Treatment[a]
Nares	Mupirocin ointment twice daily
Skin	4% Chlorhexidine wash daily
Pharynx	0.2% Chlorhexidine solution oral rinse 3 times daily
Gastrointestinal tract	Vancomycin 1 g PO twice daily
Urinary tract	Cotrimoxazole 800/160 mg PO twice daily
Genital tract	Povidone-iodine ovule once daily

[a] Five-day course of treatment.

decolonization fail, physicians should address patient compliance.

Environmental Decontamination in Chronic Furunculosis

Successful management of recurrent furunculosis requires decontamination of a patient's environment, and recommendations rely on common sense and practical measures. Universal precautions, such as regular hand washing with soap or with alcohol-based hand rubs, help contain recurrent MRSA furunculosis. To control intrafamilial furunculosis, family members should avoid direct contact with infected skin, wash contaminated clothing and bedding with the warmest temperatures recommended on the clothing label, and use disinfectants to decontaminate commonly used fomites.[67,68] Over-the-counter products or household chlorine bleach can be used (0.25 cup of regular household bleach in 1 gallon of water [1:100 dilution]) to disinfect precleaned surfaces.[69]

Similar measures should be implemented at group facilities (ie, prisons, rehabilitation centers, senior homes, schools, and athletic and day care centers). Athletes involved in contact sports should be screened for cutaneous signs of MRSA infections before competition/practice, and measures should be taken to bandage all open wounds. Sports equipment should be cleaned at least once daily and perhaps more frequently with diluted bleach solutions.

Nosocomial spread of MRSA infection in health care facilities can be reduced with use of strict infection-control measures. In hospitals, MRSA surveillance should include early identification and isolation of carriers, barrier precautions for patient care and visits (gloves, gowns, and masks), and environmental cleaning of patient rooms and fomites. Education about and surveillance for proper hand hygiene can also help reduce nosocomial spread of furuncle-inducing bacteria in facilities.

VACCINES

In the past decade, MRSA has become the most important multidrug-resistant pathogen worldwide, causing significant morbidity, appreciable mortality, and noteworthy health care expense. Given the impact of *S aureus* furunculosis and other SSTIs, efforts to develop an effective vaccination against staphylococci have been promising.[70] Active immunizations with staphylococcal polysaccharide protein conjugates are effective but have limited usefulness in functionally immunocompromised patients, who are at highest risk of infections.[6,71] Passive immunization with high-titer immunoglobulin or monoclonal antibodies offers an alternative to active immunization, but it has limited immunogenicity and protective duration, requiring repeated inoculations with suboptimal results.[72] Clinical trials investigating immunizations with a mouse-human chimeric monoclonal antibody against lipoteichoic acid (pagibaximab) and a humanized monoclonal antibody against staphylococcal clumping factors (tefamizumab) are ongoing with promising results thus far.[73]

PHAGES

An innovative new antibacterial technology involves the use of bacteriophages (or simply, phages), bacterial viruses that attack and destroy bacteria, including MRSA strands. This form of therapy has been known since the beginning of the twentieth century and is applied in several medical centers in Europe (1, 2). Phages are found widespread in nature and can appear in food and in the human body, primarily the intestines. In the experimental studies to date, phages have been successfully used in MRSA cases where antibiotic treatment did not bring improvement (eg, in patients with nonhealing postoperative wounds or difficult to manage bone, upper respiratory tract, urinary, or reproductive tract infections). Small, acid-soluble spore proteins (SASPs) are novel modified and disabled phages designed to inject an antibacterial gene into target bacteria (SASPject, Phico Therapeutics, Cambridge, UK). SASPs can inactivate bacterial DNA in a non–sequence-specific manner so their activity is unaffected by DNA mutations. Selected pathogens can be targeted, avoiding the normal flora. An *S aureus*–targeted SASPject, PT1.2, has been developed for nasal decolonization, including MRSA strains; currently a commercial version is in phase 1 clinical trials. Additional SASPs targeted against *C difficile* and multidrug-resistant gram-negative organisms are in development.

SUMMARY

Treatment of recurrent furunculosis is a difficult and challenging process. The mainstay of therapy is incision and drainage of a furuncle coupled with bacterial culture. Patients with recurrent furunculosis deserve an empiric treatment of CA-MRSA with TMP/SMX or doxycycline or with vancomycin if they require hospitalization.

For recurrent furunculosis, decolonization should be used, topically at first, and systemically if necessary, including therapy for gastrointestinal and urogenital colonization. Affected patients and their family members must practice good hygiene

predicated with regular hand washing, fomite cleaning, and avoiding contact with contaminated skin.

REFERENCES

1. Stevens DL, Bisno AL, Chambers HF, et al. Practice guidelines for the diagnosis and management of skin and soft-tissue infections. Clin Infect Dis 2005; 41(10):1373–406.
2. Taira BR, Singer AJ, Thode HC Jr, et al. National epidemiology of cutaneous abscesses: 1996 to 2005. Am J Emerg Med 2009;27(3):289–92.
3. Moran GJ, Krishnadasan A, Gorwitz RJ, et al. Methicillin-resistant *S. aureus* infections among patients in the emergency department. N Engl J Med 2006; 355(7):666–74.
4. El-Gilany AH, Fathy H. Risk factors of recurrent furunculosis. Dermatol Online J 2009;15(1):16.
5. Steele RW. Recurrent staphylococcal infection in families. Arch Dermatol 1980;116(2):189–90.
6. Shinefield HR, Ruff NL. Staphylococcal infections: a historical perspective. Infect Dis Clin North Am 2009;23(1):1–15.
7. Abrahamian FM, Talan DA, Moran GJ. Management of skin and soft-tissue infections in the emergency department. Infect Dis Clin North Am 2008;22(1): 89–116, vi.
8. Stewart GT, Holt RJ. Evolutio of natural resistance to the newer penicillins. Br Med J 1963;1(5326): 308–11.
9. Graffunder EM, Venezia RA. Risk factors associated with nosocomial methicillin-resistant *Staphylococcus aureus* (MRSA) infection including previous use of antimicrobials. J Antimicrob Chemother 2002;49(6):999–1005.
10. Whitman TJ. Community-associated methicillin-resistant *Staphylococcus aureus* skin and soft tissue infections. Dis Mon 2008;54(12):780–6.
11. Seybold U, Kourbatova E, Johnson J, et al. Emergence of community-associated methicillin-resistant *Staphylococcus aureus* USA300 genotype as a major cause of health care–associated blood stream infections. Clin Infect Dis 2006;42(5):647–56.
12. Fridkin SK, Hageman JC, Morrison M, et al. Methicillin-resistant *Staphylococcus aureus* disease in three communities. N Engl J Med 2005;352(14): 1436–44.
13. Baba T, Takeuchi F, Kuroda M, et al. Genome and virulence determinants of high virulence community-acquired MRSA. Lancet 2002;359(9320):1819–27.
14. Wisplinghoff H, Rosato AE, Enright MC, et al. Related clones containing SCCmec type IV predominate among clinically significant *Staphylococcus epidermidis* isolates. Antimicrob Agents Chemother 2003;47(11):3574–9.
15. Francis JS, Doherty MC, Lopatin U, et al. Severe community-onset pneumonia in healthy adults caused by methicillin-resistant *Staphylococcus aureus* carrying the Panton-Valentine leukocidin genes. Clin Infect Dis 2005;40(1):100–7.
16. Meunier O, Falkenrodt A, Monteil H, et al. Application of flow cytometry in toxinology: pathophysiology of human polymorphonuclear leukocytes damaged by a pore-forming toxin from *Staphylococcus aureus*. Cytometry 1995;21(3):241–7.
17. Hedstrom SA. Recurrent staphylococcal furunculosis. Bacteriological findings and epidemiology in 100 cases. Scand J Infect Dis 1981;13(2):115–9.
18. Cohen PR. Community-acquired methicillin-resistant *Staphylococcus aureus* skin infections: implications for patients and practitioners. Am J Clin Dermatol 2007;8(5):259–70.
19. Leonard FC, Markey BK. Meticillin-resistant *Staphylococcus aureus* in animals: a review. Vet J 2008; 175(1):27–36.
20. Hoeger PH. Antimicrobial susceptibility of skin-colonizing *S. aureus* strains in children with atopic dermatitis. Pediatr Allergy Immunol 2004;15(5):474–7.
21. Demircay Z, Eksioglu-Demiralp E, Ergun T, et al. Phagocytosis and oxidative burst by neutrophils in patients with recurrent furunculosis. Br J Dermatol 1998;138(6):1036–8.
22. Dissemond J. Methicillin resistant *Staphylococcus aureus* (MRSA): diagnostic, clinical relevance and therapy. J Dtsch Dermatol Ges 2009;7(6):544–51 [quiz: 552–3].
23. Murakami K, Minamide W, Wada K, et al. Identification of methicillin-resistant strains of staphylococci by polymerase chain reaction. J Clin Microbiol 1991;29(10):2240–4.
24. Lee MC, Rios AM, Aten MF, et al. Management and outcome of children with skin and soft tissue abscesses caused by community-acquired methicillin-resistant *Staphylococcus aureus*. Pediatr Infect Dis J 2004;23(2):123–7.
25. Krucke GW, Grimes DE, Grimes RM, et al. Antibiotic resistance in *Staphylococcus aureus*-containing cutaneous abscesses of patients with HIV. Am J Emerg Med 2009;27(3):344–7.
26. Rohana AR, Rosli MK, Nik Rizal NY, et al. Bilateral ophthalmic vein thrombosis secondary to nasal furunculosis. Orbit 2008;27(3):215–7.
27. Cosgrove SE, Sakoulas G, Perencevich EN, et al. Comparison of mortality associated with methicillin-resistant and methicillin-susceptible *Staphylococcus aureus* bacteremia: a meta-analysis. Clin Infect Dis 2003;36(1):53–9.
28. Paydar KZ, Hansen SL, Charlebois ED, et al. Inappropriate antibiotic use in soft tissue infections. Arch Surg 2006;141(9):850–4 [discussion: 855–6].
29. Moellering J, Robert C. Current treatment options for community-acquired methicillin-resistant *Staphylococcus aureus* infection. Clin Infect Dis 2008;46(7): 1032–7.

30. Garau J, Bouza E, Chastre J, et al. Management of methicillin-resistant *Staphylococcus aureus* infections. Clin Microbiol Infect 2009;15(2):125–36.
31. Daum RS. Clinical practice. Skin and soft-tissue infections caused by methicillin-resistant *Staphylococcus aureus*. N Engl J Med 2007;357(4):380–90.
32. Morgan MS. Diagnosis and treatment of Panton–Valentine Leukocidin (PVL)-associated staphylococcal pneumonia. Int J Antimicrob Agents 2007; 30(4):289–96.
33. Ruhe JJ, Monson T, Bradsher RW, et al. Use of long-acting tetracyclines for methicillin-resistant *Staphylococcus aureus* infections: case series and review of the literature. Clin Infect Dis 2005; 40(10):1429–34.
34. Minuth JN, Holmes TM, Musher DM. Activity of tetracycline, doxycycline, and minocycline against methicillin-susceptible and -resistant staphylococci. Antimicrob Agents Chemother 1974;6(4):411–4.
35. Han LL, McDougal LK, Gorwitz RJ, et al. High frequencies of clindamycin and tetracycline resistance in methicillin-resistant *Staphylococcus aureus* pulsed-field type USA300 isolates collected at a Boston ambulatory health center. J Clin Microbiol 2007;45(4):1350–2.
36. Kaka AS, Rueda AM, Shelburne SA 3rd, et al. Bactericidal activity of orally available agents against methicillin-resistant *Staphylococcus aureus*. J Antimicrob Chemother 2006;58(3):680–3.
37. Loeb M, Main C, Walker-Dilks C, et al. Antimicrobial drugs for treating methicillin-resistant *Staphylococcus aureus* colonization. Cochrane Database Syst Rev 2003;(4):CD003340.
38. Besier S, Ludwig A, Brade V, et al. Molecular analysis of fusidic acid resistance in *Staphylococcus aureus*. Mol Microbiol 2003;47(2):463–9.
39. Tenover FC, Moellering RC Jr. The rationale for revising the Clinical and Laboratory Standards Institute vancomycin minimal inhibitory concentration interpretive criteria for *Staphylococcus aureus*. Clin Infect Dis 2007;44(9):1208–15.
40. Moellering RC. Linezolid: the first oxazolidinone antimicrobial. Ann Intern Med 2003;138(2):135–42.
41. Li Z, Willke RJ, Pinto LA, et al. Comparison of length of hospital stay for patients with known or suspected methicillin-resistant *Staphylococcus* species infections treated with linezolid or vancomycin: a randomized, multicenter trial. Pharmacotherapy 2001;21(3):263–74.
42. Taylor JJ, Estes LL, Wilson JW. Linezolid and serotonergic drug interactions. Clin Infect Dis 2006;43(10): 1371.
43. Fowler VG Jr, Boucher HW, Corey GR, et al. Daptomycin versus standard therapy for bacteremia and endocarditis caused by *Staphylococcus aureus*. N Engl J Med 2006;355(7):653–65.
44. Rose WE, Leonard SN, Sakoulas G, et al. Daptomycin activity against *Staphylococcus aureus* following vancomycin exposure in an in vitro pharmacodynamic model with simulated endocardial vegetations. Antimicrob Agents Chemother 2008;52(3):831–6.
45. Mangili A, Bica I, Snydman DR, et al. Daptomycin-resistant, methicillin-resistant *Staphylococcus aureus* bacteremia. Clin Infect Dis 2005;40(7): 1058–60.
46. Drew RH, Perfect JR, Srinath L, et al. Treatment of methicillin-resistant *Staphylococcus aureus* infections with quinupristin-dalfopristin in patients intolerant of or failing prior therapy. For the Synercid Emergency-Use Study Group. J Antimicrob Chemother 2000;46(5):775–84.
47. Chopra I. Glycylcyclines: third-generation tetracycline antibiotics. Curr Opin Pharmacol 2001;1(5):464–9.
48. Jauregui LE, Babazadeh S, Seltzer E, et al. Randomized, double-blind comparison of once-weekly dalbavancin versus twice-daily linezolid therapy for the treatment of complicated skin and skin structure infections. Clin Infect Dis 2005;41(10):1407–15.
49. Smith WJ, Drew RH. Telavancin: a new lipoglycopeptide for gram-positive infections. Drugs Today (Barc) 2009;45(3):159–73.
50. Mercier RC, Hrebickova L. Oritavancin: a new avenue for resistant Gram-positive bacteria. Expert Rev Anti Infect Ther 2005;3(3):325–32.
51. Stryjewski ME, Corey GR. New treatments for methicillin-resistant *Staphylococcus aureus*. Curr Opin Crit Care 2009;15(5):403–12.
52. Gorwitz R, Kruszon-Moran D, McAllister S, et al. Changes in the prevalence of nasal colonization with *Staphylococcus aureus* in the United States, 2001–2004. J Infect Dis 2008;197(9):1226–34.
53. Navarro MB, Huttner B, Harbarth S. Methicillin-resistant *Staphylococcus aureus* control in the 21st century: beyond the acute care hospital. Curr Opin Infect Dis 2008;21(4):372–9.
54. Andrews JI, Fleener DK, Messer SA, et al. Screening for *Staphylococcus aureus* carriage in pregnancy: usefulness of novel sampling and culture strategies. Am J Obstet Gynecol 2009; 201(4):396 e1–5.
55. Ringberg H, Cathrine Petersson A, Walder M, et al. The throat: an important site for MRSA colonization. Scand J Infect Dis 2006;38(10):888–93.
56. Simor AE, Phillips E, McGeer A, et al. Randomized controlled trial of chlorhexidine gluconate for washing, intranasal mupirocin, and rifampin and doxycycline versus no treatment for the eradication of methicillin-resistant *Staphylococcus aureus* colonization. Clin Infect Dis 2007;44(2):178–85.
57. Harbarth S, Dharan S, Liassine N, et al. Randomized, placebo-controlled, double-blind trial to evaluate the efficacy of mupirocin for eradicating carriage of methicillin-resistant *Staphylococcus aureus*. Antimicrob Agents Chemother 1999;43(6): 1412–6.

58. Okano M, Noguchi S, Tabata K, et al. Topical gentian violet for cutaneous infection and nasal carriage with MRSA. International Journal of Dermatol 2000; 39(12):942–4.
59. Loveday HP, Pellowe CM, Jones SR, et al. A systematic review of the evidence for interventions for the prevention and control of meticillin-resistant *Staphylococcus aureus* (1996–2004): report to the Joint MRSA Working Party (Subgroup A). J Hosp Infect 2006;63(Suppl 1):S45–70.
60. Walsh TJ, Standiford HC, Reboli AC, et al. Randomized double-blinded trial of rifampin with either novobiocin or trimethoprim-sulfamethoxazole against methicillin-resistant *Staphylococcus aureus* colonization: prevention of antimicrobial resistance and effect of host factors on outcome. Antimicrob Agents Chemother 1993;37(6):1334–42.
61. Lipsky BA, Pecoraro RE, Ahroni JH, et al. Immediate and long-term efficacy of systemic antibiotics for eradicating nasal colonization with *Staphylococcus aureus*. Eur J Clin Microbiol Infect Dis 1992;11(1):43–7.
62. Boyce JM, Havill NL, Maria B. Frequency and possible infection control implications of gastrointestinal colonization with methicillin-resistant *Staphylococcus aureus*. J Clin Microbiol 2005;43(12): 5992–5.
63. Maraha B, van Halteren J, Verzijl JM, et al. Decolonization of methicillin-resistant *Staphylococcus aureus* using oral vancomycin and topical mupirocin. Clin Microbiol Infect 2002;8(10):671–5.
64. Silvestri L, Milanese M, Oblach L, et al. Enteral vancomycin to control methicillin-resistant *Staphylococcus aureus* outbreak in mechanically ventilated patients. Am J Infect Control 2002;30(7):391–9.
65. Reichman O, Sobel JD. MRSA infection of buttocks, vulva, and genital tract in women. Curr Infect Dis Rep 2009;11(6):465–70.
66. Buehlmann M, Frei R, Fenner L, et al. Highly effective regimen for decolonization of methicillin-resistant *Staphylococcus aureus* carriers. Infect Control Hosp Epidemiol 2008;29(6):510–6.
67. Elston DM. How to handle a CA-MRSA outbreak. Dermatol Clin 2009;27(1):43–8.
68. Elston DM. Practical management tips for methicillin-resistant *Staphylococcus aureus*. Cutis 2008; 81(4):311–3.
69. CDC Guidelines. Community-associated methicillin resistant *Staphylococcus aureus* (CA-MRSA). 2009. Available at: http://www.cdc.gov/ncidod/dhqp/ar_mrsa.html. Accessed November 2, 2009.
70. Schaffer AC, Lee JC. Staphylococcal vaccines and immunotherapies. Infect Dis Clin North Am 2009; 23(1):153–71.
71. Shinefield H, Black S, Fattom A, et al. Use of a *Staphylococcus aureus* conjugate vaccine in patients receiving hemodialysis. N Engl J Med 2002;346(7): 491–6.
72. Bloom B, Schelonka R, Kueser T, et al. Multicenter study to assess safety and efficacy of INH-A21, a donor-selected human staphylococcal immunoglobulin, for prevention of nosocomial infections in very low birth weight infants. Pediatr Infect Dis J 2005;24(10):858–66.
73. Weisman LE, Fischer GW, Thackray HM, et al. Safety and pharmacokinetics of a chimerized anti-lipoteichoic acid monoclonal antibody in healthy adults. Int Immunopharmacol 2009;9(5): 639–44.

Innovative Management of Lupus Erythematosus

Haydee M. Knott, MD[a], José Darío Martínez, MD, IFAAD[b,*]

KEYWORDS

• Lupus • Cutaneous lupus • Management

Systemic lupus erythematosus (SLE) is a chronic autoimmune disease that may affect any tissue or organ system, but most often involves the skin and joints. SLE affects women much more commonly than men (9:1), with a lifetime prevalence of 25 to 64 cases per 100,000 people, mainly among people of Afro-Caribbean origin.[1] Its clinical course is episodic, and can range from an indolent cutaneous disease with occasional flares to a fulminant systemic course with significant mortality. Furthermore, primary dermatologic lupus may herald the progression of the indolent cutaneous manifestation to systemic internal disease. Many important topical and systemic therapies have been developed recently to better manage this life-threatening disease.

No specific genetic cause for SLE has heretofore been identified; however, multiple large demographic studies have highlighted genetic, racial, hormonal, and environmental factors associated with this disorder. Given multiorgan involvement, the diagnosis of SLE rests on the recognition of the relationship of disparate features. There are 11 criteria from the American College of Rheumatology (ACR) for the diagnosis of SLE and 3 of these are cutaneous lesions: malar rash, photosensitivity, and discoid rash (**Table 1**).[2]

Cutaneous involvement occurs in 90% of patients with SLE. A new system that standardizes disease scoring in cutaneous lupus has been spearheaded by Dr Victoria Werth. This system is similar to the Psoriasis Area Severity Index (PASI) and is called the Cutaneous Lupus Erythematosus Disease Area and Severity Index (CLASI). This system scores skin damage and disease activity separately, thereby enabling investigators to standardize assessment of therapeutic response (**Table 2**).[3,4]

The cutaneous presentation of lupus can be divided into 3 distinct groups:

1. Lupus erythematosus (LE) specific skin lesions
   - acute cutaneous LE (ACLE) or "Butterfly rash"
   - subacute cutaneous LE (SCLE)
   - chronic cutaneous LE (CCLE) or discoid LE (DLE)
   - LE panniculitis and LE tumidus
2. LE nonspecific skin disease: vasculitis, urticaria, and livedo reticularis
3. Cutaneous complications of drug therapy for LE.

This article focuses on the management of DLE, SCLE, and SLE when the usual therapeutic arsenal such as oral antimalarial drugs and topical/oral steroids fail or provide insufficient treatment efficacy (**Table 3**). Many of the treatments listed are the same or similar to each other because of similarities in the pathogenesis of various subtypes of cutaneous lupus. The clinical challenge is to determine the indications for topical versus systemic

Financial disclosure: no conflict of interest.
[a] Department of Dermatology, Cleveland Clinic, 9500 Euclid Avenue, A-61, Cleveland, OH 44195, USA
[b] Internal Medicine and Dermatology, Internal Medicine Clinic, University Hospital, University Autonomus of Nuevo León, Madero y Gonzalitos s/n, Colonia Mitras Centro, Monterrey, Nuevo León, México 64460
* Corresponding author.
E-mail address: jdariomtz@yahoo.com.mx

Dermatol Clin 28 (2010) 489–499
doi:10.1016/j.det.2010.03.007
0733-8635/10/$ – see front matter © 2010 Elsevier Inc. All rights reserved.

derm.theclinics.com

Table 1
1997 Update of the 1982 American College of Rheumatology revised criteria for classification of systemic lupus erythematosus[a]

Malar rash	Fixed erythema, flat or raised, over the malar eminences, tending to spare the nasolabial folds
Discoid rash	Erythematous raised patches with adherent keratotic scaling and follicular plugging; atrophic scarring may occur in older lesions
Photosensitivity	Skin rash as a result of unusual reaction to sunlight by patient history or physician observation
Oral ulcers	Oral or nasopharyngeal ulceration, usually painless, observed by physician
Arthritis	Nonerosive arthritis involving 2 or more peripheral joints, characterized by tenderness, swelling or effusion
Serositis	1. Pleuritis-convincing history of pleuritic pain, rubbing heard by a physician, or evidence of pleural effusion OR 2. Pericarditis-documented by ECG, rub, or evidence of pericardial effusion
Renal disorder	1. Persistent proteinuria greater than 0.5 g/d or greater than 3+ if quantitation not performed OR 2. Cellular casts—may be red cell, hemoglobin, granular, tubular, or mixed
Neurologic disorder	1. Seizures—in the absence of offending drugs or known metabolic derangements, eg, uremia, ketoacidosis, or electrolyte imbalance OR 2. Psychosis—in the absence of offending drugs or known metabolic derangements, eg, uremia, ketoacidosis, or electrolyte imbalance
Hematologic disorder	1. Hemolytic anemia with reticulocytosis OR 2. Leukopenia—less than 4000/mm^3 total white blood cells on 2 or more occasions OR 3. Lymphopenia—less than 1500/mm^3 on 2 or more occasions OR 4. Thrombocytopenia—less than 100 000/mm^3 in the absence of offending drugs

Immunologic disorder	1. Anti-DNA antibody to native DNA in abnormal titer OR 2. Anti-Sm: presence of antibody to Sm nuclear antigen OR 3. Positive finding of antiphospholipid antibodies based on (1) an abnormal serum level of immunoglobulin (Ig)G or IgM anticardiolipin antibodies; (2) a positive test result for lupus anticoagulant using standard methods; or (3) a false-positive serologic test for syphilis known to be positive for at least 6 months and confirmed by treponema pallidum immobilization or fluorescent treponemal antibody absorption test (FTA-ABS)
Antinuclear antibody	An abnormal titer of antinuclear antibody by immunofluorescence (or an equivalent assay) at any point in time and in the absence of drugs known to be associated with "drug-induced lupus" syndrome

Abbreviation: ECG, electocardiogram.

[a] The proposed classification is based on 11 criteria. For the purpose of identifying study patients for clinical studies of systemic lupus erythematosus if any 4 or more of the 11 criteria are present, serially or simultaneously, during any interval of observation.

From Tan EM, Cohen AS, Fries JF, Masi AT, McShane DJ, Rothfield NF, et al. The 1982 revised criteria for the classification of systemic lupus erythematosus. Arthritis Rheum 1982;25:1271–7; and Hochberg MC. Updating the American College of Rheumatology revised criteria for the classification of systemic lupus erythematosus [letter]. Arthritis Rheum 1997;40:1725; with permission.

therapy, and to also identify the scenarios when combined therapy is necessary.

For more information on current clinical trials and innovative ideas we refer you to the following Web site sponsored by the National Institutes of Health: http://ClinicalTrials.gov. ClinicalTrials.gov is a registry of federally and privately supported clinical trials conducted in the United States and around the world. http://ClinicalTrials.gov gives information about a trial's purpose, who may participate, locations, and contact numbers.

DLE

DLE is the most common manifestation of chronic cutaneous LE, and is characterized by single or multiple persistent, well-defined plaques with hyperkeratosis, scaling, telangiectasia, atrophy, scarring, follicular plugging, and peripheral hyperpigmentation with central hypopigmentation (**Fig. 1**A). **Fig. 1**B shows illustration of histopathology demonstrating follicular plugging. Female/male ratio is 3:1. Localized involvement of the head and scalp accounts for 70% of DLE, whereas the disseminated form involves the chest, upper back, and extensor surfaces of the arms. High-titer antinuclear antibodies (ANAs) occur in 5% of patients, but generally no anti-double-stranded DNA (anti-dsDNA) antibodies are present. It is associated with photosensitivity in 50% of cases, and a small minority of patients (<5%) eventually develop SLE. Largely because of its chronicity and cosmetic sequelae, DLE severely affects quality of life.

Current treatment options include topical and systemic glucocorticoids, sunscreens, antimalarials, retinoids, dapsone, thalidomide, methotrexate, azathioprine, immunoglobulins, and cyclophosphamide. In a Cochrane database review, treatment of DLE with topical 0.05% fluocinonide was more effective than the use of 1% hydrocortisone. Likewise, a comparison between the use of acitretin and hydroxychloroquine showed no significant differences in treatment efficacy. Nevertheless, treatment-related adverse effects were more frequent and severe with acitretin. The review concluded that there was not enough reliable evidence to support the use of other drugs that are commonly used to treat DLE such as azathioprine, chloroquine, clofazamine, dapsone, gold, interferon alpha-2a, methotrexate, phenytoin, retinoids, sulphasalazine, thalidomide, topical calcineurin blockers, and biologic agents.[5] Despite the paucity of high-quality evidence, some of these interventions have become commonplace and will be reviewed herein.

Table 2
New approaches to cutaneous lupus

CLASI (Cutaneous Lupus Erythematosus Disease Area and Severity Index)	
Activity	**Damage**
-Erythema	-Dyspigmentation
-Scale/Hypertrophy	-Scarring
-Nonscarring alopecia	-Scarring alopecia

Data from Victoria P. Werth, MD. Available at: http://www.dermatologyfoundation.org, Summer 2009.

NEW THERAPIES FOR DLE

Topical Calcineurin Inhibitors

Licensed for the treatment of moderate and severe atopic dermatitis in children and adults, topical calcineurin inhibitors are effective and have fewer severe side effects than topical steroids. The most frequent adverse events are irritation, burning, and erythema.[6]

Pimecrolimus

This topical calcineurin inhibitor is an immunomodulator closely related to tacrolimus. Both inhibit T-cell proliferation and the production and release of proinflammatory cytokines such as interleukin-2 (IL-2), IL-4, and tumor necrosis factor-alpha (TNF-alpha). In contrast to tacrolimus, pimecrolimus has no effect on dendritic cells. Pimecrolimus does not induce skin atrophy or telangectasias because it does not affect endothelial cells and fibroblasts. It has comparable efficacy to betamethasone valerate.[7] The use of pimecrolimus has correlated well with an improved quality of life in a number of studies.[8]

Pimecrolimus is not approved by the Food and Drug Administration (FDA) for DLE.

Tacrolimus

Tacrolimus is a calcineurin inhibitor that may be used topically to block cutaneous T-cell activation. Skin infiltrating T lymphocytes play a major role in CCLE (DLE). Many small studies and case reports have established both the efficacy and safety of tacrolimus in the treatment of DLE. It has an advantage in safety over clobetasol concerning the development of skin telangiectasias.[6] Additionally, one small study showed that tacrolimus compounded in clobetasol ointment was more effective than tacrolimus ointment or clobetasol ointment alone for the treatment of cutaneous lupus erythematosus.[9]

Tacrolimus is not FDA approved for DLE.

Table 3
Summary of novel therapies for cutaneous lupus erythematosus

	Discoid Lupus Erythematosus	Subacute Cutaneous Lupus Erythematosus	Systemic Lupus Erythematosus
Topical:	Pimecrolimus, tacrolimus, R-salbutamol	Sunscreens—anti UVA and UVB, pimecrolimus, tacrolimus	Pimecrolimus, tacrolimus
Systemic:	Hydroxychloroquine, chloroquine, quinacrine, lenalidomide, abatacept, efalizumab,[a]	Hydroxychloroquine, thalidomide, leflunomide, mycophenolate mofetil, intravenous immunoglobulin, efalizumab,[a] rituximab calcipotriene	Vitamin D supplementation Cyclophosphamide + azathioprine, intravenous immunoglobulin, mycophenolate mofetil, rituximab, belimumab, abatacept, epratuzumab
Other:	Pulse dye laser	Intralesional triamcinolone	

[a] Withdrawn from market as of June 8, 2009.

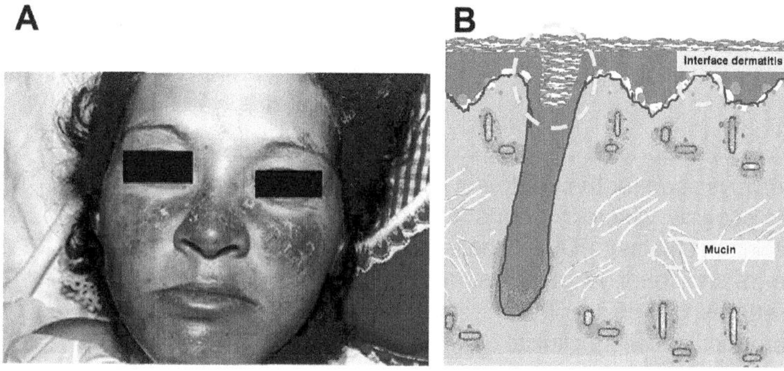

Fig. 1. (*A*) Patient with DLE. (*Courtesy of* Michelle Tarbox, MD.) (*B*) Illustration of DLE skin biopsy. Histopathology demonstrating follicular plugging "carpet tacking or cat's tongue," vacuolar interface changes, thickened basement membrane, dermal mucin deposition, and superficial and deep perivascular and periadnexal infiltrate (predominantly lymphocytic).

R-salbutamol

R-salbutamol sulfate, a topical anti-inflammatory preparation, was tested successfully on patients with treatment-resistant DLE. An R-enantiomer of salbutamol, formulated as a cream for topical treatment of cutaneous lupus, it holds promising therapeutic potential in cutaneous lupus treatment (DLE). A double-blinded, randomized controlled trial of 37 patients with DLE showed significant improvement on scaling/hypertrophy, induration, pain, and itching. It was found to be safe and well tolerated.[10–12]

Hydroxychloroquine, Chloroquine, and Quinacrine

Quinacrine (Qn), chloroquine (CQ), and hydroxychloroquine (HCQ) are antimalarial drugs routinely used to treat autoimmune diseases such as SLE and rheumatoid arthritis (RA). Their therapeutic impact on lupus treatment derives from their immunomodulating and photoprotective properties. A recent study on CQ showed a reduction of skin lesions via inhibition of angiogenesis.[13] Qn leads to inhibition of neovascularization in mice during experimentally provoked inflammation, thereby impairing pathologic angiogenesis.[14] The association of HCQ (dosage up to 5 mg/kg/d) and Qn (100 mg/d) appears to be safe and effective in DLE lesions when HCQ (200 mg twice a day or dosage up to 6.5 mg/kg/d) alone fails.[15]

Lenalidomide

A thalidomide analog developed in the mid-1990s and FDA approved for multiple myeloma and myelodysplastic syndrome, lenalidomide is 2000-fold more potent than thalidomide in blocking the formation of TNF-alpha. Lenalidomide has fewer side effects (sedation, constipation, neuropathy, and teratogenicity) than its precursor thalidomide. Its most important side effects are myelosuppresion (neutropenia and thrombocytopenia) and an increased risk of deep venous thrombosis. In a recent report, 2 African American female patients were treated with low-dosage lenalidomide (5 mg/d), with 1 responding to treatment in the first month. This oral drug may be a good alternative for severe recalcitrant generalized DLE.[16]

Abatacept

Abatacept is a fully human recombinant fusion protein that selectively modulates T-cell activation by blocking costimulation via the B7:CD28 pathway. This results in decreased T-cell activation, proliferation, cytokine secretion, and subsequent autoantibody production without depletion of T or B cells. It has effectively prevented SLE onset in several murine models.[17,18] It has been used to treat lupus flares, mainly discoid lesions, pericarditis, and pluritis/pleurisy. Treatment consists of 4 monthly intravenous boluses of 10 mg/kg.

Efalizumab

Efalizumab is an anti-CD-11 monoclonal antibody, which is no longer available because of an association with the development of progressive multifocal leukoencephalopathy (PML) in 3 patients who took this drug over 3 years. It had been used to treat a small group of patients with DLE with good results. Usmani and Goodfield[19] reported treatment success at 5.5 weeks among 12 of 13 patients treated with a weekly subcutaneous dosage of 1 mg/kg efalizumab. An additional report claimed almost complete remission in one 50-year-old male with DLE treated with subcutaneous efalizumab.[20] Unfortunately, because of the possible etiologic association with progressive multifocal encephalopathy, this agent has been withdrawn from the American, Canadian, and European Union marketplaces.

Pulsed Dye Laser

Pulsed dye laser (PDL) is used for the treatment of benign skin lesions such as vascular lesions (eg, port wine stains, telangiectasias). PDL is considered to be the laser of choice for vascular lesions, because at wavelengths of 585 to 595 nm, the laser is known to produce excellent clinical results at minimal risk to patients. PDL is designed to deliver an intense but gentle burst of laser light to the skin. The light is absorbed by the erythrocytes, while leaving the surrounding tissue undamaged.

Treatment of DLE lesions with PDL was first described in 1999 by Raulin and colleagues.[21] In a new study, 12 patients with active DLE demonstrated overall improvement when treated with the 585 nm PDL (fluence 5.5 J/cm^2) with a pulse duration of 0.45 milliseconds over a spot size diameter of 7 mm, and a treatment interval of 6 weeks. PDL may be effective and safe in cases of refractory DLE, and may be considered for the treatment of stable, solitary, active chronic DLE lesions when topical or systemic therapies have failed.[22]

SCLE

Subacute cutaneous lupus erythematosus is characterized by highly photosensitive papulosquamous or annular polycyclic lesions on sun-exposed areas, mainly on the upper back, upper chest, shoulders, and upper arms, which tend to last for weeks or months and heal without scarring (**Fig. 2**). In SCLE, there is a paucity of systemic manifestations, and the most common extracutaneous symptoms are arthritis and myalgias. Approximately 10% to 15% of patients develop a moderately severe form of SLE. Most patients have anti-Ro (70%–90%) and/or anti-La (30%–50%) antibodies, most commonly occurring in the annular-polycyclic subgroup. Routine treatment options consist of sunscreens and antimalarial drugs.

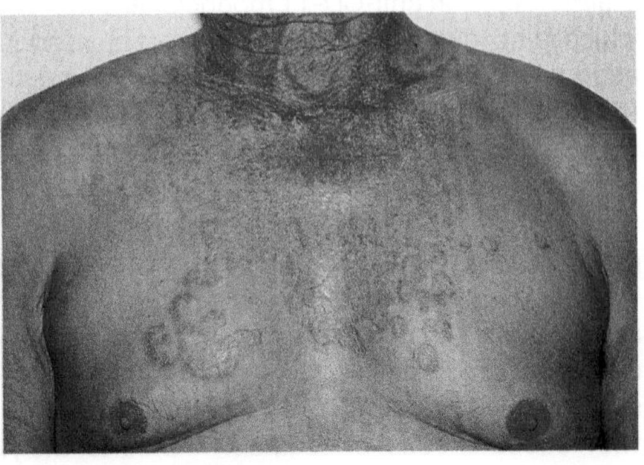

Fig. 2. Patient with SCLE.

NEW THERAPIES FOR SCLE

Sunscreens

Both UVB and UVA play a role in the pathogenesis of cutaneous LE. Protection from solar radiation is of outmost importance in patients with photosensitivity.[23,24] Mexoryl is the highest photostable sunblock currently available, providing good anti-UVA and anti-UVB protection.

Mexoryl acts as a normal filter, but becomes highly energized by absorbing the energy of UV photons, thereby preventing cutaneous photon penetration. The stimulated mexoryl molecule rapidly deactivates and releases the absorbed energy to the environment as harmless energy, and then repeats the process.

Vitamin D Plus Calcium

Corticosteroid-induced osteoporosis with subsequent pathologic fractures contributes to significant morbidity among patients with SLE. The use of high-SPF sunscreens may accentuate this problem, leading to even greater levels of vitamin D deficiency. Supplements of calcium and vitamin D should be the standard of care in all corticosteroid-treated patients.[25] Calcipotriene has been found to be beneficial in diseases such as scleroderma and may show good effects in cutaneous LE.[26]

Corticosteroids: Topical/Intralesional

A minority of patients with SCLE fail to respond to topical corticosteroids. These patients may be candidates for subcutaneous steroid therapy. Intralesional triamcinolone (3–5 mg/mL) is particularly useful in the treatment of chronic, recalcitrant, hyperkeratotic lesions, particularly those located in the scalp. Side effects include skin atrophy and depigmentation.[27]

Antimalarials

Most patients respond well to antimalarials. Cigarette smoking is usually the primary reason for poor treatment response. Smoking cessation in these patients is usually beneficial, and may allow for a successful treatment. In patients who do not respond to a trial of hydroxychloroquine, the addition of quinacrine at 6 to 8 weeks of therapy may add to the efficacy of hydroxychloroquine.[3]

Thalidomide

In selected cases, thalidomide may represent an excellent alternative among patients with treatment refractory SCLE. The potent anti-inflammatory properties and the immunosuppressive effects of thalidomide are of value in the treatment of SCLE. The dosage used in most studies ranges between 50 and 200 mg/d; 15% to 20% of patients achieve remission and 90% achieve some benefit. The main side effects are teratogenicity, somnolence, and neuropathy.[28]

Leflunomide

This novel drug exerts anti-inflammatory and immunomodulatory effects through the inhibition of pyrimidine synthesis, thereby impairing the proliferation of B and T lymphocytes. Common side effects include elevation of hepatic enzymes, anemia, and an exfoliative dermatitis. There are few reports that this drug can improve SCLE when other standard therapies fail. In one report there was both a remission and deterioration of SCLE.[29]

Pimecrolimus

This calcineurin inhibitor can improve the cutaneous lesions in SCLE. Topical pimecrolimus can improve 50% or more the skin lesions, and may also improve quality of life. Pimecrolimus 1% cream twice daily for 3 weeks under semiocclusive conditions has led to the regression of skin lesions and 57% improvement on clinical severity score.[30]

Tacrolimus

Tacrolimus inhibits T-cell activation and cytokine release. It is an immunomodulatory macrolide isolated form a soil microbe, *Streptomyces tsukubaensis*. Application of 0.1% topical tacrolimus ointment in 12 patients with cutaneous LE resistant to standard therapies, of whom 4 had SCLE of 6 weeks' duration, resulted in regression for 2 patients and improvement for 2 others. Therefore, topical tacrolimus 1% ointment may be an effective alternative in severe recalcitrant cutaneous LE.[31]

Mycophenolate Mofetil

Mycophenolate mofetil (MMF) is a potent immunosuppressive used extensively to prevent rejection in solid organ transplantation, particularly among renal transplant recipients. MMF is a purine analog similar to azathioprine but with more specific inhibition of the de novo pathway in lymphocytes. This characteristic allows for potentially greater efficacy and less toxicity in treating severe, recalcitrant SCLE, which is consistent with clinical studies.

MMF has demonstrated efficacy in the treatment of SLE nephritis, and it is used to treat SCLE skin lesions refractory to systemic corticosteroid and antimalarial therapy. The standard treatment dosage is 2 g/d, with good response in a few weeks. One study used a mycophenolate sodium enteric-coated formulation of mycophenolic acid (EC-MPS), which has an equivalent efficacy and similar safety profile to mycophenolate mofetil. This was shown to be effective and safe in patients with SCLE resistant to standard therapy.[32] Likewise, it has also been shown to give poor results in refractory SLE.[33]

Intravenous Immunoglobulin

Intravenous immunoglobulin (IVIG) is a viable alternative for the treatment of SCLE refractory to other standard therapies. It has been administered in pulses of 0.4 g/kg/d for 5 days, leading to clinical improvement, and a good remission period.[34] There are various IVIG preparations, and the optimum one for SCLE has not been determined. IVIG is extremely expensive and carries some risk of nephrotoxicity. Thus, it should be reserved for the most severe and refractory cases.

Efalizumab

This biologic agent is a recombinant, humanized, monoclonal antibody against CD11a, the alpha subunit of leukocyte function-associated antigen1 (LFA-1), a protein involved in T-cell activation and trafficking. There are reports that it was effective for SCLE refractory to other standard therapies, but is no longer used because efalizumab has been associated with PML.

Rituximab

Rituximab is a monoclonal antibody with activity against CD20. It induces B-lymphocyte depletion through complement-dependent lysis. One case report has been published in which a 48-year-old woman with refractory SCLE responded successfully to rituximab.[35]

SLE

SLE affects the skin in the form of acute cutaneous LE, which generally presents with a photosensitive, symmetric, confluent erythema and edema over the malar areas called "butterfly erythema." This lesion is transient, does not lead to scarring, and spares the nasolabial folds (**Fig. 3**). Butterfly erythema occurs in 20% to 60% of patients with SLE.

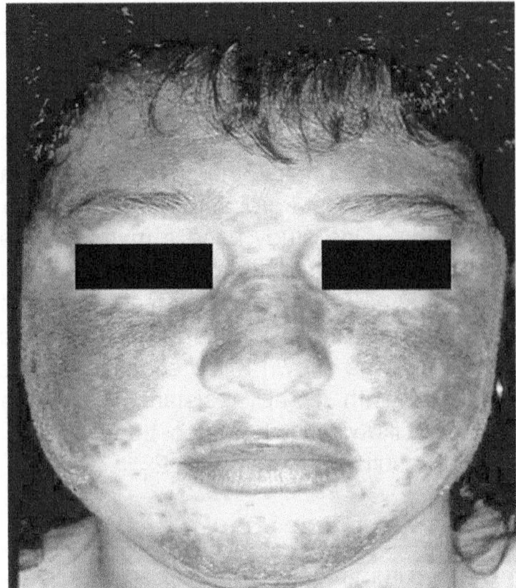

Fig. 3. "Butterfly" malar erythema.

Active SLE is strongly associated with positive ANAs and anti-dsDNA antibodies. B cells play a central role in the pathogenesis of SLE. SLE complications include lupus nephritis (LN); central nervous system (CNS) symptoms like anxiety, psychosis, and seizures; cutaneous and systemic vasculitis (**Fig. 4**); and may affect the bone marrow (cytopenias). Current treatment includes corticosteroids, antimalarials, cyclophosphamide, and azathioprine.

NEW THERAPIES FOR ACTIVE SLE

Tacrolimus and Pimecrolimus

Both tacrolimus and pimecrolimus are calcineurin inhibitors as described previously. Several studies have shown that tacrolimus has a higher tolerability when compared with corticosteroids. Their efficacy is greatest with cutaneous lesions of SLE. Their efficacy in treating the lesions associated with DLE and SCLE is lower, which is believed to be secondary to the chronicity of these lesions.[36]

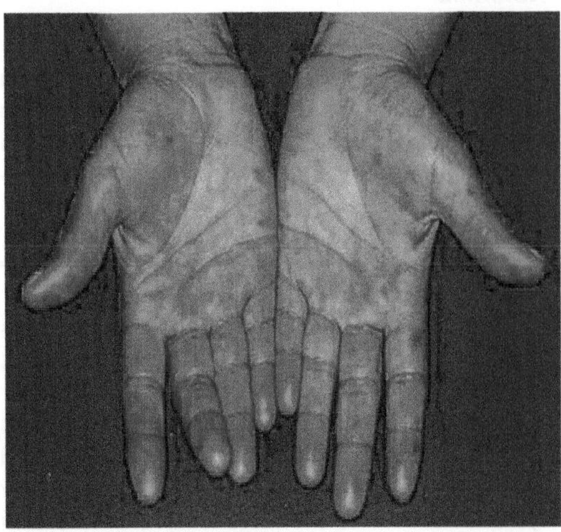

Fig. 4. SLE vasculitis of the hands.

Vitamin D

At the time of this writing, vitamin D is the vogue topic of investigation. Vitamin D deficiency has been correlated with cancers as well as increased incidence of autoimmunity.[37] Vitamin D produces and maintains self-immunologic tolerance.[38] A recent report in the literature shows that vitamin D deficiency was more common in Saudi patients with SLE as compared with a control group.[39] It is important that the clinician is mindful of the possibility of vitamin D deficiency. Given that photoprotection is of paramount importance in this patient population, vitamin D supplementation assumes a critical role. Dietary supplementation with Vitamin D with at least 400 IU daily may be beneficial.[40] Recent trends suggest that even higher dosages may be required to achieve pharmacologic effect (1000–2000 IU daily in adults).

Cyclophosphamide Plus Azathioprine

For many years, intermittent intravenous cyclophosphamide (IVC) has been the standard therapy for proliferative lupus nephritis. This regimen involves the use of IVC in dosages of 0.05 to 1.00 g/m^2 body surface area (BSA), monthly, for 6 months. The toxicity of IVC includes risk of infection, malignancy, and gonadal failure.[41]

In some centers in Europe, the dose of IVC has been lowered and azathioprine (daily dosage 1 mg/kg) has been added for maintenance with good remission rates. Before giving azathioprine, the enzyme activity of thiopurine methyltransferase (TMPT) should be evaluated to avoid fatal neutropenia.

As novel therapies and biologic agents are more widely used, it is likely that IVC use will decline because of the high potential for adverse events.[42]

Intravenous Immunoglobulin

IVIG has been used in cases of severe SLE with pulmonary hemorrhage, neurologic involvement, leukocytoclastic vasculitis, and polyradiculopathy. The mechanism of action of IVIG in SLE includes suppression of the expansion of autoreactive B lymphocytes through signaling of the FcgRIIB, idiotype-mediated inhibition of B-cell receptors, and neutralization of cytokines such as the B-cell survival factors. The dosage used is 2 g/kg over 5 days. In case reports and in open trial, high-dose IVIG has consistently been shown to be a beneficial and safe adjunct therapeutic agent.[43]

As noted previously, cost may be a limiting factor in administration of IVIG off-label.

Mycophenolate Mofetil

Mycophenolate mofetil (MMF) is a reversible inhibitor of inosine monophosphate dehydrogenase, the rate-limiting step in de novo purine synthesis. MMF has been studied in patients with lupus nephritis and has shown better results than IVC. Five randomized trials enrolled patients with World Health Organization (WHO) class III, IV, or V (mostly IV) lupus nephritis, predominantly comparing MMF (1 to 3 g daily) with IVC and steroid. In the trials that compared IVC with MMF, MMF had a complete/partial response in 80% of patients, lowered the mortality from 7.8% to 1.7%, and lowered hospital admissions from 15.0% to 1.7%. In addition, MMF had lower serious infections related to the therapy.[44]

Rituximab

Rituximab is an anti-CD20 monoclonal antibody used in SLE to treat refractory lupus nephritis. Rituximab targets CD20+ B cells, causing cell lysis. Lupus nephritis occurs in 30% of patients with SLE, and conventional therapy controls approximately 52% to 71% of these patients. There is a 45% risk of frequent relapse. Three cases of severe class IV (WHO) lupus nephritis were successfully treated with rituximab for both induction and maintenance.[45]

In a systematic review of 188 patients with SLE treated with rituximab, 91% showed significant improvement in one or more systemic SLE manifestations. Also, among the 103 patients with lupus nephritis, 91% reported a good response. This biologic agent is typically used in a dose of 375 mg/m^2 in weekly infusions and then monthly for maintenance. No adverse reactions have been reported, and this therapy may be used for long-term control.[46] Rituximab has been used in patients with SLE who have neurologic and neuropsychiatric complications, as this biologic agent may reduce brain lesions while maintaining a good safety profile. Although 2 cases of PML have been described among patients with SLE receiving rituximab, causation has not been demonstrated, as there have also been reports of PML in patients with SLE with no exposure to rituximab.

Belimumab

Belimumab (BLyS), a humanized monoclonal antibody, binds to the common growth factor B-lymphocyte stimulator (BLyS), and is a novel strategy for the treatment of inflammatory diseases like SLE. Belimumab is an investigational human monoclonal antibody drug that specifically recognizes and inhibits the biologic activity of B-lymphocyte stimulator, or BLyS. In lupus and certain other autoimmune diseases, elevated levels of BLyS are believed to contribute to the production of autoantibodies, antibodies that attack and destroy the body's own healthy tissues.[47]

BLyS, a B-lymphocyte stimulator, is a cytokine member of the TNF family. BLyS is made by monocytes and macrophages with subsequent release when the monocytes and macrophages are activated. BlyS binds to a receptor on the B cells, which stimulates maturation into antibody-secreting plasma cells. Belimumab inhibits the biologic activity of BLyS.

It has been used to treat SLE flares with a dosage of 10 mg/kg monthly, and has resulted in sustained improvement in SLE disease activity for years. As compared with standard of care, the reduction of SLE disease activity or flares was not significant.[48]

Abatacept

Abatacept is a fusion protein, a cytotoxic T-lymphocyte-associated antigen 4-immunoglobulin (CTL4), and inhibits T cells. Abatacept has been used to treat patients with SLE flares such as discoid lesions, pericarditis, pleurisy/pleuritis, and arthritis. This drug, which is approved to treat rheumatoid arthritis, has been evaluated along with prednisone in a phase IIb clinical trial for SLE, and a phase III trial for SLE is currently recruiting patients. The dosage used is 10 mg/kg, intravenous, once a month, and prednisone has been added in a dosage of 30 mg/d as adjuvant therapy.[49]

Epratuzumab

This biologic agent is an anti-CD22 humanized monoclonal antibody, which depletes circulating B cells. It has been used to treat patients with SLE with mild to moderate muco-cutaneous and musculoskeletal symptoms. The dosage is 360 mg/m^2, IV, every 2 weeks, for 4 doses, with good outcome and safety profile.[50]

SUMMARY

Cutaneous lupus erythematosus is a challenging dermatologic disorder that is mainly photosensitive. Standard ladder of therapy should be tried and include the education of patients on sunscreens, photoprotective clothing, and behavior modification. Treatment modalities, as new topical and systemic drugs are available, will allow us to make a mental algorithm of therapy on our patients, moving cautiously from the safest to the most aggressive agent. Several B-cell-targeted therapies are noted, eg, rituximab, belimumab, epratuzumab, but as published in Looney and colleagues[51] recent article, results have been disappointing in SLE. Still, there are current and ongoing clinical trials so it remains to be seen if these hold as much promise as anticipated.

ACKNOWLEDGMENTS

We would like to thank the following individuals for their help with electronic information retrieval: Griselda Izabal, MD, Christus Muguerza Hospital, Monterrey, Michelle Gatica and Alan Burguete, Instituto Tecnólogico y de Estudios Superiores de Monterrey, Monterrey, Mexico.

REFERENCES

1. Jacobson DL, Gange SJ, Rose NR, et al. Epidemiology and estimated population burden of selected autoimmune diseases in the United States. Clin Immunol Immunopathol 1997;84:223–43.
2. Kuhn A, Sticherling M, Bonsmann G. Clinical manifestations of cutaneous lupus erythematosus. J Dtsch Dermatol Ges 2007;5:1124–40.
3. Werth VP. New approaches to cutaneous lupus. Dermatology focus, DF Clinical Symposia: Proceedings 2009-Part II, Summer 2009 Vol. 28 NO.2. Naples, Florida, January 28–February 1, 2009.
4. Pelle MT. Issues and advances in the management and pathogenesis of cutaneous lupus erythematosus. Adv Dermatol 2006;22:55–65.
5. Jessop S, Whitelaw DA, Delamere FM. Drugs for discoid lupus erythematosus. Cochrane Database Syst Rev 2009;4:CD002954.
6. Sárdy M, Ruzicka T, Kuhn A. Topical calcineurin inhibitors in cutaneous lupus erythematosus. Arch Dermatol Res 2009;301(1):93–8.
7. Barikbin B, Givrad S, Yousefi M, et al. Pimecrolimus 1% cream versus betamethasone 17-valerate 0.1% cream in the treatment of facial discoid lupus erythematosus: a double-blind, randomized pilot study. Clin Exp Dermatol 2009;34(7):776–80.
8. Tlacuilo-Parra A, Guevara-Gutiérrez E, Gutiérrez-Murillo F, et al. Pimecrolimus 1% cream for the treatment of discoid lupus erythematosus. Rheumatology 2005;44:1564–8.
9. Madan V, August PJ, Chalmers RJ. Efficacy of topical tacrolimus 0.3% in clobetasol propionate 0.05% ointment in therapy-resistant cutaneous lupus erythematosus: a cohort study. Clin Exp Dermatol 2010;35(1):27–30.
10. Jemec GB, Ullman S, Goodfield M, et al. A randomized controlled trial of R-salbutamol for topical treatment of discoid lupus erythematosus. Br J Dermatol 2009;161:1365–70.
11. Wulf HC, Ullman S. Discoid and subacute lupus erythematosus treated with 0.5% R-salbutamol cream. Arch Dermatol 2007;143(12):1589–90.
12. Available at: http://www.astion.com/default.asp?side=ASF-1096&side_id=5574&topmenu_id=1615&submenu_id=3492. Accessed April 6, 2010.
13. Lesiak A, Narbutt J, Kobos J, et al. Systematic administration of chloroquine in discoid lupus erythematosus reduces skin lesions via inhibition of angiogenesis. Clin Exp Dermatol 2009;34(5):570–5.
14. Illanes J, Dabancens A, Acuña O, et al. Effects of betamethasone, sulindac and quinacrine drugs on the inflammatory neoangiogenesis response induced by polyurethane sponge implanted in mouse. Biol Res 2002;35(3-4):339–45.
15. Cavazzana I, Sala R, Bazzani C, et al. Treatment of lupus skin involvement with quinacrine and hydroxychloroquine. Lupus 2009;18:735–9.
16. Shah A, Albrecht J, Bonilla Martínez Z, et al. Lenalidomide for the treatment of resistant discoid lupus erythematosus. Arch Dermatol 2009;145(3):303–6.
17. Dall'Era M, Davis J. CTLA4Ig: a novel inhibitor of costimulation. Lupus 2004;13(5):372–6.
18. Dubois EA, Cohen AF. Abatacept. Br J Clin Pharmacol 2009;68(4):480–1.
19. Usmani N, Goodfield M. Efalizumab in the treatment of discoid lupus erythematosus. Arch Dermatol 2007;143(7):873–7.
20. Booken N, Schumann T, Fuchslocher M, et al. [Successful therapy of discoid lupus erythematosus with efalizumab]. Hautlarzt 2010;61(3):246–9 [in German].
21. Raulin C, Schimdt C, Hellwig S. Cutaneous lupus erythematosus—treatment with pulsed dye laser. Br J Dermatol 1999;141:1046–50.
22. Erceg A, Bovenschen HJ, van de Kerkhof PC, et al. Efficacy and safety of pulsed dye laser treatment for cutaneous discoid lupus erythematosus. J Am Acad Dermatol 2009;60(4):626–32.
23. Bens G. Photosensitivity in lupus erythematosus. Rev Med Interne 2009;30(10):857–65.
24. Obermoser G, Zelger B. Triple need for photoprotection in lupus erythematosus. Lupus 2008;17(6):525–7.
25. Vasudevan AR, Ginzler EM. Established and novel treatments for lupus. J Muscoskel Med 2009;26:291–300.
26. Callen JP. Cutaneous lupus erythematosus: a personal approach to management. Australas J Dermatol 2006;47:13–27.
27. Callen JP. Management of skin disease in patients with lupus erythematosus. Best Pract Res Clin Rheumatol 2002;16(2):245–64.
28. Pelle MT, Werth VP. Thalidomide in cutaneous lupus erythematosus. Am J Clin Dermatol 2003;4(6):379–87.

29. Suess A, Sticherling M. Leflunomide in subacute cutaneous lupus erythematosus—two sides of a coin. Int J Dermatol 2008;47(1):83–6.
30. Kreuter A, Gambichler T, Breuckmann F, et al. Pimecrolimus 1% cream for cutaneous lupus erythematosus. J Am Acad Dermatol 2004;51:407–10.
31. Lampropoulus CE, Sangle S, Harrison G, et al. Topical tacrolimus therapy of resistant cutaneous lesions in lupus erythematosus: a possible alternative. Rheumatology 2004;43:1383–5.
32. Kreuter A, Tomi NS, Weiner SM, et al. Mycophenolate sodium for subacute cutaneous lupus erythematosus resistant to standard therapy. Br J Dermatol 2007;156(6):1321–7.
33. Pisoni CN, Obermoser G, Cuadrado MJ, et al. Skin manifestations of systemic lupus erythematosus refractory to multiple treatment modalities: poor results with mycophenolate mofetil. Clin Exp Rheumatol 2005;23(3):393–6.
34. Lampropoulos CE, Hughes GR, D'Cruz DP. Intravenous immunoglobulin in the treatment of resistant subacute cutaneous lupus erythematosus: a possible alternative. Clin Rheumatol 2007;26(6): 981–3.
35. Kieu V, O'Brien T, Yap LM, et al. Refractory subacute cutaneous lupus erythematosus successfully treated with rituximab. Australas J Dermatol 2009; 50(3):202–6.
36. Tzellos TG, Kouvelas D. Topical tacrolimus and pimecrolimus in the treatment of cutaneous lupus erythematosus: an evidence-based evaluation. Eur J Clin Pharmacol 2008;64:337–41.
37. Adorini L, Penna G. Control of autoimmune diseases by the vitamin D endocrine system. Nat Clin Pract Rheumatol 2008;4(8):404–12.
38. Ginanjar E, Sumariyono, Setiati S, et al. Vitamin D and autoimmune disease. Acta Med Indones 2007; 39(3):133–41.
39. Damanhouri LH. Vitamin D deficiency in Saudi patients with systemic lupus erythematosus. Saudi Med J 2009;30(10):1291–5.
40. Cusack C, Danby C, Fallon JC, et al. Photoprotective behaviour and sunscreen use: impact on vitamin D levels in cutaneous lupus erythematosus. Photodermatol Photoimmunol Photomed 2008;24(5):260–7.
41. Baskin E, Ozen S, Cakar N, et al. The use of low-dose cyclophosphamide followed by AZA/MMF treatment in childhood lupus nephritis. Pediatr Nephrol 2010;25(1):111–7.
42. D'Cruz DP, Houssiau FA. The Euro-Lupus nephritis trial: the development of the sequential treatment protocol. Lupus 2009;18(10):875–7.
43. Zandman-Goddard G, Blanck M, Shoenfeld Y. Intravenous immunoglobulins in systemic lupus erythematosus: from the bench to the bedside. Lupus 2009;18(10):884–8.
44. Moore RA, Derry S. Systematic review and meta-analysis of randomized trials and cohort studies of mycophenolate mofetil in lupus nephritis. Arthritis Res Ther 2006;8(6):R182.
45. Camous L, Melander C, Vallet M, et al. Complete remission of Lupus Nephritis with Rituximab and steroids for induction and Rituximab alone for maintenance therapy. Am J Kidney Dis 2008;52:346–52.
46. Ramos-Casals M, Soto MJ, Cuadrado MJ, et al. Rituximab in systemic lupus erythematosus: a systematic review of off-label use in 188 cases. Lupus 2009;18(9):767–76.
47. Available at: http://www.hgsi.com/belimumab.html. Accessed April 6, 2010.
48. Wallace DJ, Stohl W, Furie RA, et al. A phase II, randomized, double-blind, placebo-controlled, dose-ranging study of belimumab in patients with active systemic lupus erythematosus. Arthritis Rheum 2009;61(9):1168–78.
49. Monneaux F, Muller S. Molecular therapies for systemic lupus erythematosus: clinical trials and future prospects. Arthritis Res Ther 2009;11: 234–43.
50. Dòrner T, Kaufmann J, Wegener WA, et al. Initial clinical trial of epratuzumab (humanized anti-CD22 antibody) for immunotherapy of systemic lupus erythematosus. Arthritis Res Ther 2006;8(3):R74.
51. Looney RJ, Anolik J, Sanz I. A perspective on B-cell-targeting therapy for SLE. Mod Rheumatol 2010;20: 1–10.

Innovative Therapy of Cutaneous T-Cell Lymphoma: Beyond Psoralen and Ultraviolet Light and Nitrogen Mustard

Brian Poligone, MD, PhD[a,b,*], Peter Heald, MD[c]

KEYWORDS

- Mycosis fungoides • Cutaneous T-cell lymphoma
- Therapeutics • Phototherapy • Laser • Imiquimod

The incidence of cutaneous T-cell lymphoma (CTCL) in the United States continues to rise.[1] Although CTCL has come to encompass a broad group of cutaneous lymphomas, mycosis fungoides (MF) and Sezary syndrome (SS) remain the most common forms of CTCL. The staging system for CTCL applies only to MF/SS.[2,3] Additionally, most of the literature on therapy and the treatments discussed in this article are focused on these variants. As the number of patients with MF/SS increases, so do the therapy problems that arise in their management.

Two dichotomies must help position available treatments (**Table 1**). One is whether the treatment is localized or generalized. The second is whether the goal of therapy is to achieve remission or to achieve palliation. The initial therapies—topical nitrogen mustard (NM) and photochemotherapy with psoralen and ultraviolet A light (PUVA)—published for the treatment of MF/SS would be considered as generalized and intended for remission. NM was first applied topically to MF in 1959.[4] Perhaps the most widely used generalized remittive therapy, phototherapy, has been in use for treatment of the disease since the 1970s.[5] Undoubtedly the highest response rates for remission are with radiotherapy whether generalized (total skin electron beam[6]) or localized.[7] Whereas the use of NM and PUVA has remained stable, there has been an expansion in the variety of therapies in the categories of localized ablative, generalized palliative, and generalized remittive (as outlined in **Table 1**). When lesions do not therapeutically respond to the first course of conventional therapy, then the innovative new therapies need to be considered. This article discusses some innovative therapies that are being used to treat MF/SS. Although randomized controlled trials are needed to verify the preliminary results, a patient's predicament may benefit from the promising therapies reviewed.

Dr Poligone is supported by the Wilmot Cancer Research Fellowship Program and the Dermatology Foundation Career Development Award.
Financial Disclosure: None reported.
[a] Department of Dermatology, University of Rochester School of Medicine, Rochester, NY, USA
[b] James P. Wilmot Cancer Center, University of Rochester School of Medicine, Rochester, NY, USA
[c] Department of Dermatology, Yale University School of Medicine, New Haven, CT, USA
* Corresponding author. Department of Dermatology, University of Rochester School of Medicine, Rochester, NY.
E-mail address: brian_poligone@urmc.rochester.edu

Dermatol Clin 28 (2010) 501–510
doi:10.1016/j.det.2010.03.010
0733-8635/10/$ – see front matter © 2010 Elsevier Inc. All rights reserved.

Table 1
Two dichotomies that help position therapies

	Palliative	Remittive
Localized	Steroid cream	Radiograph Bexarotene gel Excimer laser Imiquimod Cryotherapy Surgical excision
Generalized	Prednisone Chlorambucil Methotrexate Photopheresis Oral bexarotene Oral vorinostat Denileukin diftitox Romidepsin Liposomal doxorubicin Alemtuzumab	Nitrogen mustard Total skin electron beam Phototherapy Allogeneic stem cell transplantation

The dichotomies are based on properties of the therapy. One is whether the therapy is localized or generalized. The latter includes both systemic and total skin treatments. The second property is whether the treatment is administered with a primary intent of reducing tumor burden to zero (remittive) or whether it is to improve quality of life (palliative). Although there have been infrequent remissions with some of the palliative therapies, a cut off of 50% remission rate was used to define the treatments in the far right column.

LOCALIZED ABLATIVE THERAPIES

Photodynamic Therapy

Photosensitizers in photochemotherapy have been used to treat skin disease for centuries. The use of PUVA has been a key strategy in the treatment of MF for decades. With the application of photodynamic therapy (PDT), which uses aminolevulinic acid (ALA) and its derivatives in the presence of light, a new topical photosensitizing strategy has been used for the treatment of cutaneous malignancies.[8] Topical PDT is activated in the visible light spectrum (580–720 nm). The specificity for PDT is still under investigation but it is known that only cells within the epidermis and epidermal appendages initially become photoreactive. Interestingly, tumors of epidermal origin are also photosensitive, even when located within the dermis, suggesting that the depth of ALA absorption or light penetration are not the only factors determining which cells may be targeted by this treatment.[9] Activated T lymphocytes, as observed in skin lymphoma, can absorb ALA, whereas unactivated T lymphocytes can not.[10] Therefore, the use of PDT in MF has a physiologic basis. Malignant T cells localized in plaques or tumors of CTCL can be bathed in ALA and thereafter photoactivated, causing cell death through the production of reactive oxygen species and apoptosis.

The use of PDT in CTCL dates back to 1994 when Svanberg and colleagues[11] and Wolf and colleagues,[12] each described patients with CTCL treated with PDT. Svanberg and colleagues[11] treated two patients, once or twice for a year or less, showing a complete response. Wolf and colleagues[12] also reported complete remission in two patients with 4 to 5 courses of PDT over 6 months. Later Orenstein and colleagues[13] treated one patient with tumor-stage MF who showed a complete response confirmed by biopsy with 2 years of follow-up. In 2001, a larger case series was performed that showed the first histologic confirmation of clearance of MF with PDT.[14] Ten patients with MF, 8 with plaque stage and 2 with tumor stage, were treated. They had all failed previous therapies, including etretinate, PUVA, and radiotherapy. In lesions that showed a clinical response to PDT, there was a decrease in CD3+ CD4+ cells in the epidermis and dermis, although a few foci remained. In a patient that did not respond, a longer incubation time with the ALA (18 hours instead of 5–6 hours), did not change the clinical or histologic appearance of the lesions after two treatments. The patient who had previously received radiotherapy had some baseline fibrosis and required 11 cycles of treatment to respond.

Various forms of ALA and various light sources have been used (**Table 2**). There have been over 30 patients reported and the results have been favorable. Because there has been no consistency in methodology, response rates cannot be obtained; however, multiple studies have shown response in both plaques and tumors of MF. Although recurrence may occur, many remissions lasted at least 1 to 2 years during follow-up. Application time varied but most studies used a range of 3 to 6 hours. Light sources have also been variable although all were within the visible light spectrum. The various light sources, doses, and dose rate used in PDT have been reviewed elsewhere, and those used in CTCL are shown in **Table 2**.[15] For lesions of CTCL that are refractory to standard therapies, PDT is an emerging therapy with an extensive history awaiting further exploration.

PDT may be considered in cases of oligolesional persistent disease or for patients where a radiation-sparing therapy is needed due to prior sun, phototherapy, or radiotherapy.

Table 2
PDT

	Photosensitizer	Application Time (hours)	Source	Dose (J cm^{-2})	Follow-up (months)	Patients
Wolf et al, 1994[12]	20% dALA	4–6	Modified slide projector	40	8–14	2
Svanberg et al, 1994[11]	20% dALA	5–18	Doubled pulsed frequency Nd:YAG dye laser	60	6–14	2
Orenstein et al, 2000[13]	20% dALA	16	Broad band red light (580–720 nm)	170–380	24–27	2
Edstrom et al, 2001[14]	20% dALA	5–6	Waldmann PDT 1200 (600–730 nm)	50–180	4–21	10
Markham et al, 2001[39]	20% dALA	4	Waldmann PDT 1200	20	12	1
Paech et al, 2002[40]	20% dALA	4	Waldmann PDT 1200	180	12	1
Leman et al, 2002[41]	20% dALA	6–24	Xenon short arc discharge lamp	100	12	1
Coors et al, 2004[42]	20% dALA	6	Waldmann PDT 1200	96–144	14–18	4
Umegaki et al, 2004[43]	20% dALA	6	SUS66 illuminator	120	NR	1
Zane et al, 2006[44]	20% mALA	3	Aktilite CL128 lamp	37.5	12–34	5
Recio et al, 2008[45]	20% ALA	4	585 nm pulsed dye laser	8	24	2
Hegyi et al, 2008[46]	20% mALA	3	Aktilite lamp (635 nm red light)	100[a]	16	1

Abbreviations: dALA, delta-aminolevulinic acid; mALA, methyl-aminolevulinic acid; Nd:YAG, Neodymium: Yttrium-Aluminum-Garnet; NR, not reported.

[a] 200 J cm^{-2} caused ulceration.

Cryotherapy

Cryosurgery is a readily available and overlooked modality in treating CTCL. The freeze-thaw cycle causes localized tissue injury that can destroy all living cells, leading to necrosis.[16] Freezing should be fast and thawing should be slow. Most dermatologists use cryotherapy for the treatment of benign and premalignant lesions, including warts and actinic keratoses and, less commonly, malignancy. Nevertheless, there is little evidence in the medical literature to direct the physician regarding the exact procedural method. This is especially true for treating malignant T cells. There has been no study showing the optimal temperature for killing lymphocytes in human skin. Nevertheless, there is little doubt that cryotherapy can be used to destroy benign and malignant cells in the skin, including T cells.

In general most experts report that multiple freezes are better for malignant lesions than a single freeze-thaw cycle.[16] It can be used to treat any part of the body, so is particularly useful for small lesions that have resisted previous therapies. As with other malignancies, a greater amount of necrosis is required to destroy a malignant lesion.[17] A tissue temperature of −50° to −60°C will destroy malignant lesions.[16] Because the depth of damage is determined by the freeze time, thaw time, and area treated, experience is needed to properly deliver the cryogen. However, malignant lymphocytes in the skin, even when within a tumor, can be readily killed with freezing. One guide is to choose a thaw time that is at least twice the freeze time. Although a lateral margin of normal skin should be treated, there is no data regarding its size. Topical and injected anesthetics can be used for treating larger lesions.

Patients with CTCL who are treated with cryosurgery have a typical tissue reaction that includes crusting and occasionally bulla formation. Weeping and sloughing of the skin are also common. Melanocytes are more sensitive to freezing than most other cell types in the skin and, therefore, patients should be warned about possible hypo- and depigmentation after treating the malignant lesion. As mentioned, although it has not been established in all cell types, destruction of malignant cells often requires colder temperatures. Therefore, the use of higher temperatures to protect melanocytes may ultimately lead to failure in adequately treating the malignancy.

Cryotherapy may be considered in cases of oligolesional persistent disease and for patients where a radiation sparing-therapy is needed due to prior sun, phototherapy, or radiotherapy.

Surgery

Surgery with steel can be an overlooked modality in treating CTCL. Although commonly used in the treatment of cutaneous B-cell lymphoma, the use of primary excision in T-cell lymphoma is infrequent.[18] There have been reports of treating variants of MF including unilesional MF with surgical excision.[19] Case reports have suggested that lesions do not recur.[20] It is more natural to consider surgical excision in a patient presenting with one small lesion. However, surgical excision should also be considered as an option in patients who have failed first line therapies or have had a recurrence or nonresponse to treatment of a solitary lesion.

Surgery may be considered for patients with unilesional MF, pagetoid reticulosis, or small, solitary recurrent lesions.

Excimer Laser

The US Federal Drug Administration approval of the excimer laser for psoriasis and vitiligo has increased access to this therapeutic option. The xenon-chloride laser emits monochromatic light in the UV range at a wavelength of 308 nm. This wavelength is within the UV B spectrum (UVB) (320 nm–280 nm), which suggests that the excimer laser light would be effective in MF. There have been a number of case reports or series and open trials showing benefit. It has a safety profile similar to phototherapy because local phototoxicity is the major adverse event. However, the ability to localize treatment to lesional skin helps minimize this.

In 2004, Nistico and colleagues[21] treated five patients with Stage IA patch-plaque MF, and 10 lesions in total, with excimer laser with one year of follow-up. All 10 lesions had a complete response without recurrence over 1 year (**Table 3**). Five patients with patch-plaque disease were treated by Passeron and colleagues.[22] All showed a clinical response, and four of five showed a complete response. At the end of the trial, all five had maintained the response, including the partial responder who had "minimal residual activity." Mori and colleagues[23] also presented a case series in four patients with Stage IA disease. Seven lesions were treated and showed complete response with follow-up between 3 and 28 months. One patient developed a new lesion in a different, untreated site during follow-up, while the other three remained disease free. In one case series of two patients, recurrence of MF after excimer laser was observed. The patient had patch-plaque disease and previously developed recurrence following a complete response with PUVA 15 months prior.[24] Because the patient had previously experienced nausea with psoralen, excimer laser was used after disease recurrence. Several lesions showed a partial or complete response, but she continued to develop new plaques after discontinuation of therapy. Finally, two patients have been presented who had individual lesions treated with excimer laser while undergoing narrow-band (NB)UV light therapy for other lesions.[25] One patient had a complete response to both NB-UVB and excimer laser-treated lesions. The other patient had a partial and incomplete response to her lesions with both NB-UVB and excimer laser.

Excimer laser may be considered for patients with unilesional MF—especially those patients that have had good success with phototherapy or have not used phototherapy. This would be a good modality for a patient successfully treated with phototherapy who has sanctuary lesions that are not well exposed during UV treatments such as those on the feet, inguinal area, or parts of the face.

Imiquimod

Imiquimod is a nucleoside analog and agonist of toll-like receptor (TLR) 7 and 8. It was originally developed while looking for antiviral drugs; however, it does not have direct antiviral properties. Imiquimod does stimulate the release of interferon and cytokines, which have antiviral as well as antitumor responses.[26,27] The exact mechanism

Table 3
Excimer laser therapy

	Starting Dose ($J\ cm^{-2}$)	Further Dosing ($J\ cm^{-2}$)	Frequency	Treatments	MED Testing	Follow-up (Months)	Patients	Side Effects	Recurrence	Complete Response
Nistico et al, 2004[21]	0.5–1 (Twice MED)	0.15–0.5/session	q 7 to 10 d	10	Yes	12	5	Transient hyperpigmentation, itch	None	5
Passeron et al, 2004[22]	0.17–0.5 (50 mJ below MED)	0.1/per week	Twice weekly	21	Yes	3	5	Erythema, blistering	None	5
Mori et al, 2004[23]	0.5–1 (2–3 time MED)	0.15–0.5/session	Weekly	8	Yes	28	4	Erythema, itch	None	3 of 4
Meisenheimer, 2006[24]	0.1–0.15	0.3/session	Twice weekly	14 to >38	Yes	6	2	Persistent erythema	1 of 2	1 of 2
Kontos et al, 2006[25]	NR	NR	Thrice weekly	14 to 22	NR	NR	2	Erythema, itch, blisters, erosions, hyperpigmentation	1 of 2	1 of 2

Abbreviations: MED, minimal erythema dose; NR, not reported.

behind the antitumor response is still unknown; however, there are several possibilities, including activation of innate immunity as well as the stimulation of dendritic cells, which directs a cell-mediated antitumor response.[28] The central role of the nuclear transcription factor -κB also requires further exploration because it mediates TLR signaling. Finally, because CTCL is generally composed of Th2 T lymphocytes, the production of interferon correcting the Th1 and Th2 imbalance may be important in the treatment of CTCL.

Although larger clinical trials are needed, there is mounting evidence from case reports and series that imiquimod cream has activity against CTCL (**Table 4**). One current limitation in the United States is that the cream is distributed in small packets, which are difficult to use over larger areas of the body. A recent review of the currently published cases has shown imiquimod has been applied with good success at many centers. In Suchin and colleagues[29] initial report, the cream was applied daily, which led to the patient having redness, vesiculation, erosion, and pruritus of the lesion. This led to a 2-day discontinuation of treatment, but the patient was then able to restart daily application. The inflammation decreased gradually over the 4-month course of treatment. Deeths and colleagues[30] reported a case series of six patients, who were allowed to continue photochemotherapy or interferon during imiquimod treatment. This trial also allowed patients to decrease frequency of dosing to once a week if they experienced irritation with 3 times weekly application. Despite the decreased frequency, four of six patients experienced some localized irritation, including one patient with ulceration and suspected cellulitis requiring oral antibiotic therapy.

Two studies have shown synergy of imiquimod with systemic interferon.[30,31] Imiquimod has been used to treat unilesional MF on the penis and buttock.[32,33] In most case reports to date, the patient had failed at least one standard first-line topical therapy, suggesting imiquimod may be beneficial in treatment resistant MF. Recently, Coors and colleagues[34] obtained a complete response with imiquimod in one patient with CD30+ anaplastic, large cell lymphoma (ALCL), suggesting that imiquimod may have applicability beyond MF. Didona and colleagues[35] has also examined imiquimod in three patients with ALCL with complete response. Martinez-Gonzalez and colleagues[31] reported four patients treated with imiquimod showing a complete response. However, during the study period, one patient developed new lesions outside of the treatment area.

There is ample data supporting the effect of imiquimod in certain patients with MF. Larger studies will provide better efficacy data, but the 20 patients that have been reported thus far show some level of activity. One important question will be whether imiquimod can provide long-term remission. It is always important to consider this when choosing therapies in CTCL because some treatments provide temporary responses but do not provide solid remissions. For example, plaques of MF will disappear after treatment with ultrapotent topical corticosteroids; however, experience shows that many of these patients have recurrence or new lesions. On the other hand, photochemotherapy can provide longer term remissions and is generally a preferred therapy when looking for such remission compared with topical corticosteroids. It will be important to determine if imiquimod can provide long-term remission.

Finally, the studies reported to date included patients who had failed more standard therapies such as topical carmustine and NM; topical corticosteroid; systemic interferon; PUVA; low-dose retinoids; and radiation. With the positive response to date, there is data to support imiquimod for the topical treatment of localized MF that has failed standard therapies.

Imiquimod may be considered for patients who have failed topical corticosteroid, bexarotene gel, NM-carmustine, or phototherapy—yet have residual or new isolated plaques; or for patients with plaques, genital lesions, or unilesional MF.

GENERALIZED THERAPY FOR PALLIATION

Romidepsin

Many of the modalities currently approved for CTCL are primarily palliative: denileukin diftitox, oral bexarotene, and oral vorinostat. Any systemic therapy that has its success determined by quality of life indices must have an acceptable level of side effects. With CTCL, there can be improvement of disease using drugs that inhibit histone deacetylase (HDAC). The recently approved romidepsin provides an innovative approach to HDAC inhibition with a weekly pulsing regimen that is relatively free of severe adverse events.[36] Fewer than half of the patients achieved a significant response, but those who did had a marked reduction in pruritus. The side-effect profile was markedly similar to the oral HDAC inhibitor vorinostat. Many patients had mild gastrointestinal upset, mild asthenia, and anorexia. The most common laboratory abnormality was bone marrow suppression that was mild. As with vorinostat, the electrocardiographic changes of romidepsin can be striking but appear to be inconsequential.[37]

Table 4
Imiquimod therapy

	Stage	Patients	Length of Treatment	Frequency	Response	Side Effects	Recurrence	F/U
Suchin et al, 2002[29]	IA	1	4 months	Daily	CR	Vesicles, erythema, erosions, pruritus	NR	4 months
Dummer et al, 2003[47]	NR	1	8 weeks	Daily	CR	Ulceration	No	12 months
Chong et al, 2004[48]	IB	3	NR	Daily	NR	Mild Irritation	NR	32 weeks
Deeths et al, 2005[30]	IA to IIB	6	12 weeks	1–3 times per week	3 of 6 had CR, 1 of 6 had PR, 2 of 6 had minimal or no response	Erythema, irritation, erosion and ulceration	NR	16 weeks to 2 years
Chiam and Chan, 2006[33]	IA	1	4.5 months	Every other day	CCR	Pain, ulceration	No	6 months
Ardigo et al, 2006[32]	IA	1	24 weeks	5×/week	CR	Erythema, edema	No	6 months
Coors et al, 2006[34]	IA to IB	4	8–24 weeks	3×/week	50% CCR	Erythema, papules, pruritus	NR	6 to 45 months
Martinez-Gonzalez et al, 2008[31]	IA to IIB	4	3–14 months	3×/week	100% CR	Localized inflammation	Yes	NR

Abbreviations: CCR, clinical complete response (no histologic confirmation); CR, complete response; F/U, follow-up; NR, not reported; PR, partial response.

GENERALIZED THERAPY FOR REMISSION

Stem Cell Transplant

Although the number of patients treated with stem cell transplantation remains small, there are a number of centers throughout the United States that have experience with transplantation in CTCL.

Reduced-intensity allogeneic stem cell transplants cause less immunosuppression while still allowing for a graft versus lymphoma response. Reduced-intensity allogeneic stem cell transplants have been performed with increasing frequency in all lymphomas and have made their way into use for CTCL. There is less morbidity associated with the reduced conditioning treatment; therefore, it allows for older patients and those who are less fit to be considered for transplant. Both allogeneic and autologous stem cell transplants have recently been reviewed elsewhere.[38]

Allogeneic stem cell transplants have shown better success; however, there is an increased morbidity associated with the procedure. Of 21 patients treated to date with allogeneic stem cell transplant, 15 were reported alive without evidence of disease at variable follow-up times. Although standard intensity regimens were initially used, more recently reduced-intensity regimens have been used. Each has shown good success. Although the number of reported transplants for CTCL remains low, there have been complete, durable responses in patients who have failed standard therapies and who have the most aggressive disease.

Stem cell transplant may be considered in cases of aggressive disease such as transformed MF, lymph node involvement, erythroderma, or widespread tumors; or for patients under the age of 70, especially with sibling donors.

SUMMARY

The treatment modalities available to treat CTCL have been expanding in recent years. Targeted biologic therapies, molecular targets that cause T-lymphocyte apoptosis, and new application of established therapies, have allowed for a greater armamentarium in treating CTCL. Moreover, as we develop better biomarkers for the disease, we will be able to predict whether a particular patient will respond to a particular treatment modality.

However, for patients currently suffering from CTCL, treatments are required today. There are a number of moderately effective standard therapies for CTCL. Nevertheless, failures are common. Moreover, partial responses are common and these require additional therapy. A number of available therapies that can be used strategically to treat CTCL have been described. In some cases, such as excimer laser or imiquimod, the therapy has a well-understood safety profile and can be helpful for recalcitrant patch-plaque MF. In others, such as PDT, excision, and cryotherapy, the treatment can be used not only for patch-plaque stage disease, but also for limited tumor-stage disease. Finally, stem cell transplant has a role in treating patients with advanced-stage disease who have failed at least one standard therapy and who have a health status and age that would allow stem cell transplant. The therapies presented here are the most recent ones to join the ranks of treatments listed in **Table 1**. New therapies will still employ old strategies of remission or palliation. As these therapies are considered, their success will be determined by improvement in the quality of life or the ability to induce durable remissions. Both of these goals represent significant impacts that the treating physician can have when managing MF/SS.

REFERENCES

1. Criscione VD, Weinstock MA. Incidence of cutaneous T-cell lymphoma in the United States, 1973–2002. Arch Dermatol 2007;143(7):854–9.
2. Olsen E, Vonderheid E, Pimpinelli N, et al. Revisions to the staging and classification of mycosis fungoides and Sezary syndrome: a proposal of the International Society for Cutaneous Lymphomas (ISCL) and the cutaneous lymphoma task force of the European Organization of Research and Treatment of Cancer (EORTC). Blood 2007;110(6): 1713–22.
3. Willemze R, Jaffe ES, Burg G, et al. WHO-EORTC classification for cutaneous lymphomas. Blood 2005;105(10): 3768–85.
4. Haserick J, Richardson J, Grant J. Remission of lesions in mycosis fungoides following topical application of nitrogen mustard. Cleve Clin Q 1959;26: 144–7.
5. Gilchrest BA, Parrish JA, Tanenbaum L, et al. Oral methoxsalen photochemotherapy of mycosis fungoides. Cancer 1976;38(2):683–9.
6. Jones G, Wilson LD, Fox-Goguen L. Total skin electron beam radiotherapy for patients who have mycosis fungoides. Hematol Oncol Clin North Am 2003;17(6):1421–34.
7. Wilson LD, Kacinski BM, Jones GW. Local superficial radiotherapy in the management of minimal stage IA cutaneous T-cell lymphoma (mycosis fungoides). Int J Radiat Oncol Biol Phys 1998;40(1): 109–15.

8. Kennedy JC, Pottier RH, Pross DC. Photodynamic therapy with endogenous protoporphyrin IX: basic principles and present clinical experience. J Photochem Photobiol B 1990;6(1–2):143–8.
9. Krammer B, Plaetzer K. ALA and its clinical impact, from bench to bedside. Photochem Photobiol Sci 2008;7(3):283–9.
10. Rittenhouse-Diakun K, Leengoed H, Morgan J, et al. The role of transferrin receptor (CD71) in photodynamic therapy of activated and malignant lymphocytes using the heme precursor delta-aminolevulinic acid (ALA). Photochem Photobiol 1995; 61(5):523–8.
11. Svanberg K, Andersson T, Killander D, et al. Photodynamic therapy of non-melanoma malignant tumours of the skin using topical delta-amino levulinic acid sensitization and laser irradiation. Br J Dermatol 1994;130(6):743–51.
12. Wolf P, Fink-Puches R, Cerroni L, et al. Photodynamic therapy for mycosis fungoides after topical photosensitization with 5-aminolevulinic acid. J Am Acad Dermatol 1994;31(4):678–80.
13. Orenstein A, Haik J, Tamir J, et al. Photodynamic therapy of cutaneous lymphoma using 5-aminolevulinic acid topical application. Dermatol Surg 2000; 26(8):765–70.
14. Edstrom DW, Porwit A, Ros AM. Photodynamic therapy with topical 5-aminolevulinic acid for mycosis fungoides: clinical and histological response. Acta Derm Venereol 2001;81(3):184–8.
15. Taub AF. Photodynamic therapy in dermatology: history and horizons. J Drugs Dermatol 2004; 3(Suppl 1):S8–25.
16. Gage AA. History of cryosurgery. Semin Surg Oncol 1998;14(2):99–109.
17. Kuflik EG. Cryosurgery updated. J Am Acad Dermatol 1994;31(6):925–44 [quiz: 944–6].
18. Pandolfino TL, Siegel RS, Kuzel TM, et al. Primary cutaneous B-cell lymphoma: review and current concepts. J Clin Oncol 2000;18(10):2152–68.
19. Cerroni LMD, Fink-Puches RMD, El-Shabrawi-Caelen LMD, et al. Solitary skin lesions with histopathologic features of early mycosis fungoides. Am J Dermatopathol 1999;21(6):518–24.
20. Lambert WC, Cohen PJ, Schwartz RA. Surgical management of mycosis fungoides. J Med 1997; 28(3–4):211–22.
21. Nistico S, Costanzo A, Saraceno R, et al. Efficacy of monochromatic excimer laser radiation (308 nm) in the treatment of early stage mycosis fungoides. Br J Dermatol 2004;151(4):877–9.
22. Passeron T, Zakaria W, Ostovari N, et al. Efficacy of the 308-nm excimer laser in the treatment of mycosis fungoides. Arch Dermatol 2004;140(10):1291–3.
23. Mori M, Campolmi P, Mavilia L, et al. Monochromatic excimer light (308 nm) in patch-stage IA mycosis fungoides. J Am Acad Dermatol 2004;50(6):943–5.
24. Meisenheimer JL. Treatment of mycosis fungoides using a 308-nm excimer laser: two case studies. Dermatol Online J 2006;12(7):11.
25. Kontos AP, Kerr HA, Malick F, et al. 308-nm excimer laser for the treatment of lymphomatoid papulosis and stage IA mycosis fungoides. Photodermatol Photoimmunol Photomed 2006;22(3): 168–71.
26. Sauder DN. Immunomodulatory and pharmacologic properties of imiquimod. J Am Acad Dermatol 2000; 43(1 Pt 2):S6–11.
27. Schon MP, Schon M. Imiquimod: mode of action. Br J Dermatol 2007;157(Suppl 2):8–13.
28. Stanley MA. Imiquimod and the imidazoquinolones: mechanism of action and therapeutic potential. Clin Exp Dermatol 2002;27(7):571–7.
29. Suchin KR, Junkins-Hopkins JM, Rook AH. Treatment of stage IA cutaneous T-Cell lymphoma with topical application of the immune response modifier imiquimod. Arch Dermatol 2002;138(9):1137–9.
30. Deeths MJ, Chapman JT, Dellavalle RP, et al. Treatment of patch and plaque stage mycosis fungoides with imiquimod 5% cream. J Am Acad Dermatol 2005;52(2):275–80.
31. Martinez-Gonzalez MC, Verea-Hernando MM, Yebra-Pimentel MT, et al. Imiquimod in mycosis fungoides. Eur J Dermatol 2008;18(2):148–52.
32. Ardigo M, Cota C, Berardesca E. Unilesional mycosis fungoides successfully treated with imiquimod. Eur J Dermatol 2006;16(4):446.
33. Chiam LY, Chan YC. Solitary plaque mycosis fungoides on the penis responding to topical imiquimod therapy. Br J Dermatol 2007;156(3):560–2.
34. Coors EA, Schuler G, Von Den Driesch P. Topical imiquimod as treatment for different kinds of cutaneous lymphoma. Eur J Dermatol 2006; 16(4):391–3.
35. Didona B, Benucci R, Amerio P, et al. Primary cutaneous CD30+ T-cell lymphoma responsive to topical imiquimod (Aldara). Br J Dermatol 2004;150(6): 1198–201.
36. Piekarz R, Frye R, Wright J, et al. Update of the NCI multiinstitutional phase II trial of romidepsin, FK228, for patients with cutaneous or peripheral T-cell lymphoma. 2007 ASCO Annual Meeting Proceedings Part I. J Clin Oncol 2007;25(18S):8027.
37. Piekarz RL, Frye AR, Wright JJ, et al. Cardiac studies in patients treated with depsipeptide, FK228, in a phase II trial for T-cell lymphoma. Clin Cancer Res 2006;12(12):3762–73.
38. Duarte RF, Schmitz N, Servitje O, et al. Haematopoietic stem cell transplantation for patients with primary cutaneous T-cell lymphoma. Bone Marrow Transplant 2008;41(7):597–604.
39. Markham T, Collins P. Topical 5-aminolaevulinic acid photodynamic therapy for extensive scalp actinic keratoses. Br J Dermatol 2001;145(3):502–4.

40. Paech V, Lorenzen T, Stoehr A, et al. Remission of a cutaneous Mycosis fungoides after topical 5-ALA sensitisation and photodynamic therapy in a patient with advanced HIV-infection. Eur J Med Res 2002; 7(11):477–9.
41. Leman JA, Dick DC, Morton CA. Topical 5-ALA photodynamic therapy for the treatment of cutaneous T-cell lymphoma. Clin Exp Dermatol 2002; 27(6):516–8.
42. Coors EA, von den Driesch P. Topical photodynamic therapy for patients with therapy-resistant lesions of cutaneous T-cell lymphoma. J Am Acad Dermatol 2004;50(3):363–7.
43. Umegaki N, Moritsugu R, Katoh S, et al. Photodynamic therapy may be useful in debulking cutaneous lymphoma prior to radiotherapy. Clin Exp Dermatol 2004;29(1):42–5.
44. Zane C, Venturini M, Sala R, et al. Photodynamic therapy with methylaminolevulinate as a valuable treatment option for unilesional cutaneous T-cell lymphoma. Photodermatol Photoimmunol Photomed 2006;22(5):254–8.
45. Recio ED, Zambrano B, Alonso ML, et al. Topical 5-aminolevulinic acid photodynamic therapy for the treatment of unilesional mycosis fungoides: a report of two cases and review of the literature. Int J Dermatol 2008;47(4):410–3.
46. Hegyi J, Frey T, Arenberger P. The treatment of unilesional mycosis fungoides with methyl aminolevulinate-photodynamic therapy. J Eur Acad Dermatol Venereol 2008;22(9):1134–5.
47. Dummer R, Urosevic M, Kempf W, et al. Imiquimod induces complete clearance of a PUVA-resistant plaque in mycosis fungoides. Dermatology 2003; 207(1):116–8.
48. Chong A, Loo WJ, Banney ML, et al. Imiquimod 5% cream in the treatment of mycosis fungoides–a pilot study. J Dermatolog Treat 2004;15(2):118–9.

Biologic Drugs for the Treatment of Hidradenitis Suppurativa: An Evidence-Based Review

Fareesa Shuja, MD, C. Stanley Chan, MD, Ted Rosen, MD*

KEYWORDS

• Hidradenitis suppurativa • Biologics • Nodules • Abscesses

Hidradenitis suppurativa (HS) is a recurrent and suppurative disease with an insidious onset. It is characterized by deep furuncles, abscesses, fistulas, sinus tracts, and scarring and has a prevalence of 0.3% to 4% of the general population.[1] The average age of onset is 23 but may fall anywhere between postpubertal age to middle age.[2] HS is more prevalent in women than men by a ratio of between 2:1 and 5:1, with genitofemoral lesions found more often in women and anogenital lesions found more often in men.[2,3] The most commonly affected site, the axilla, is involved in an equal proportion of men and women. Other affected areas may include the areola, inframammary folds, periumbilical skin, scalp, zygomatic and malar face, buttocks, thighs, popliteal fossa, ear canal, and eyelids.[1,4] Patients with active disease generally develop 2 furuncles per month with an average disease duration of 19 years.[4]

The initial symptoms of HS are localized erythema, pruritus, and hyperhidrosis followed by the spontaneous development of painful and tender red nodules and abscesses with incessant purulent drainage, open comedones, sinus tracts, and scarring.[1,3] The pathologic event that culminates in full-blown HS is hyperkeratosis of the terminal hair follicle that leads to an occlusive keratin plug.[5] Eventual rupture of the lower end of the occluded follicle leads to an acute inflammatory infiltrate. This inflammation can be confined to the hair follicle leading to a granulomatous reaction and limited disease. If the inflammation is not confined or if nearby perifollicular inflammatory nodules coalesce, however, a large abscess forms, extends to, and destroys the adnexal apocrine glands.[6] Follicular epithelium may proliferate in an attempt to confine the inflammation and form sinus tracts, which can secondarily become infected with bacteria. Multiple abscesses and sinus tracts in the dermis and subcutaneous tissues form a reticulated network that can extend to the fascia and muscle.[1,5] HS

Dr Rosen has received honoraria and travel reimbursements as a member of the Speaker's Bureau for Abbott, Amgen, Centocor, and Genentech. None of the other authors has any affiliation with or financial involvement in any organizations with a direct financial interest in the subject matter or materials discussed in this article. This includes employment, honoraria, consultancies, and relevant stock ownership.
Department of Dermatology, Baylor College of Medicine, 6620 Main Street, Suite 1425, Houston, TX 77030, USA
* Corresponding author.
E-mail address: vampireted@aol.com

Dermatol Clin 28 (2010) 511–524
doi:10.1016/j.det.2010.03.012
0733-8635/10/$ – see front matter © 2010 Elsevier Inc. All rights reserved.

is thus a misnomer, because the pathogenesis does not involve sweat gland dysfunction as originally thought. Because of the similarities in their development, HS, dissecting cellulitis, acne conglobata, and pilonidal sinus are known as the follicular occlusion tetrad.[1] Other names for HS include apocrinitis, hidradenitis axillaries, and acne inversa, with the latter rapidly gaining in popularity and acceptance. Although 1 study found 34% of first-degree relatives of probands had HS, a specific genetic locus or specific HLA association has yet to be elucidated.[7]

The diagnosis of HS is based on clinical findings and is substantiated by a history of recurrence, onset after puberty, poor response to antimicrobials, and overall disease duration greater than 6 months.[1,3] Biopsy may be performed to exclude cutaneous Crohn disease or the development of squamous cell carcinoma.[8] Laboratory findings, such as elevated erythrocyte sedimentation rate, leukocytosis, decreased serum iron, and alterations in the serum protein electrophoresis, are reflective of chronic inflammation and thereby nonspecific.[1] Complications include anemia of chronic disease, septicemia, decreased mobility from scars, anal strictures, urethral fistulas, disfiguring genital edema, amyloidosis, locally aggressive squamous cell carcinoma, and malignancy in general.[2,3] These complications, along with the significant morbidity related to pain and disability from the disease, emphasize the urgent need for reliably effective treatment.

TRADITIONAL THERAPIES FOR HS

Although there are various treatment options for HS, none of the traditional therapies is wholly satisfactory or uniformly effective. Therapy varies based on the severity of disease, although there is considerable overlap between treatment groups. Mild HS consists of solitary nodules and abscesses, and treatment is generally conservative.[3] Mainstays of treatment are nonsteroidal anti-inflammatory drugs for pain and inflammation, antiseptics, antibacterial soaps, warm compresses, hydrotherapy, and antibiotics.[8] Bacteria may lead to secondary infection but this is not likely central to the pathogenesis of the disease. Staphylococcus aureus and coagulase-negative Staphylococci are the 2 most commonly cultured organisms, although Streptococcus, gram-negative rods, and anaerobes are also frequently isolated.[6] Antimicrobial treatment generally consists of topical clindamycin or oral antistaphylococcal agents for axillary disease, whereas more broad-spectrum coverage is called for in those with perineal disease.[3] The average duration of a HS nodule is 6.9 days, which is approximately the same duration as a course of antibiotics, making it difficult to determine if antibiotics are rally effective.[8] Oral contraceptive pills with a high estrogen:progesterone ratio as well as immunosuppressive drugs, such as cyclosporine, azathioprine, and prednisone, are occasionally successful.[9] Single nodules may be injected with intralesional triamcinolone (3–5 mg/mL) to decrease inflammation.[3] Topical and oral retinoids inhibit keratinization and have been used with some success in mild to moderate HS. Acitretin and isotretinoin are more often used to decrease inflammation before surgery than as definitive treatments.[3,4] Although there is no definitive evidence linking hyperandrogenism and HS, antiandrogens, such as cyproterone acetate and the 5α-reductase inhibitor, finasteride, also have been used with varying degrees of success.[6] Incision and drainage of abscesses is not recommended because it is only transiently beneficial and does nothing to halt progression of the disease.[8] On an individual basis, however, incision and drainage might be indicated to relieve excessive lesional pain. Weight loss and avoidance of heat and humidity can help reduce maceration and irritation of the affected sites.[2,3] Other measures, such as avoidance of shaving affected areas, eliminating tight synthetic clothing, lowering stress, and smoking cessation, have only anecdotally been associated with amelioration of the disease.[8,9]

Moderate disease is characterized by multiple nodules and abscesses with purulent discharge.[3] It can be treated with similar therapies as for mild disease with the addition of limited excision if needed. Unroofing and marsupialization of individual nodules or tracts may also be performed, although such limited extent surgical intervention is less beneficial in the long term than en bloc excision.[9] Carbon dioxide laser treatment is a less-invasive method of removing affected skin than traditional scalpel surgery. Disadvantages of carbon dioxide laser treatment and cryotherapy, another modality used to treat mild to severe HS, are substantial increases in healing time and pain. Radiotherapy has also been used for HS, but the long-term side effects make it less popular and probably less safe.[2]

Severe HS is comprised of multiple sites of draining abscesses and sinuses with associated scarring.[3] In this case as well as some moderate cases of HS, local excision with wide margins has traditionally been the only effective therapy. Nevertheless, there is still a risk of recurrence adjacent to the excision site or even at a distant site.[8]

Screening for depression and psychological support is an important dimension of treatment, because patients with moderate to severe HS become progressively unable to interact socially or maintain employment due to pain, odor, and shame.[6] It is important to stress to patients that HS is neither caused by poor hygiene nor contagious. Because surgical intervention can be disfiguring and not entirely curative, clinicians have pursued alternative treatment modalities. Biologic drugs, although not yet approved for treatment of HS, offer a potentially promising solution.

EVIDENCE-BASED GRADING OF BIOLOGIC DRUGS

Many of the studies discussed in this review use scoring systems to measure the efficacy of the drug being discussed. The Sartorius scale, one of the most commonly used scoring systems for HS, tallies points based on the number of regions involved, lesion types (ulcers, fistulas, nodules, or scars), and number, size of individual lesions, and separation of affected tissue from normal tissue.[10] The Dermatology Life Quality Index (DLQI) assesses the effect of the disease on 6 separate categories, including daily activities, work and school, leisure activities, and personal relations.[11] Another often-mentioned tool is the visual analog scale (VAS), which is used by patients to grade their own perception of disease severity.[12]

Although many reports on the efficacy of biologic drugs for off-label treatment of HS have surfaced, to the authors' knowledge, this is the first in-depth review of the published evidence on this topic. The authors compiled data via a PubMed search of each of the 5 biologic agents and HS. Then a systematic review was performed of the evidence and each relevant article assigned an evidence level based on the type of study and its quality. Evidence levels range from 1 to 4 with stratification standards borrowed from Harbour and Miller's system of evidence-based grading.[13] The endpoint was a final recommendation as to the efficacy of each drug for the treatment of HS based on the amassed evidence. A grade A recommendation corresponds to studies rated as 1 (randomized controlled trials and meta-analyses); a grade B recommendation is based on evidence characterized as level 2+ (case-control studies, cohort studies, and systematic review of anything other than a randomized controlled trial); a grade C recommendation is reserved for level 2 evidence (open-label clinical trials, retrospective analyses, and extrapolated evidence from level 2+ studies); and finally, a grade D recommendation is conferred on level 3 studies (case reports and case series) and level 4 studies (anecdotal evidence and expert opinion).[13,14] This grading system was chosen to clearly and consistently judge the strength of the available evidence and transparently display how recommendations were arrived at.

BIOLOGIC DRUGS

The 5 biologic drugs included in this review are adalimumab (Humira), alefacept (Amevive), efalizumab (Raptiva), etanercept (Enbrel), and infliximab (Remicade). Adalimumab, etanercept, and infliximab are tumor necrosis factor (TNF)-α inhibitors whereas alefacept and efalizumab are T-cell–specific agents.[15] To date, the data on the efficacy of the latter 2 drugs for treatment of HS are sparse. Efalizumab was recently withdrawn from the marketplace due to perceived increased risk of progressive multifocal leukoencephalopathy, making the usefulness of this agent a moot point.

Although mostly produced by monocytes and macrophages, TNF-α is also produced in the skin by keratinocytes, melanocytes, Langerhans cells, activated T cells, natural killer cells, and mast cells in response to infection or keratinocyte death.[16] Soluble TNF-α monomers form a trimer, which binds to the TNF-α receptor 1 or TNF-α receptor 2, entities found in most cells of the body excluding erythrocytes and unstimulated lymphocytes.[16,17] Cross-linked receptors induce signal transduction cascades that ultimately influence cell differentiation, mitogenesis, regulation of cytotoxic responses, inflammation, immunomodulation, and wound healing. Specifically, TNF-α receptor activation upregulates vascular cell leukocyte adhesion molecule 1, intercellular adhesion molecule 1 (ICAM-1), E-selectins, and metalloproteinases 1 and 3, all of which promote cellular infiltration.[16–18] It also increases vascular endothelial growth factor, increases production of proinflammatory cytokines, increases keratinocyte production of transforming growth factor α causing epidermal proliferation, inhibits melanocyte activity, promotes growth of fibroblasts, and releases acute phase reactants from hepatocytes.

Most available data on the TNF-α inhibitors are related to studies of rheumatoid arthritis, but use for dermatologic conditions is increasingly common. TNF-α, via its induction of proinflammatory cytokines and accretion of an inflammatory infiltrate, is necessary for granuloma development and maintenance.[14] Although HS is not primarily a granulomatous disease, granulomas have been observed in histologic examination of the skin surrounding HS sites.[19] Inhibiting TNF-α is also thought to inhibit the keratinocyte activation cycle and to downregulate keratin 6, thereby preventing hyperkeratinization.[20] High levels of TNF-α often go hand in hand with interleukin-1α, which has been shown to cause hypercornification of the follicular infundibulum and may be involved in the perpetuation of HS in its chronic state.[21] Some of the current treatments of HS are also immunosuppressive or anti-inflammatory drugs, lending further credence to the hypothesis that immune dysregulation is at least partially responsible for the development of this disorder.[19]

Side effects of TNF-α inhibitors include injection site reactions, reactivation of latent tuberculosis (TB), increased risk of sundry bacterial and fungal infections, demyelinating disease, worsening of congestive heart failure, hepatotoxicity, reactivation of hepatitis B virus, hypersensitivity reactions, pancytopenia and aplastic anemia, and autoimmune diseases.[18] Although the most common infections associated with biologic treatment are upper respiratory tract infections, bronchitis, and urinary tract infections, deep fungal infections and TB are also documented.[14] Contraindications to treatment are active TB, known active and serious infections, hepatitis B, and heart failure classified as New York Heart Association (NYHA) level III or level IV.[18] Caution is advised for patients with latent TB, malignancy, heart failure classified as NYHA level I or II, or a hematologic disorder.

Adalimumab (Humira)

Adalimumab is a monoclonal immunoglobulin G1 antibody to soluble and membrane-bound TNF-α.[12] Because it is fully human, it is hoped it will prove less immunogenic than the other TNF-α inhibitors on the market. Adalimumab is administered subcutaneously and is absorbed slowly, reaching peak concentration in approximately 5 days with a mean half-life of 2 weeks.[18] It is delivered via an autoinjectable pen device or prefilled syringe, thus allowing for home administration.[22] Adalimumab is currently approved by the Food and Drug Administration for treatment of rheumatoid arthritis, psoriatic arthritis and psoriasis, polyarticular juvenile idiopathic arthritis, ankylosing spondylitis, and Crohn disease.[14] There are no dosage guidelines for the off-label use of adalimumab in the treatment of HS, but 40 mg per week to 40 mg every other week is the norm. Adalimumab has the fewest data available of all the TNF-α inhibitors because it is the newest, available on the commercial market only since 2003.[18]

A review of the data on use of adalimumab for the treatment of HS yielded the following: 2 case reports, 1 case series, and 1 open-label clinical trial (summary in **Table 1**).[12,22–24] The first report was published in 2005 by Scheinfeld and showed improved ambulation and decreased flocculence of axillary nodules within 2 months of treatment with adalimumab.[23] When treatment was halted for insurance reasons, the patient experienced a flare; when the medication was later restarted, symptoms abated. The next case was reported by Moul and Korman[24] in 2006. This report describes severe HS in a patient with inflammatory bowel disease who had resolution of all pain and significant improvement of HS severity after 1 month of treatment with adalimumab. He improved further with continued treatment at the 4-month follow-up visit. Lastly, in 2009, a small case series was published by Yamauchi and Mau[22] pertaining to patients with HS successfully treated with adalimumab. All 3 cases showed significant improvement 1 year after initiation of adalimumab therapy with the first 2 cases showing 70% to 80% improvement from baseline. Unfortunately, due to the confounding administration of other drugs in the third patient in this series, it is difficult to ascribe resolution of the patient's condition to any 1 particular medication.

The most substantial report on patients treated with adalimumab for HS was an open-label clinical trial published in 2008, studying 3 patients treated with adalimumab for 3 months.[12] A greater than 50% reduction in disease severity according to the objective Sartorius scale was achieved in all patients after 2 months of treatment, but 3 months after discontinuation of adalimumab, relapse was the rule. Despite this, the mean disease severity after relapse was still lower than at baseline for all patients. During the study, 2 patients had mild pain at the injection site. Because the majority of the evidence concerning adalimumab treatment of HS consists of case reports with only 1 small open-label, nonrandomized, noncontrolled trial, the authors recommendation for adalimumab is currently grade D. The results reported thus far are remarkable enough to warrant further appropriate investigation.

Although injection site reactions were the only adverse events reported in the study and cases the authors found, patients on adalimumab are at risk for any of the sundry adverse events common to all TNF-α inhibitors (discussed previously). Three percent to 13% of patients treated with adalimumab develop antinuclear and anti–double-stranded DNA antibodies, but few go on to develop drug-induced lupus.[18] It is too early for reliable long-term data on malignancy to be generated, but a meta-analysis published in 2006 on patients with rheumatoid arthritis treated with high-dose versus low-dose adalimumab or etanercept found a significant increase in malignancies with high-dose biologic treatment.[25] Patients should not take adalimumab concomitantly with Anakinra or with live vaccines and are advised not to breastfeed for 5 months after completion of treatment.[18] The biggest obstacle to overcome for many patients is the approximately $16,000 per year that an injection of adalimumab every other week costs on the open market without insurance coverage.[24]

Alefacept (Amevive)

Alefacept is a fusion protein of human leukocyte function-associated antigen-3 (LFA-3) and IgG that prevents T-cell activation via blockage of LFA-3 binding to CD2 on T cells.[15] Alefacept is known to cause lymphopenia and therefore requires weekly monitoring of CD4 T-cell counts. To the best of the authors' knowledge, there are no published reports or studies on the use of alefacept in patients with HS.

Efalizumab (Raptiva)

Efalizumab, like alefacept, prevents T-cell activation. It is a humanized murine monoclonal antibody to LFA-1, preventing its binding to ICAM-1.[15,26] Ultimately, efalizumab prevents activation of T cells, adhesion of T cells to the endothelium, and the migration of T cells to sites of inflammation.[26] The authors found only 1 study regarding the use of this drug for the treatment of HS.[26] Of the 5 participants, only 2 finished the study and none showed improvement in disease severity. The authors confer a grade C recommendation against the use of efalizumab for treatment of HS because there is no evidence-based proof of its efficacy as such a treatment. Because the drug has been withdrawn from the American, Canadian, and European marketplaces due to its association with progressive multifocal leukoencephalopathy, no further work in this area is anticipated.[27]

Etanercept (Enbrel)

Etanercept is a fusion protein of human IgG and the extracellular component of the TNF-α receptor.[15] By binding unbound TNF-α, etanercept acts as a competitive inhibitor. Etanercept has Food and Drug Administration approval for treatment of rheumatoid arthritis, psoriasis and psoriatic arthritis, polyarticular juvenile idiopathic arthritis, and ankylosing spondylitis.[14,28] It is administered subcutaneously (generally 25–50 mg

Table 1
Evidence for Adalimumab

Name	Number of Patients	Age range	Dosage Regimen	Success Rate	Comments
Scheinfeld[23]	1	41	40 mg EOW for 2 mo, 40 mg QW thereafter	Significant improvement	
Moul[24]	1	67	40 mg EOW	Significant improvement	IBD
Yamauchi[22]	3	34–44	40 mg EOW (2 patients required increase to 40 mg QW)	70%–80% improvement	Concomitant IL steroids, MTX, and levofloxacin
Sotiriou[12]	3	Mean age 35.3	40 mg EOW for 3 mo	Over 50% decrease in disease severity within 2 mo	

Abbreviations: EOW, every other week, IBD, inflammatory bowel disease; IL, intralesional; MTX, methotrexate; QW, weekly.

weekly to twice weekly). Via a literature search of etanercept and HS, the authors found 2 relevant case reports and 4 open-label clinical trials (summary in **Table 2**).[10,11,19,28–30] The most common dosage regimen used was 50 mg weekly; only 1 study involved the use of the higher dose of 50 mg twice weekly, the currently approved induction dose for psoriasis in the United States.

In both case reports, improvement was seen within 1 month.[20,29] Unfortunately, oral and topical antibiotics were also being given to the patient (discussed by Henderson).[29] A weakness of the case report by Zangrilli and colleagues[30] is that although the baseline scores on the DLQI and VAS were given, no subsequent scores were reported, making it difficult to objectively assess the degree of improvement.

The first interventional study done on patients with HS treated with etanercept was in 2006 with 6 female patients.[11] The average decreases in disease activity and DLQI scores at 6 months of treatment were by 61% and 64%, respectively. All patients who finished the trial claimed it was their most effective treatment to date. In a subsequent prospective open-label clinical trial by Giamarellos-Bourboulis and colleagues,[10] etanercept was given for 12 weeks in 10 patients with HS. Most patients relapsed within 4 to 8 weeks after discontinuation of treatment; nevertheless, 7 patients had a greater than 50% reduction in disease severity compared with baseline assessed by their Sartorius scale at week 24. Another single-armed, open-label, clinical trial published in 2008 was conducted on 4 patients who, after 6 months of treatment, had a 66.5% decrease in their DLQI scores and a 68.7% decrease in their Sartorius scale on average.[19] Three months after ending treatment, 3 of the 4 patients had relapsed and had commenced a second course of etanercept. The only adverse events reported in these studies were mild injection site reactions.[10,19]

The most recent study was published by Lee and colleagues.[28] Response was defined as a greater than 50% decrease on the physician's global assessment (PGA) scale by week 12; only 3 of the 15 patients qualified as responders. No patient experienced complete remission, 29% had moderate improvement, and 57% had some improvement. Etanercept was generally well tolerated, although 2 patients discontinued treatment due to skin infections and 1 patient discontinued treatment due to worsening carpal tunnel syndrome. This last study demonstrated only minimal efficacy of etanercept for treatment of HS.

The cases and studies discussed in this article have no standardized dose or duration for treatment with etanercept. None of the studies had controls or a second arm of intervention, and none were blinded. The evidence is in support of etanercept for the treatment of HS with the notable exception of the last study discussed wherein only 20% of subjects responded. This study used a different scoring system for disease severity; perhaps the use of the PGA instead of the Sartorius scale played a role in the discrepancy between results. Also, there was an overall high relapse rate after discontinuation of treatment. Possibly, the strength of etanercept lies in the potential of reducing disease activity and not in ultimate eradication of HS. Based on the evidence, the authors give a grade C recommendation for use of etanercept for HS. Larger and more long-term studies are needed to fully elucidate the usefulness of this drug for HS and to help determine an optimal dosing regimen.

The side-effect profile of etanercept is similar to that of other TNF-α inhibitors. Most commonly reported side effects of etanercept are injection site reactions and infections.[11] A few cases have been reported of an increase in antinuclear and anti–double-stranded DNA antibodies, drug-induced lupus, discoid lupus erythematosus, and necrotizing vasculitis due to cryglobulins. The authors also found a case report of a patient with an indwelling intravenous catheter taking etanercept and corticosteroids for HS who subsequently developed candidal septicemia and bilateral chorioretinitis.[31] Similar precautions should be taken as for adalimumab to prevent treatment morbidity from adding to inherent disease morbidity.

Infliximab (Remicade)

Infliximab is a chimeric monoclonal antibody to TNF-α, part murine antihuman TNF-α and part human IgG.[32] It is administered intravenously at doses between 3 and 10 mg/kg, with 5 mg/kg the norm; doses are given at weeks 0, 2, and 6 with the option of maintenance infusions 8 weeks thereafter. Of the biologics, only infliximab induces complement-mediated lysis and apoptosis of TNF-α bound cells in vitro. Also, because it does not affect lymphotoxin (TNF-β), it is more specific than etanercept.[17] Infliximab has Food and Drug Administration approval for the treatment of Crohn disease, ulcerative colitis, ankylosing spondylitis, rheumatoid arthritis, and psoriasis and psoriatic arthritis.[14,32] A search of the literature yielded 9 case reports,[20,33–40] 2

Table 2
Evidence for Etanercept

Name	Number of Patients	Age Range	Dosage Regimen	Success Rate	Comments
Henderson[29]	1	24	50 mg QW	Significant improvement	Topical and oral antibiotics
Zangrilli[30]	1	32	50 mg twice weekly, later decreased to 25 mg twice weekly	Significant improvement	A 48-wk study
Cusack[11]	6	16–43	25 mg twice weekly	At 24 wk, mean decrease in disease activity and DLQI by 61% and 64%, respectively	
Giamarellos-Bourboulis[10]	10	18–59	50 mg QW for 12 wk	At 24 wk, 7/10 had a greater than 50% decrease in Sartorius scale	
Sotiriou[19]	4	25–43	25 mg BIW for 6 mo (1 patient required increase to 50 mg BIW)	At 6 mo, mean decrease in DLQI and Sartorius scale by 66.5% and 68.7%, respectively	
Lee[28]	15	Mean age of 42	50 mg QW for an 18-wk trial	At wk 12, 3 patients had greater than 50% improvement according to the PGA	

Abbreviations: BIW, twice weekly; QW, weekly.

case series,[41,42] 4 retrospective analyses,[43–46] and 3 prospective observational studies[47–49] on the usefulness of infliximab for the treatment of HS.

Of the 9 case reports, 7 showed marked improvement with infliximab treatment whereas 2 showed no change. Of the 7 responders, 2 cases did not specify if there was follow-up, and 1 of these cases was treated with concomitant antibiotics.[36,39] Another 2 of the 7 responders remained in remission until the 2-year follow-up; unfortunately, 1 of these patients was on rifampicin and methotrexate and the other was on methylprednisolone, azathioprine, and isotretinoin, making it difficult to assess efficacy of any particular drug.[35,40] Martinez and colleagues[37] described a case where the patient ended treatment after 2 infusions of infliximab with concomitant azathioprine due to rash and dyspnea; despite this, the patient remained in remission 6 months later. A case reported by Adams and colleagues[33] that succeeded in achieving total resolution of HS was also complicated by use of azathioprine and sulfasalazine. In the final case of the 7 cases described by Montes-Romero and colleagues,[38] the patient received a total of 4 infusions, thereafter noting improvement within 1 month and maintaining remission at the 9-month follow-up.

Table 3
Level 3 Evidence for Infliximab

Name	Number of Patients	Age Range	Dosage Regimen	Success Rate	Comments
Pedraz[20]	1	36	5 mg/kg at 0, 2, 6 wk	No improvement 4 wk after last infusion	Pachyonychia congenita
Adams[33]	1	17	5 mg/kg at 0, 2, 6 wk	Complete resolution after 5 wk	UC; concomitant AZA, sulfasalazine
Goertz[34]	1	54	5 mg/kg for 7 infusions	No improvement after 14 mo of treatment	CD; concomitant MTX
Katsanos[35]	1	39	Not specified	Complete resolution after 2 y of treatment	CD; concomitant AZA, isotretinoin, methylprednisolone
Lebwohl[36]	1	21	Not specified	Complete re-epithelialization of lesions	
Martinez[37]	1	30	5 mg/kg at 0, 2 wk	Significant improvement	CD; concomitant AZA
Montes-Romero[38]	1	39	5 mg/kg at 0, 2, 6, 14 wk	Significant improvement	Secondary amyloidosis
Rosi[39]	1	30	5 mg/kg at 0,2,6 wk	At 5 wk, no evidence of active inflammation	CD; concomitant aztreonam and levofloxacin
Thielen[40]	1	48	5 mg/kg at 0, 2, 6 wk and q 2 mo thereafter	At 2 y, 80% improvement of DLQI from baseline	Concomitant MTX
Moschella[41]	3	24–46	5 mg/kg for 7–11 infusions	Remission achieved in all patients	2/3 had CD; 1 patient received concomitant minocycline
Antonucci[42]	2	34–39	5 mg/kg at 0, 2, 6 wk and then q 8 wk for the first patient	50% of patients responded to treatment	Patient 1 also received amoxicillin-clavulanate

Abbreviations: AZA, azathioprine; CD, Crohn disease; MTX, methotrexate; UC, ulcerative colitis.

Table 4
Level 2 Evidence for Infliximab

Name	Number of Patients	Age Range	Dosage Regimen	Success Rate	Comments
Fardet[44]	7	24–76	5 mg/kg at 0, 2, 6 wk with 5 patients receiving an infusion at 10 wk	5/7 improved by wk 6. After the fourth infusion, only 2/5 had improved from baseline	Significant adverse events
Fernández-Vozmediano[46]	6	27–45	5–10 mg/kg at 0, 2, 6 wk and q 4 wk thereafter	100% improved after the first infusion, but 50% showed decreased efficacy more than a 6-mo period	
Sullivan[43]	5	28–57	5 mg/kg times 1; 3/5 required a second infusion 4–6 wk later	100% reported marked or moderate improvement after each infusion	Multiple and varied concomitant medications
Usmani[45]	4	27–53	5 mg/kg for 3–12 infusions	50% responded to treatment	Various concomitant medications; significant adverse events
Brunasso[49]	7	35–46	5 mg/kg at 0, 2, 6 wk and q 8 wk thereafter	At 3 mo, 96.2% decrease in pain, 69.5% decrease in discharge, 7% decrease in surface area, 52% decrease in DLQI	Concomitant MTX
Mekkes[48]	10	Mean age of 41	5 mg/kg at 0, 2, 6 wk	All improved by 2–6 wk. 3 maintained improvement at 2 y	
Pedraz[47]	3	28–41	5 mg/kg at 0, 2, 6 wk and q 8 wk thereafter	At 6 wk, 2/3 of patients had improvement via Skindex-29 whereas 1/3 worsened	

Abbreviation: MTX, methotrexate.

Of the 2 cases that reported no change in disease severity or symptoms, 1 patient had initial improvement at 2 months, but by 14 months, despite maintenance infusions, there was no longer there was any change from baseline.[34] This patient was also receiving low-dose methotrexate. In the other case reported by Pedraz and colleagues,[20] the patient had no improvement after 3 infusions of infliximab and subsequently ended treatment.

In summary, of the 9 total case reports on infliximab and HS, only 3 cases did not involve confounding treatment.[20,36,38] Follow-up ranged from 4 weeks to 2 years. Four patients had concomitant Crohn disease, 1 patient had ulcerative colitis, 1 had cystic acne, 1 had a HS-induced case of amyloidosis, and 1 patient had pachyonychia congenita. Only 1 case report did not involve a concomitant disease process.[40] Overall, 3 of the 4 cases of Crohn disease with HS responded to treatment with infliximab whereas 1 did not.[34,35,37,39] Side effects reported in these 9 cases included 1 case of rash with dyspnea and 1 herpes zoster outbreak treated with valcyclovir.[37,40]

A series of 3 cases published in 2007 by Moschella[41] supports the use of infliximab as treatment of HS, although the second case in this series involved the concomitant administration of minocycline. Another case series published in 2008 showed conflicting outcomes.[42] The first patient responded well to treatment but also received concomitant amoxicillin-clavulanate. In the second case, the patient discontinued treatment after 3 infusions due to lack of improvement. Because of the complexity and subtle differences between these cases, a summary of the level 3 evidence for infliximab is provided in **Table 3**.

A retrospective 2003 chart review involved 5 patients who received only 1 to 2 infusions of infliximab.[43] All patients showed marked or moderate improvement after infusions. Unfortunately, all of these patients were on various concomitant medications at the time. A retrospective analysis conducted in 2007 by Fardet and colleagues[44] analyzed 7 patients who received 3 to 4 infliximab infusions. By week 6, 5 patients showed improvement based on the Sartorius scale, Skindex-29 quality-of-life scale, and a physician and patient overall assessment. By week 10, however, only 2 of the 5 patients continuing treatment showed improvement. Adverse events included a severe allergic reaction (bronchospasm and urticaria), severe pain from a previously undiagnosed colon cancer, and multifocal motor neuropathy with conduction block. Another retrospective analysis from 2007 disclosed somewhat discouraging results.[45] Of the 4 patients studied, 2 had no improvement after 3 infusions. Of the responders, 1 developed drug-induced lupus and the other suffered an acute hypersensitivity reaction after an on-demand infusion. Participants in this study were also receiving various concomitant medications during infliximab treatment. Fernandez-Vozmediano and Amario-Hita[46] published the most recent retrospective analysis of 6 patients with severe HS. All patients had improvement after 1 dose, but relapse invariably occurred. Three patients had a decrease in efficacy of infliximab with subsequent infusions. Aside from headache, no adverse events were observed in this study.

A prospective observational study was conducted in 2007 of 3 female patients by Pedraz and colleagues,[47] 2 of whom showed mild to moderate improvement with infliximab whereas 1 patient showed no change; 1 patient in this study had arthralgias. Another study conducted in 2008 of 10 patients who received 3 doses of infliximab scored patients based on the DLQI, patient-rated efficacy, and the Sartorius scale.[48] All patients improved within 2 to 6 weeks in all areas. Unfortunately, only 3 of the 10 patients achieved long-lasting improvement at a 2-year follow-up. Adverse effects seen were

Table 5
Recommendation Grade of Biologics for HS

	Adalimumab	Alefacept	Efalizumab	Etanercept	Infliximab
Grade	D		C	C	C
For/against	For		Against	For	For

paresthesias, myalgia, fever, and acute anaphylactic shock. The most recent clinical trial showed variable long-term efficacy.[49] Seven patients with severe HS were assessed with the DLQI and VAS during treatment with low-dose methotrexate and infliximab. Four patients quit treatment due to lack of benefit, 1 patient quit due to exacerbation of premenstrual symptoms, and 1 patient switched to a different biologic agent. Recurrences were not uncommon and response to treatment decreased linearly with time. After 3 months of treatment, pain had decreased by 96.2%, discharge by 69.5%, surface area involvement by 7%, and DLQI scores by 52%. By contrast, at 24 months, pain was only 34.8% decreased from baseline, discharge was down by 30.5%, area involvement decreased by 1.25%, and DLQI decreased by 14.7%. A summary of the level 2 evidence for infliximab as treatment of HS is in **Table 4**.

In summary, short-term effects of treatment with infliximab for HS seem encouraging, although long-term efficacy seems highly variable. Many studies described a progressive decline in efficacy of infliximab treatment, suggesting tachyphylaxis. There were only a few instances of total resolution, but the longest follow-up was 2 years, making a definitive statement impossible at this time. Also, a large proportion of patients in all of these studies were receiving sundry concomitant medications. The precise implications of this are not known but may be confounding. For instance, tetracyclines may inhibit metalloproteinases; TNF-α converting enzyme is a metalloproteinase that converts pro–TNF-α to TNF-α.[48] Therefore, use of tetracyclines may enhance efficacy of infliximab and make judgments on infliximab as a monotherapeutic modality difficult to confer. Based on the cumulative evidence, the authors give a grade C recommendation for the use of infliximab for the treatment of HS. Nonetheless, the available data indicate that protracted remission is unusual and that adverse events are frequent. An optimal dosing regimen (including any optimizing effects of concomitant medications) remains undetermined.

Three percent to 22% of patients treated with infliximab for psoriasis reported an infusion reaction, although usually mild or moderate, versus 2% of patients taking a placebo.[50] Acute reactions occur within the first 24 hours, although most commonly within the first 2 hours. Symptoms include flushing, chest tightness, shortness of breath, headache, changes in blood pressure, nausea, sweating, increase in temperature, urticaria, and bronchospasm. These usually respond to a decrease in the speed of the infusion or a temporary halt in infusion. Delayed reactions occur within 24 hours to 14 days and include arthralgias, myalgias, flu-like symptoms, headache, tiredness, and urticaria. The mechanism of action of these reactions may be anaphylactic, serum sickness–like, or due to the development of antibodies to infliximab. The rationale behind concomitant low-dose methotrexate administration is to prevent the formation of these antibodies.[17,41] The same idea is behind the 0, 2-, and 6-week loading dose regimen because it is thought less immunogenic, although this has yet to be proved.[50] On-demand treatment is also thought more likely to precipitate infusion reactions than maintenance therapy. The adverse effects common to the biologic agents do not spare infliximab, making proper pretreatment screening imperative. Infliximab, like the other biologic agents, is an expensive treatment but unlike the other agents, requires intravenous infusion, making it a less convenient treatment choice for some patients.

SUMMARY

The use of biologic drugs for the treatment of HS has thus far proved to have variable long-term results and is laden with significant adverse effects. Nevertheless, enough evidence of efficacy has been provided to make further, detailed, and systematic investigation of these drugs for the treatment of HS advisable. At this point, an evidence-based decision on whether or not to use these agents for the treatment of HS lacks evidence of level 1 or 2 quality. The authors' recommendations are based on case reports and series, retrospective analyses, and small open-label clinical trials, stressing that a low-grade recommendation does not reflect low efficacy of the drug studied but rather the quality of available evidence. **Table 5** provides a summary of the recommendation grades given to each drug reviewed. Because clinical trials are currently under way to evaluate biologics for treatment of HS, this grade is subject to change pending accumulation and publication of new evidence. Randomized, double-blinded, placebo-controlled trials are needed to better elucidate the future of these drugs for the treatment of HS.

Aside from an evidence-based global recommendation, for a given patient with hidradenitis who has already failed conventional treatments, the use of any of the 3 anti-TNF biologic agents might be considered a potentially life-altering maneuver.

Self-assessment

1. HS is
   - A. Is a recurrent disease
   - B. Is a suppurative disease
   - C. May have an insidious onset
   - D. All of the above
2. Which treatment modality for HS is most likely to result in decreased activity of HS?
   - A. Oral antibiotics
   - B. Antiandrogens
   - C. Incision and drainage
   - D. Surgical excision
3. Adalimumab is
   - A. Chimeric monoclonal antibody to TNF-α
   - B. The oldest TNF-α inhibitor on the market
   - C. Approved for treatment of HS
   - D. Administered via weekly or bimonthly self-injections
4. Patients taking adalimumab
   - A. Often develop drug-induced lupus
   - B. May have reactivation of latent TB
   - C. Do not have to worry about effects of the drug on their CHF
   - D. Have an increased risk of developing psoriasis
5. Alefacept
   - A. Has been proved an effective treatment of HS
   - B. Is a TNF-α inhibitor
   - C. May cause lymphopenia
   - D. Prevents B-cell activation
6. Etanercept
   - A. Is a competitive inhibitor of TNF-α
   - B. Is a fusion protein of IgG and TNF-α
   - C. Is administered intravenously
   - D. As a treatment of HS is inefficacious based on evidence to date
7. Which of the following is true of etanercept?
   - A. Injection site reactions are fairly common
   - B. Necrotizing vasculitis due to cryoglobins has been reported as an adverse effect of treatment
   - C. May result in a demyelinating process
   - D. All of the above
8. Which of the following is correct?
   - A. Both infliximab and etanercept induce apoptosis of TNF-α bound cells in vitro
   - B. Infliximab is a less specific agent for TNF-α than etanercept
   - C. Complete resolution is the rule for treatment of HS with infliximab
   - D. The concomitant administration of other medications in many of these studies and cases makes judgment on the efficacy of infliximab difficult
9. Infusion reactions caused by infliximab are attributable to
   - A. Anaphylactic/anaphylactoid reactions
   - B. Serum-sickness–like reactions
   - C. Antibody formation against infliximab
   - D. Any or all of the above
10. All of the following are true except:
    - A. Grade A and B recommendations for treatment of HS with biologics are justified by the available evidence
    - B. Biologics can be considered as treatment for patients with HS who have failed conventional therapy
    - C. The use of biologic drugs as treatment of HS has proved to have variable long-term results
    - D. Randomized, double-blinded, placebo-controlled trials are needed to better determine the role of biologic drugs for the treatment of HS

Self-assessment (*continued*)

Answers

1. D
2. D
3. D
4. B
5. C
6. A
7. D
8. D
9. D
10. A

REFERENCES

1. Brown TJ, Rosen T, Orengo IF. Hidradenitis suppurativa. South Med J 1998;91:1107–14.
2. Wiseman MC. Hidradenitis suppurativa: a review. Dermatol Ther 2004;17:50–4.
3. Krbec AC. Current understanding and management of hidradenitis suppurativa. J Am Acad Nurse Pract 2007;19:228–34.
4. Ather S, Chan DS, Leaper DJ, et al. Surgical treatment of hidradenitis suppurativa: case series and review of the literature. Int Wound J 2006;3:159–69.
5. Sellheyer K, Krahl D. "Hidradenitis suppurativa" is acne inversa! An appeal to (finally) abandon a misnomer. Int J Dermatol 2005;44:535–40.
6. Buimer MG, Wobbes T, Klinkenbijl JH. Hidradenitis suppurativa. Br J Surg 2009;96:350–60.
7. Fitzsimmons JS, Guilbert PR. A family study of hidradenitis suppurativa. J Med Genet 1985;22:367–73.
8. Shah N. Hidradenitis suppurativa: a treatment challenge. Am Fam Physician 2005;72:1547–52.
9. Mitchell KM, Beck DE. Hidradenitis suppurativa. Surg Clin North Am 2002;82:1187–97.
10. Giamarellos-Bourboulis EJ, Pelekanou E, Antonopoulou A, et al. An open-label phase II study of the safety and efficacy of etanercept for the therapy of hidradenitis suppurativa. Br J Dermatol 2008;158:567–72.
11. Cusack C, Buckley C. Etanercept: effective in the management of hidradenitis suppurativa. Br J Dermatol 2006;154:726–9.
12. Sotiriou E, Apalla Z, Vakirlis E, et al. Efficacy of adalimumab in recalcitrant hidradenitis suppurativa. Eur J Dermatol 2009;19:180–1.
13. Harbour R, Miller J. A new system for grading recommendations in evidence based guidelines. BMJ 2001;323:334–6.
14. Doherty CB, Rosen T. Evidence-based therapy for cutaneous sarcoidosis. Drugs 2008;68:1361–83.
15. Weller R, Hunter J, Savin J, et al. Psoriasis. In: Weller R, Hunter J, Savin J, et al, editors. Clinical dermatology. 4th edition. Malden(MA): Blackwell Publishing; 2008. p. 68–9.
16. Trent JT, Kerdel FA. Tumor necrosis factor alpha inhibitors for the treatment of dermatologic diseases. Dermatol Nurs 2005;17:97–107.
17. Gupta AK, Skinner AR. A review of the use of infliximab to manage cutaneous dermatoses. J Cutan Med Surg 2004;8:77–89.
18. Traczewski P, Rudnicka L. Adalimumab in dermatology. Br J Clin Pharmacol 2008;66:618–25.
19. Sotiriou E, Apalla Z, Ioannidos D. Etanercept for the treatment of hidradenitis suppurativa. Acta Derm Venereol 2009;89:82–3.
20. Pedraz J, Penas PF, Garcia-Diez A. Pachyonychia congenita and hidradenitis suppurativa: no response to infliximab therapy. J Eur Acad Dermatol Venereol 2008;22:1500–1.
21. Sellheyer K, Krahl D. What causes acne inversa (or hidradenitis suppurativa)?—the debate continues. J Cutan Pathol 2008;35:795–7.
22. Yamauchi PS, Mau N. Hidradenitis suppurativa managed with adalimumab. J Drugs Dermatol 2009;8:181–3.
23. Scheinfeld N. Treatment of coincident seronegative arthritis and hidradentis supprativa with adalimumab. J Am Acad Dermatol 2006;55:163–4.
24. Moul DK, Korman NJ. The cutting edge. Severe hidradenitis suppurativa treated with adalimumab. Arch Dermatol 2006;142:1110–2.
25. Bongartz T, Sutton AJ, Sweeting MJ, et al. Anti-TNF antibody therapy in rheumatoid arthritis and the risk of serious infections and malignancies: systematic review and meta-analysis of rare harmful effects in randomized controlled trials. JAMA 2006;295:2275–85.
26. Strober BE, Kim C, Siu K. Efalizumab for the treatment of refractory hidradenitis suppurativa. J Am Acad Dermatol 2007;57:1090–1.
27. Pugashetti R, Koo J. Efalizumab discontinuation: a practical strategy. J Dermatolog Treat 2009;20:132–6.
28. Lee RA, Dommasch E, Treat J, et al. A prospective clinical trial of open-label etanercept for the treatment of hidradenitis suppurativa. J Am Acad Dermatol 2009;60:565–73.
29. Henderson RL Jr. Case reports: treatment of atypical hidradenitis suppurativa with the tumor necrosis factor receptor-Fc fusion protein etanercept. J Drugs Dermatol 2006;5:1010–1.
30. Zangrilli A, Esposito M, Mio G, et al. Long-term efficacy of etanercept in hidradenitis suppurativa. J Eur Acad Dermatol Venereol 2008;22:1260–2.
31. Arriola-Villalobos P, Diaz-Valle D, Alejandre-Alba N, et al. Bilateral Candida chorioretinitis following etanercept treatment for hidradenitis suppurativa. Eye 2008;22:599–600.
32. Alexis AF, Strober BE. Off-label dermatologic uses of anti-TNF-α therapies. J Cutan Med Surg 2005;9:296–302.

33. Adams DR, Gordon KB, Devenyi AG, et al. Severe hidradenitis suppurativa treated with infliximab infusion. Arch Dermatol 2003;139:1540–2.
34. Goertz RS, Konturek PC, Naegel A, et al. Experiences with a long-term treatment of a massive gluteal acne inversa with infliximab in Crohn's disease. Med Sci Monit 2009;15:CS14–8.
35. Katsanos KH, Christodoulou DK, Tsianos EV. Axillary hidradenitis suppurativa successfully treated with infliximab in a Crohn's disease patient. Am J Gastroenterol 2002;97:2155–6.
36. Lebwohl B, Sapadin AN. Infliximab for the treatment of hidradenitis suppurativa. J Am Acad Dermatol 2003;49:S275–6.
37. Martinez F, Nos P, Benlloch S, et al. Hidradenitis suppurativa and Crohn's disease: response to treatment with infliximab. Inflamm Bowel Dis 2001;7:323–6.
38. Montes-Romero JA, Callejas-Rubio JL, Sanchez-Cano D, et al. Amyloidosis secondary to hidradenitis suppurativa. Exceptional response to infliximab. Eur J Intern Med 2008;19:e32–3.
39. Rosi YL, Lowe L, Kang S. Treatment of hidradenitis suppurativa with infliximab in a patient with Crohn's disease. J Dermatolog Treat 2005;16:58–61.
40. Thielen AM, Barde C, Saurat JH. Long-term infliximab for severe hidradenitis suppurativa. Br J Dermatol 2006;155:1105–7.
41. Moschella SL. Is there a role for infliximab in the current therapy of hidradenitis suppurativa? A report of three treated cases. Int J Dermatol 2007;46:1287–91.
42. Antonucci A, Negosanti M, Negosanti L, et al. Acne inversa treated with infliximab: different outcomes in 2 patients. Acta Derm Venereol 2008;88:274–5.
43. Sullivan TP, Welsh E, Kerdel FA, et al. Infliximab for hidradenitis suppurativa. Br J Dermatol 2003;149: 1046–9.
44. Fardet L, Dupuy A, Kerob D, et al. Infliximab for severe hidradenitis suppurativa: transient clinical efficacy in 7 consecutive patients. J Am Acad Dermatol 2007;56:624–8.
45. Usmani N, Clayton TH, Everett S, et al. Variable response of hidradenitis suppurativa to infliximab in four patients. Clin Exp Dermatol 2007;32:204–5.
46. Fernández-Vozmediano JM, Armario-Hita JC. Infliximab for the treatment of hidradenitis suppurativa. Dermatology 2007;215:41–4.
47. Pedraz J, Dauden E, Perez-Gala S, et al. Hidradenitis suppurativa [Response to treatment with infliximab]. Actas Dermosifiliogr 2007;98:325–31 [in Spanish].
48. Mekkes JR, Bos JD. Long-term efficacy of a single course of infliximab in hidradenitis suppurativa. Br J Dermatol 2008;158:370–4.
49. Brunasso AM, Delfino C, Massone C. Hidradenitis suppurativa: are tumour necrosis factor-alpha blockers the ultimate alternative? Br J Dermatol 2008;159:761–3.
50. Lecluse LL, Piskin G, Mekkes JR, et al. Review and expert opinion on prevention and treatment of infliximab-related infusion reactions. Br J Dermatol 2008; 159:527–36.

Innovative Use of Topical Metronidazole

Catherine M. Zip, MD

KEYWORDS

- Topical metronidazole • Off-label use • Rosacea
- Innovative use

Metronidazole is a synthetic nitroimidazole derivative with antimicrobial and antiinflammatory properties. It was the first topical therapy approved solely for rosacea and remains a cornerstone of rosacea management. This article reviews the optimal use of topical metronidazole in the treatment of rosacea and other innovative but off-label dermatologic uses reported in the literature.

MECHANISM OF ACTION

The exact mechanism of action of metronidazole remains unknown. The drug possesses demonstrable antibacterial and antiprotozoal effects but no activity against Demodex folliculorum,[1] staphylococci, Propionibacterium, and Malassezia species.[2] It also has direct antiinflammatory effects that may be key to its efficacy in several dermatologic conditions. Metronidazole inhibits inflammatory mediators generated by neutrophils, inhibits lymphocyte chemotaxis, and suppresses aspects of cell-mediated immunity.[3] It decreases reactive oxygen species (ROS) in the skin and hence acts as an antioxidant by decreasing ROS production and scavenging existing free radicals.[4]

PHARMACOLOGY

Topical metronidazole is minimally absorbed after topical application to the skin, with either undetectable or trace serum concentrations reported after topical use.[5,6] It is classified as US Food and Drug Administration (FDA) pregnancy risk category B. FDA-approved uses of topical metronidazole include, in addition to inflammatory lesions of rosacea, Grade III or IV anaerobically infected decubitus ulcers, perioral dermatitis, and bacterial vaginosis.

OPTIMAL USE OF METRONIDAZOLE IN THE TREATMENT OF ROSACEA

Topical metronidazole was FDA approved for the treatment of rosacea in 1988 and remains a first-line therapy. Its effectiveness in the treatment of moderate to severe rosacea has been shown in several placebo-controlled trials.[6–8] Although studies have demonstrated a significant reduction in papulopustular lesions and perilesional erythema, topical metronidazole has no effect on telangiectasias. The medication is well tolerated, with local reactions, such as stinging, dryness, and burning, reported in up to 2% of patients.[9] Allergic contact dermatitis to metronidazole has rarely been reported.[10] One study comparing the cumulative irritancy potential of metronidazole 0.75% gel and cream and metronidazole 1% cream in healthy volunteers showed no significant difference in the relative irritancy of the different formulations.[11] Metronidazole 1% gel was found to be nonirritating in a 21-day cumulative irritation study.[12] Metronidazole cream, gel, and lotion formulations have similar efficacy, as have the 0.75% and 1% concentrations currently available.[13] Hence, patient preference for vehicle may be an important factor in maximizing clinical efficacy by improving patient adherence to the suggested regimen.

Although it was originally thought that the optimal frequency of application of metronidazole should be twice daily based on pharmacokinetic data for the original 0.75% gel formulation, more recent research has shown that metronidazole is

The Dermatology Centre, 124-42 Avenue South West, Calgary, Alberta T2S3B3, Canada
E-mail address: catherinezip@shaw.ca

Dermatol Clin 28 (2010) 525–534
doi:10.1016/j.det.2010.03.015
0733-8635/10/$ – see front matter © 2010 Elsevier Inc. All rights reserved.

degraded into active metabolites that may prolong the clinical efficacy of the parent drug.[14] Jorizzo and colleagues[15] studied the efficacy of metronidazole 1% cream when applied once compared with twice daily and found both treatment regimens to be of equal efficacy. Metronidazole 1% gel is FDA approved for once daily use. More studies are necessary to determine if twice-daily dosing of other available formulations of metronidazole is truly more effective than once-daily use.

Several studies have compared metronidazole to other topical therapies in the treatment of rosacea (**Table 1**). Comparative studies have shown topical metronidazole and azelaic acid to be of similar efficacy. Elewski and colleagues[16] compared azelaic acid 15% gel to metronidazole 0.75% gel in subjects with moderate papulopustular rosacea, and found azelaic acid to be superior in improving lesion counts and erythema. Maddin[17] compared azelaic acid 20% cream and metronidazole 0.75% cream in a double-blind split-face comparative trial of subjects with papulopustular rosacea. Both groups had similar reductions in lesions but better global improvement was seen with azelaic acid. More recently, Wolf and colleagues[18] compared once-daily metronidazole 1% gel to twice-daily azelaic acid 15% gel in subjects with moderate rosacea. The efficacies of the two medications were similar. Azelaic acid 15% gel has more potential for irritation compared with metronidazole 0.75% and 1% gel.[19] Topical sodium sulfacetamide 10% with sulfur 5% is also FDA approved for the treatment of rosacea and has been compared with topical metronidazole treatment.

An investigator-blinded study comparing sodium sulfacetamide 10% and sulfur 5% cream with sunscreens to metronidazole 0.75% cream showed a greater reduction in lesions and erythema with sodium sulfacetamide/sulfur, but also more treatment-related adverse effects with this medication compared with treatment with topical metronidazole.[20] A recent, small, open-label study compared topical pimecrolimus 1% cream and metronidazole 1% cream in subjects with papulopustular rosacea.[21] Both treatments were equally effective and well tolerated. Clearly lacking in the literature are studies evaluating the efficacy of combination topical therapy in the treatment of rosacea, although preliminary data suggests the potential for improved clinical outcomes.[22]

Topical metronidazole is often combined with oral tetracycline derivatives in the management of more severe rosacea. The combination of topical metronidazole and doxycycline has been shown to result in a more rapid onset of effect and to be more effective compared with topical monotherapy.[23] However, it is not clear from the literature if the combination of topical metronidazole and oral tetracycline is actually superior to an oral tetracycline alone. In one non-blinded retrospective study, relapse rates after treatment with oral tetracycline were not lower than after treatment with metronidazole 1% cream, with most subjects relapsing within 6 months.[24] There is evidence to support the efficacy of topical metronidazole in maintaining remissions of rosacea, after initial successful treatment with a combination of topical metronidazole and a tetracycline.[25] Given the frequency of relapse

Table 1
Comparative trials of metronidazole with other topical therapies in rosacea

Trial	Results	Comment
Azelaic acid 15% gel versus metronidazole 0.75% gel[16]	Azelaic acid superior in improving lesion counts and erythema	—
Azelaic acid 20% cream versus metronidazole 0.75% cream[17]	Similar reductions in lesions but better global improvement with azelaic acid	Split-face design
Azelaic acid 15% gel versus metronidazole 1% gel[18]	Similar efficacy	—
Sodium sulfacetamide 10% and sulfur 5% cream versus metronidazole 0.75% cream[20]	Greater reduction in lesions and erythema with sodium sulfacetamide/sulfur	More treatment related adverse effects with sodium sulfacetamide/sulfur
Pimecrolimus 1% cream versus metronidazole 1% cream[21]	Equal efficacy	Small, open study

after cessation of treatment, and patients' tendency to self-discontinue treatment when their rosacea is controlled,[26] maintenance therapy with topical metronidazole should be encouraged.

INNOVATIVE USES

The remainder of this article reviews novel uses of topical metronidazole that are supported in the peer-reviewed literature. The data supporting its use in the treatment of seborrheic dermatitis, periorificial dermatitis, epidermal growth factor receptor (EGFR) inhibitor-associated skin toxicity, malodorous wounds, and topical provocation of fixed drug eruption and acute generalized exanthematous pustulosis are discussed (**Box 1**).

SEBORRHEIC DERMATITIS

Four double-blind, placebo-controlled studies and two comparative studies support the use of topical metronidazole in the treatment of seborrheic dermatitis (**Table 2**). Parsad and colleagues[27] treated 44 subjects with seborrheic dermatitis involving the scalp, face, and chest with either metronidazole 1% gel or its vehicle twice daily for 8 weeks. Metronidazole gel was significantly more effective than its vehicle, with significant improvement noted as early as week two. Koca and colleagues[28] treated 84 subjects with mild to moderate facial seborrheic dermatitis with either metronidazole 0.75% gel or its vehicle gel twice daily for 8 weeks. Both treatments showed similar efficacy. Siadat and colleagues[29] compared the efficacy of metronidazole 1% gel to its vehicle gel in a double-blind clinical trial of 55 subjects with facial seborrheic dermatitis. As in the previous studies, subjects were treated twice daily for 8 weeks. Metronidazole gel was significantly more effective than its vehicle as early as week two. Finally, Ozcan and colleagues[30] treated 67 subjects with mild to moderate seborrheic dermatitis involving the scalp, face, and chest with either metronidazole 0.75% gel or its vehicle twice daily for 4 weeks. Both treatment arms showed equivalent and statistically significant improvement. Topical metronidazole gel was well tolerated in all four studies.

Box 1
Innovative uses of topical metronidazole

Seborrheic dermatitis

Periorificial dermatitis in children

Epidermal growth factor receptor inhibitor-associated papulopustular eruption

Smelly wounds

Topical provocation of fixed drug eruption and acute generalized exanthematous pustulosis

Seckin and colleagues[31] compared metronidazole 0.75% gel and ketoconazole 2% cream in a double-blind study of 60 consecutive subjects with mild to moderate facial seborrheic dermatitis. Subjects were randomized to receive either ketoconazole 2% cream and metronidazole gel vehicle or metronidazole 0.75% gel and ketoconazole cream vehicle each applied once daily for 4 weeks. Both treatments were equally effective and well tolerated. More recently, Cicek and colleagues[32] compared the efficacy and safety of pimecrolimus 1% cream, methylprednisolone aceponate 0.1% cream, and metronidazole 0.75% gel in the treatment of facial seborrheic dermatitis. In this open study, 64 consecutive subjects were randomized into one of the three treatment arms and applied their medication twice daily for 8 weeks. All three drugs were found to be effective, although pimecrolimus was significantly more effective than either methylprednisolone aceponate, or topical metronidazole. Significantly more subjects in the metronidazole group developed side effects, including erythema and burning.

Is topical metronidazole effective in the treatment of seborrheic dermatitis? Although more studies are needed, several trials support the use of metronidazole gel in the treatment of seborrheic dermatitis. Although its mechanism of action in seborrheic dermatitis is not clear, it may be acting through inherent antiinflammatory effects. Although treatment with anti-Malassezia agents, such as ketoconazole, is usually sufficient, some patients do not respond. Thus, at the very least, topical metronidazole offers a viable therapeutic alternative to reliance on topical steroids in this group of patients.

PERIORIFICIAL DERMATITIS

Periorificial dermatitis consists of monomorphous grouped erythematous papules around the mouth, nose, and eyes. The spectrum of disease includes perioral dermatitis; granulomatous periorificial dermatitis; and facial Afro-Caribbean childhood eruption (FACE).[33]

Several case series support the use of topical metronidazole in the treatment of periorificial dermatitis in children. Manders and Lucky[34] reported 14 consecutive cases of perioral dermatitis in children seen in one pediatric dermatology practice. Eight of the cases were managed with metronidazole 0.75% gel alone, applied once, or more commonly, twice daily. Five of the children were treated with metronidazole gel in combination

Table 2
Placebo-controlled trials of topical metronidazole in seborrheic dermatitis

Study	Study Design	Number of Subjects	Result
Parsad et al[27]	Metronidazole 1% gel versus vehicle BID for 8 weeks	44	More effective than vehicle
Koca et al[28]	Metronidazole 0.75% gel versus vehicle BID for 8 weeks	84	Equally effective
Siadat et al[29]	Metronidazole 1% gel versus vehicle BID for 8 weeks	55	More effective than vehicle
Ozcan et al[30]	Metronidazole 0.75% gel versus vehicle BID for 4 weeks	67	Equally effective

with other medications, including topical or oral erythromycin and hydrocortisone 1% cream. One case was treated with hydrocortisone 1% cream alone. All of the children cleared after 1 to 8 weeks of treatment, with a mean of 5 weeks to clearance. No relapses were seen in up to 16 months of follow-up. Miller and Shalita[35] reported three children with perioral dermatitis treated with metronidazole 0.75% gel twice daily. All three subjects completely cleared after 14 weeks of therapy and were significantly improved after 2 months. Boeck and colleagues[36] treated seven pediatric subjects with perioral dermatitis with metronidazole 1% emulsion. The dosage was increased to 2% emulsion applied twice daily after 2 weeks. All children completely cleared after 3 to 6 months, with significant improvement seen at 4 to 6 weeks. No side effects were noted and all subjects remained clear during 2 years of follow-up. Nguyen and Eichenfield[37] reported a retrospective chart review of 79 cases of periorificial dermatitis in children and adolescents. Treatment with metronidazole cream or gel, oral erythromycin, or both was associated with resolution of the rash, whereas treatment with a calcineurin inhibitor, sulfacetamide, hydrocortisone, or an antifungal agent was associated with persistent disease. The investigators suggest initial treatment of periorificial dermatitis in children with topical metronidazole for 1 to 2 months, with addition of oral erythromycin if the rash persists.

Veien and colleagues[38] compared the efficacy of topical metronidazole and oral tetracycline in the treatment of adults with perioral dermatitis. In a double-blind, double-dummy, randomized multicenter trial, 108 adults with perioral dermatitis were treated with metronidazole 1% cream or tetracycline 250 mg twice daily for 8 weeks. Although both treatments were effective, oral tetracycline was significantly more effective and resulted in more rapid improvement.

Weber and colleagues used guidelines of evidence-based medicine to evaluate the quality of studies on the treatment of perioral dermatitis.[39] They found only two therapeutic trials of medium-range quality; the other studies were rated as low quality. Most support was found for treatment of perioral dermatitis with oral tetracycline. There was inconsistency in the literature reviewed with respect to the efficacy of topical therapy. The data also supported avoidance of topical corticosteroids and cosmetics. Support was also found for the option of no therapy, because spontaneous clearance has been documented.

What is the role of topical metronidazole in the treatment of periorificial dermatitis? Based on the current literature, when treating children with periorificial dermatitis, an initial trial of topical metronidazole for 1 to 2 months is reasonable and justifiable. If the condition persists, oral erythromycin should be considered. For the treatment of adults with perioral dermatitis, oral tetracycline (or doxycycline) is the treatment of choice. Topical metronidazole is an option for therapy in adults if there is a compelling need to avoid tetracyclines or if patients would prefer topical treatment.

EPIDERMAL GROWTH FACTOR RECEPTOR INHIBITOR-ASSOCIATED CUTANEOUS TOXICITY

Epidermal growth factor receptor inhibitors are being used with increasing frequency to treat advanced epithelial tumors. EGFR plays an important role in control of cell growth and differentiation and is overexpressed in various epithelial cancers.[40] Currently, EGFR inhibitors are FDA approved for the treatment of non-small cell lung cancer, pancreatic cancer, colorectal cancer, and head and neck cancer. There are two main classes of agents that target EGFR (**Table 3**).

Table 3
Classification of epidermal growth factor receptor inhibitors

Type	Mechanism of Action	Examples	Skin Toxicity
Tyrosine kinase inhibitors	Bind intracellular adenosine triphosphate-binding site of tyrosine kinase, preventing activation	erlo**tinib** gefi**tinib** lapa**tinib**	Less frequent and severe
Monoclonal antibodies	Bind extracellular domain of EGFR, preventing ligand binding and activation	cetuxi**mab** panitumu**mab**	More frequent and severe

The tyrosine kinase inhibitors, which include erlotinib, gefitinib, and lapatinib, bind the intracellular protein kinase portion of the receptor and hence prevent its activation. The monoclonal antibodies, including cetuximab and panitumumab, block ligand-dependent activation of EGFR. EGFR is present in keratinocytes, the follicular epithelium, and sweat and sebaceous glands and plays an important role in normal development and function of the epidermis.[41] The most common adverse effect associated with the use of EGFR inhibitors is skin and adnexal toxicity.[42] Because cutaneous toxicity has been observed with all agents that target EGFR, it is considered a class effect. However, the monoclonal antibodies tend to be associated with more frequent and severe skin toxicity.[43]

Several dermatologic effects have been associated with use of EGFR inhibitors. These include a papulopustular eruption, xerosis, paronychia, hair loss, increased growth of eyelashes and eyebrows, hyperpigmentation, and telangiectases.[44] Cutaneous toxicity is dose dependent and several studies have shown a positive association between the presence and severity of skin toxicity and improved tumor response and survival.[43]

The remainder of this discussion focuses on the most common skin toxicity associated with the use of EGFR inhibitors, namely an acneiform or papulopustular rash. This eruption occurs in 45% to 100% of patients and consists of monomorphic erythematous follicular papules and pustules affecting primarily sebaceous areas of the central face, neck, and upper trunk.[43] Comedones are not present, and the eruption is not felt to be acne related. Pruritus and discomfort is variable, and secondary infection may occur. The eruption typically develops within the first 2 weeks of treatment and may improve with time despite ongoing treatment. Although most patients are mildly affected, in a recent survey of oncologists in the United States, 32% reported discontinuing EGFR inhibitor treatment because of rash.[45] In the same survey, only 8% of those surveyed consulted dermatology, with some reporting that they felt dermatologists had nothing to offer in therapeutic intervention of EGFR inhibitor-associated rash.

Management of this unique papulopustular eruption is largely anecdotal, based on personal experience and isolated case reports. Currently, no evidence-based treatment guidelines are available to prevent or treat EGFR inhibitor-associated skin toxicities. General measures recommended in the management of these eruptions include use of emollients, sun protective measures, and sedating antihistamines if pruritus is present.[46] Specific therapies used depend on the severity of the papulopustular rash (**Table 4**).[46] For patients with mild, localized eruptions, either no therapy or topical treatment is typically offered. Patients with moderate reactions are generally treated with topical therapy in combination with either doxycycline or minocycline. In patients who develop severe papulopustular eruptions, reduction or discontinuation of EGFR inhibitor therapy is recommended. Two placebo-controlled trials have shown that prophylactic use of either tetracycline or minocycline significantly reduces the severity of the papulopustular rash when given during the first month of treatment.[47,48]

Although several topical agents have been recommended for the treatment of EGFR inhibitor-associated papulopustular eruption, the evidence supporting their use is for the most part anecdotal. These agents include topical clindamycin, erythromycin, fusidic acid, retinoids, pimecrolimus, corticosteroids, benzyl peroxide, and metronidazole.[49] Two prospective, randomized, open-label, split-face trials failed to show benefit from use of either tazarotene 0.05% cream[48] or pimecrolimus 1% cream.[50] Segaert and Van Cutsem[51] and Galimont-Collen and colleagues[52] favor metronidazole as topical therapy in the management of papulopustular eruptions associated with EGFR inhibitors, with concomitant use of oral minocycline or doxycycline for more severe involvement. Their rationale is that the eruption is more akin to

Table 4
Treatment algorithm for the management of epidermal growth factor receptor inhibitor-associated papulopustular eruption

Severity	Description	EGFR Inhibitor	Treatment
Mild	Localized erythema/papules/pustules Minimal symptoms No impact on ADL	Continue	General measures (emollients, sun protection, antihistamines, antibiotics if infected) No therapy or topicals
Moderate	Generalized erythema/papules/pustules Mild symptoms Minimal impact on ADL	Continue	General measures Topicals and oral minocycline or doxycycline
Severe	Severe generalized erythema/papules/pustules Severe symptoms Significant impairment of ADL ± secondary infection	Dose reduction or discontinuation by oncologist	General measures Topicals and oral minocycline or doxycycline Consider systemic corticosteroids

Abbreviation: ADL, activities of daily living.

Data from Lynch TJ Jr, Kim ES, Eaby B, et al. Epidermal growth factor receptor inhibitor-associated cutaneous toxicities: an evolving paradigm in clinical management. Oncologist 2007;12(5):610–21.

inflammatory rosacea rather than acne. Anti-acne therapy, such as retinoids and benzyl peroxide, and calcineurin inhibitors may be too irritating, whereas topical corticosteroids may lead to steroid-induced acne and atrophy.

Controlled clinical trials that will help to determine the optimal approach to the prevention and management of dermatologic effects of EGFR inhibitors are currently underway. Given the potential effect of dermatologic toxicity on treatment compliance and quality of life, these trials are sorely needed. An interdisciplinary approach to the care of these patients involving oncologists and dermatologists is optimal.

SMELLY WOUNDS

Wounds often have an unpleasant odor, which can be a source of distress to patients, families, and caregivers. Aside from treating the cause of the wound, alleviating wound odor can enhance the quality of life of these patients. The anaerobic organisms flourishing in necrotic tissue create odor by producing volatile fatty acids as an end product of anaerobic metabolism.[53] In the first published cutaneous use of topical metronidazole, Jones and colleagues[54] reported the effectiveness of a 1% solution of the drug for the topical treatment of infected pressure ulcers with a putrid odor. Metronidazole likely is effective in eliminating wound odor through complete or partial eradication of etiologic anaerobic bacteria.

There are two placebo-controlled trials in the literature evaluating the use of topical metronidazole in the management of malodorous wounds. Bower and colleagues[55] reported a double-blind, placebo-controlled, randomized trial of 11 subjects with fungating tumors. Subjects were initially randomized to receive either metronidazole 0.8% gel or vehicle gel daily for 5 days, followed by treatment of all subjects with metronidazole gel daily for 5 days. Although there was a trend in favor of the active preparation during the initial double-blind phase of the study, this did not achieve statistical significance because of the small number of subjects. In view of the significant improvement seen with active treatment, it was considered unethical to continue with the placebo arm of the trial in these terminally ill subjects and the trial was stopped. Bale and colleagues[56] evaluated the effectiveness of topical metronidazole gel in the treatment of wound malodor in a randomized, placebo-controlled, double-blind study of 41 subjects with venous leg ulcers, arterial leg ulcers, pressure ulcers, and other wounds. Although wound odor significantly improved in both groups, improvement occurred faster in the treatment arm. The high success rate of the placebo arm was unanticipated and felt to be caused in part by increased frequency of dressing changes. Pain significantly decreased only in the metronidazole treated group.

Paul and Pieper[57] recently reviewed the literature regarding the use of topical metronidazole to decrease wound odor. They identified 15 studies in the literature, including seven case reports or case series, six descriptive longitudinal studies, and the two controlled clinical trials discussed earlier. Ten of the fifteen studies were small, with a sample size of between 1 and 16 subjects. The most frequent wound types were pressure ulcers, fungating malignant neoplasms, venous ulcers, and arterial ulcers. Typically, 0.75% to 0.8% metronidazole gel was applied to the wound base once or twice daily and covered with a saline-moistened or dry gauze dressing. Reported benefits of treatment included decreased wound odor, drainage, pain, necrosis, and surrounding cellulitis. The authors concluded that topical metronidazole appears to be a safe and effective treatment of wound odor although additional studies are necessary to elucidate an optimal usage pattern.

FIXED DRUG ERUPTIONS

Although there are few reports of oral metronidazole as a cause of fixed drug eruption (FDE) in the literature, it was the fifth most common cause of FDE in one series reported from India.[58] This finding may reflect the frequency of its use in developing countries. Three case reports have documented the use of topical metronidazole to confirm a diagnosis of FDE caused by oral metronidazole (**Table 5**). Gastaminza and colleagues[59] reported a 25-year-old woman who developed a FDE after treatment with Rhodogil (spiramycin and metronidazole). Topical provocation was performed using crushed tablets in petrolatum and left on for 48 hours. Topical provocation with Rhodogil and metronidazole reproduced localized erythema and itchiness in the residual lesion, which lasted for 4 to 5 days. Short and colleagues[60] reported the case of a 41-year-old woman with a history of recurrent FDE caused by oral metronidazole. Topical provocation testing was done using a commercially available formulation of metronidazole 0.8% gel. The metronidazole gel was applied to sites of previous FDE and to unaffected skin using a Finn chamber. Results showed a positive reaction only at the sites of previous FDE. A biopsy done at 72 hours from lesional skin showed histologic features consistent with FDE. The third case reported by Vila and colleagues[61] is of a 31-year-old woman who developed a FDE after taking Rhodogil. Topical provocation done on involved skin with metronidazole 10% aqueous was positive, whereas topical provocation with spiramycin was negative. These case reports support the use of topical provocation testing using topical metronidazole in cases of suspected FDE caused by oral metronidazole. Topical provocation must be done on previously affected skin and may eliminate the need for oral challenge, which would be most helpful in the setting of FDE encountered in patients receiving multiple medications, any one of which might be the culprit.

ACUTE GENERALIZED EXANTHEMATOUS PUSTULOSIS

A growing number of medications have been reported to induce acute generalized exanthematous pustulosis (AGEP) and to yield positive patch testing. Watsky reported a 41-year-old man who developed AGEP while taking oral metronidazole.[62] One month later, diagnostic closed patch testing was done using a commercially available preparation of metronidazole 0.75% cream. At the 3-day follow-up reading, the test site was erythematous, indurated, and studded with multiple microvesicles and pustules. When the subject underwent repeat patch testing several years later to metronidazole 1% in petrolatum, biopsy of the positive patch-test site showed epidermal spongiosis and a predominantly lymphocytic infiltrate rather than histologic

Table 5
Use of topical metronidazole to confirm a diagnosis of fixed drug eruption

Report	Case	Test Material	Biopsy Result
Gastaminza[59]	25-year-old woman treated with Rhodogil	Crusted tablets 50% in petrolatum	Not done
Short[60]	41-year-old woman treated with metronidazole	Metronidazole 0.8% gel	Consistent with FDE at 72 hours
Vila[61]	31-year-old woman treated with Rhodogil	Metronidazole 10% aqueous	Not done

Rhodogil (metronidazole and spiramycin).

features of AGEP.[63] This finding is consistent with the histologic findings of other positive patch-test sites in patients with a history of AGEP induced by medications other than metronidazole.[64,65] Current limitations in the use of patch testing to clarify the causative agent in AGEP include uncertain specificity and sensitivity, lack of standardized topical preparations for testing, and potential for systemic reactions, as has been reported.[66]

SUMMARY

Topical metronidazole continues to be a first-line therapy for rosacea. Metronidazole cream, gel, and lotion have similar efficacies, as do the 0.75% and 1% concentrations in current formulations. Once-daily application may be as effective as twice-daily use. Topical metronidazole is effective and important in maintaining remissions of rosacea. More studies are needed to determine if use of combinations of topical agents in the treatment of rosacea would result in improved efficacy. There is evidence to support the use of metronidazole in the treatment of several other dermatologic conditions, including seborrheic dermatitis, periorificial dermatitis, EGFR inhibitor-associated cutaneous toxicity, and malodorous wounds. It has also been used in topical provocation testing to confirm a diagnosis of FDE and AGEP caused by oral metronidazole.

REFERENCES

1. Persi A, Rebora A. Metronidazole and demodex folliculorum. Acta Derm Venereol 1981;61(2):182–3.
2. Eriksson G, Nord CE. Impact of topical metronidazole on the skin and colon microflora in patients with rosacea. Infection 1987;15(1):8–10.
3. Schmadel LK, McEvoy GK. Topical metronidazole: a new therapy for rosacea. Clin Pharm 1990;9(2): 94–101.
4. Narayanan S, Hunerbein A, Getie M, et al. Scavenging properties of metronidazole on free oxygen radicals in a skin lipid model system. J Pharm Pharmacol 2007;59(8):1125–30.
5. Neilsen PG. Treatment of rosacea with 1% metronidazole cream. A double-blind study. Br J Dermatol 1983;108(3):327–32.
6. Aronson IK, Rumsfield JA, West DP, et al. Evaluation of topical metronidazole gel in acne rosacea. Drug Intell Clin Pharm 1987;21(4):346–51.
7. Bleicher PA, Charles JH, Sober AJ. Topical metronidazole therapy for rosacea. Arch Dermatol 1987; 123(5):609–14.
8. Breneman DL, Stewart D, Hevia O, et al. A double-blind, multicenter clinical trial comparing efficacy of once-daily metronidazole 1 percent cream to vehicle in patients with rosacea. Cutis 1998;61(1):44–7.
9. Nally JB, Berson DS. Topical therapies for rosacea. J Drugs Dermatol 2006;5(1):23–6.
10. Madsen JT, Thormann J, Kerre S, et al. Allergic contact dermatitis to topical metronidazole-3 cases. Contact Dermatitis 2007;56(6):364–6.
11. Kirkland CR, Yelverton CB, Fleischer AB Jr, et al. Gel vehicles are not inherently more irritating than creams. J Drugs Dermatol 2006; 5(3):269–72.
12. Dow G, Basu S. A novel aqueous metronidazole 1% gel with hydrosolubilizing agents (HAS-3). Cutis 2006;77(4 Suppl):18–26.
13. Yoo J, Reid DC, Kimball AB. Metronidazole in the treatment of rosacea: do formulation, dosing and concentration matter? J Drugs Dermatol 2006;5(4): 317–9.
14. Lamp KC, Freeman CD, Klutman NE, et al. Pharmacokinetics and pharmacodynamics of the nitroimidazole antimicrobials. Clin Pharmacokinet 1999;36(5): 353–73.
15. Jorizzo JL, Lebwohl M, Tobey RE. The efficacy of metronidazole 1% cream once daily compared with metronidazole 1% cream twice daily and their vehicles in rosacea: a double-blind clinical trial. J Am Acad Dermatol 1998;39(3):502–4.
16. Elewski BE, Fleischer AB Jr, Pariser DM. A comparison of 15% azelaic acid gel and 0.75% metronidazole gel in the topical treatment of papulopustular rosacea: results of a randomized trial. Arch Dermatol 2003;139(11):1444–50.
17. Maddin S. A comparison of topical azelaic acid 20% cream and topical metronidazole 0.75% cream in the treatment of patients with papulopustular rosacea. J Am Acad Dermatol 1999;40(6 Pt 1):961–5.
18. Wolf JE Jr, Kerrouche N, Arsonnaud S. Efficacy and safety of once-daily metronidazole 1% gel compared with twice-daily azelaic acid 15% gel in the treatment of rosacea. Cutis 2006;77(4 Suppl):3–11.
19. Colon LE, Johnson LA, Gottschalk RW. Cumulative irritation potential among metronidazole gel 1%, metronidazole gel 0.75%, and azelaic acid gel 15%. Cutis 2007;79(4):317–21.
20. Torok HM, Webster G, Dunlap FE, et al. Combination sodium sulfacetamide 10% and sulfur 5% cream with sunscreens versus metronidazole 0.75% cream for rosacea. Cutis 2005;75(6):357–63.
21. Koca R, Altinyazar HC, Ankarali H, et al. A comparison of metronidazole 1% cream and pimecrolimus 1% cream in the treatment of patients with papulopustular rosacea: a randomized open-label clinical trial. Clin Exp Dermatol 2009;35(3):251–6.
22. Del Rosso JQ, Bikowski J. Topical metronidazole combination therapy in the clinical management of rosacea. J Drugs Dermatol 2005;4(4):473–80.

23. Del Rosso JQ. Anti-inflammatory dose doxycycline in the treatment of rosacea. J Drugs Dermatol 2009;8(7):664–8.
24. Nielsen PG. The relapse rate for rosacea after treatment with either oral tetracycline or metronidazole cream [letter]. Br J Dermatol 1983;109(1):122.
25. Dahl MV, Katz HI, Krueger GG, et al. Topical metronidazole maintains remissions of rosacea. Arch Dermatol 1998;134(6):679–83.
26. Elewski BE. Results of a national rosacea patient survey: common issues that concern rosacea suffers. J Drugs Dermatol 2009;8(2):120–3.
27. Parsad D, Pandhi R, Negi KS, et al. Topical metronidazole in seborrheic dermatitis-a double-blind study. Dermatology 2001;202(1):35–7.
28. Koca R, Altinyazar HC, Esturk E. Is topical metronidazole effective in seborrheic dermatitis? A double-blind study. Int J Dermatol 2003;42(8):632–5.
29. Siadat AH, Iraji F, Shahmoradi Z, et al. The efficacy of 1% metronidazole gel in facial seborrheic dermatitis: a double-blind study. Indian J Dermatol Venereol Leprol 2006;72(4):266–9.
30. Ozcan H, Seyhan M, Yologlu S. Is metronidazole 0.75% gel effective in the treatment of seborrheic dermatitis? A double-blind, placebo controlled study. Eur J Dermatol 2007;17(4):313–6.
31. Seckin D, Gurbuz O, Akin O. Metronidazole 0.75% gel vs. ketoconazole 2% cream in the treatment of facial seborrheic dermatitis: a randomized, double-blind study. J Eur Acad Dermatol Venereol 2007; 21(3):345–50.
32. Cicek D, Kandi B, Bakar S, et al. Pimecrolimus 1% cream, methylprednisolone aceponate 0.1% cream and metronidazole 0.75% gel in the treatment of seborrheic dermatitis: a randomized clinical study. J Dermatolog Treat 2009;20(2):1–6.
33. Laude TA, Salvemini JN. Perioral dermatitis in children. Semin Cutan Med Surg 1999;18(3):206–9.
34. Manders SM, Lucky AW. Perioral dermatitis in childhood. J Am Acad Dermatol 1992;27(5 Pt 1):688–92.
35. Miller SR, Shalita AR. Topical metronidazole gel (0.75%) for the treatment of perioral dermatitis in children. J Am Acad Dermatol 1994;31(5 Pt 2): 847–8.
36. Boeck K, Abeck D, Werfel S, et al. Perioral dermatitis in children-clinical presentation, pathogenesis-related factors and response to topical metronidazole. Dermatology 1997;195(3):235–8.
37. Nguyen V, Eichenfield LF. Periorificial dermatitis in children and adolescents. J Am Acad Dermatol 2006;55(5):781–5.
38. Veien NK, Munkvad JM, Nielsen AO, et al. Topical metronidazole in the treatment of perioral dermatitis. J Am Acad Dermatol 1991;24(2 Pt 1):258–60.
39. Weber K, Thurmayr R. Critical appraisal of reports on the treatment of perioral dermatitis. Dermatology 2005;210(4):300–7.
40. Mendelsohn J. Targeting the epidermal growth factor receptor for cancer therapy. J Clin Oncol 2002;20(18 Suppl):1S–13S.
41. Nanney LB, McKanna JA, Stoscheck CM, et al. Visualization of epidermal growth factor receptors in human epidermis. J Invest Dermatol 1984;82(2):165–9.
42. Lacouture ME, Basti S, Patel J, et al. The SERIES clinic: an interdisciplinary approach to the management of toxicities of EGRF inhibitors. J Support Oncol 2006;4(5):236–8.
43. Li T, Perez-Soler R. Skin toxicities associated with epidermal growth factor receptor inhibitors. Target Oncol 2009;4(2):107–19.
44. Lorusso P. Toward evidence-based management of the dermatologic effects of EGRF inhibitors. Oncology 2009;23(2):186–93.
45. Boone SL, Rademaker A, Liu D, et al. Impact and management of skin toxicity associated with anti-epidermal growth factor receptor therapy: survey results. Oncology 2007;72(3-4):152–9.
46. Lynch TJ Jr, Kim ES, Eaby B, et al. Epidermal growth factor receptor inhibitor-associated cutaneous toxicities: an evolving paradigm in clinical management. Oncologist 2007;12(5):610–21.
47. Jatoi A, Rowland K, Sloan JA, et al. Does tetracycline prevent/palliate epidermal growth factor receptor (EGRF) inhibitor-induced rash? A phase III trial from the North Central Cancer Treatment Group (N03CB) (abstract LBA9006). J Clin Oncol 2007;25(18S):494s.
48. Scope A, Agero AL, Dusza SW, et al. Randomized double-blind trial of prophylactic oral minocycline and topical tazarotene for cetuximab-associated acne-like eruption. J Clin Oncol 2007;25(34): 5390–6.
49. Agero AL, Dusza SW, Benvenuto-Andrade C, et al. Dermatologic side effects associated with the epidermal growth factor receptor inhibitors. J Am Acad Dermatol 2006;55(4):657–70.
50. Scope A, Lieb JA, Dusza SW, et al. A prospective randomized trial of topical pimecrolimus for cetuximab-associated acne-like eruption. J Am Acad Dermatol 2009;61(4):614–20.
51. Segaert S, Van Cutsem E. Clinical management of EGRFI dermatologic toxicities: the European perspective. Oncology 2007;21(11 Suppl 5):22–6.
52. Galimont-Collen AF, Vos LE, Lavrijsen AP. Classification and management of skin, hair, nail and mucosal side-effects of epidermal growth factor receptor (EGFR) inhibitors. Eur J Cancer 2007;43(5):845–51.
53. Sapico FL, Ginunas VJ, Thornhill-Joynes M, et al. Quantitative microbiology of pressure sores in different stages of healing. Diagn Microbiol Infect Dis 1986;5(1):31–8.
54. Jones PH, Willis AT, Ferguson IR. Treatment of anaerobically infected pressure sores with topical metronidazole. Lancet 1978;1(8057):213–4.

55. Bower M, Stein R, Evans TR, et al. A double-blind study of the efficacy of metronidazole gel in the treatment of malodorous fungating tumours. Eur J Cancer 1992;28A(4-5):888–9.
56. Bale S, Tebbie N, Price P. A topical metronidazole gel used to treat malodorous wounds. Br J Nurs 2004;13(11):S4–11.
57. Paul JC, Pieper BA. Topical metronidazole for the treatment of wound odor: a review of the literature. Ostomy Wound Manage 2008;54(3):18–27.
58. Sharma VK, Dhar S, Gill AN. Drug related involvement of specific sites in fixed eruptions: a statistical evaluation. J Dermatol 1996;23(8):530–4.
59. Gastaminza G, Anda M, Audicana MT, et al. Fixed-drug eruption due to metronidazole with positive topical provocation. Contact Dermatitis 2001;44(1):36.
60. Short KA, Fuller LC, Salisbury JR. Fixed drug eruption following metronidazole therapy and the use of topical provocation testing in diagnosis. Clin Exp Dermatol 2002;27(6):464–6.
61. Vila JB, Bernier MA, Gutierrez JV, et al. Fixed drug eruption caused by metronidazole. Contact Dermatitis 2002;46(2):122.
62. Watsky KL. Acute generalized exanthematous pustulosis induced by metronidazole: the role of patch testing. Arch Dermatol 1999;135(1):93–4.
63. Girardi M, Duncan KO, Tigelaar RE, et al. Cross-comparison of patch test and lymphocyte proliferation responses in patients with a history of acute generalized exanthematous pustulosis. Am J Dermatopathol 2005;27(4):343–6.
64. Jan V, Machet L, Gironet N, et al. Acute generalized exanthematous pustulosis induced by diltiazem: value of patch testing. Dermatology 1998;197(3):274–5.
65. Britschgi M, Steiner UC, Schmid S, et al. T-cell involvement in drug-induced acute generalized exanthematous pustulosis. J Clin Invest 2001;107(11):1433–41.
66. Mashiah J, Brenner S. A systemic reaction to patch testing for the evaluation of acute generalized exanthematous pustulosis. Arch Dermatol 2003;139(9):1181–3.

Innovative Use of Topical Calcineurin Inhibitors

Andrew N. Lin, MD, FRCPC

KEYWORDS

• Calcineurin inhibitors • Tacrolimus • Pimecrolimus

Topical tacrolimus and pimecrolimus are calcineurin inhibitors (TCI) that are indicated and approved for the treatment of atopic dermatitis in patients 2 years of age or older. This article reviews the many studies that have assessed their efficacy in disorders other than atopic dermatitis (ie, off-label uses), focusing on disorders for which efficacy was assessed in double-blind studies. These include oral lichen planus, psoriasis, and vitiligo, in which double-blind studies have shown efficacy for tacrolimus and pimecrolimus. The efficacy of TCI in contact dermatitis, seborrheic dermatitis, rosacea, cutaneous lupus erythamatosus, perioral dermatitis, cutaneous Crohn disease, and other dermatoses is also examined.

ORAL LICHEN PLANUS

Oral lichen planus is 1 of the best studied off-label uses for topical calcineurin inhibitors. Investigators have shown that tacrolimus and pimecrolimus are effective in double-blind studies.

Tacrolimus

In one head to head study involving 32 patients, tacrolimus 0.1% ointment and clobetasol propionate 0.05% ointment showed significant improvement from baseline, and, notably, tacrolimus was significantly better than clobetasol ($P<.001$).[1] Medication was applied four times a day for 4 weeks, and patients were not allowed to eat or drink for 30 minutes after application. In another study of 30 patients with oral erosive/ulcerative lichen planus, tacrolimus 0.1% ointment was as effective as topical clobetasol propionate 0.05% ointment, both showing significant improvement from baseline.[2] In 1 open study of 50 patients with oral erosive/ulcerative lichen planus, tacrolimus 0.1% ointment resulted in complete resolution in 14% of patients, partial resolution in 80%, and no benefit in 6%.[3] Whole blood tacrolimus was detected in 27 patients, with mean maximum of 2.7 μg/L (range up to 11 μg/L). This level compares with the lower therapeutic level for renal transplant patients of 5 to 10 μg/L. No adverse clinical events related to systemic tacrolimus absorption were observed. Favorable results were also seen in 4 other open studies.[4–7] Another open study showed initial results that were better than triamcinolone acetonide ($P = .007$).[8] Favorable results were also seen in 2 retrospective reviews,[9,10] and 1 questionnaire survey of 37 patients.[11]

Pimecrolimus

In 2 double-blind studies, pimecrolimus 1% cream was superior to placebo in oral erosive lichen planus.[12,13] In another double-blind study, pimecrolimus 1% cream and triamcinolone acetonide 0.1% paste showed significant improvement from baseline, but there was no significant difference between the 2 treatments ($P = .70, .38, .86$).[14]

Summary

Tacrolimus and pimecrolimus have a definite place in the treatment of oral lichen planus. Open studies have shown that tacrolimus 0.1% ointment can be effective in oral erosive lichen planus, but double-blind studies have shown that it may be more

Dr Lin has been a paid speaker for Astellas Pharma Canada, Inc.
Division of Dermatology and Cutaneous Sciences, University of Alberta, 2-104 Clinical Sciences Building, Edmonton, Alberta, T6G 2G3, Canada
E-mail address: anlin00@yahoo.com

Dermatol Clin 28 (2010) 535–545
doi:10.1016/j.det.2010.03.008
0733-8635/10/$ – see front matter © 2010 Elsevier Inc. All rights reserved.

effective, or as effective, as clobetasol 0.05%. In 1 study, blood tacrolimus was detected in up to 54% of patients, but there were no signs of systemic toxicity. Double-blind studies showed that pimecrolimus 1% cream is superior to vehicle, and is equal in efficacy to triamcinolone acetonide paste, especially in oral erosive lichen planus.

VITILIGO

Double-blind studies have shown that tacrolimus and pimecrolimus are effective in vitiligo.

Tacrolimus

In 1 double-blind study, tacrolimus 0.1% ointment plus excimer laser resulted in greater than 75% repigmentation in areas in which vitiligo is generally considered to be UV resistant (bony prominences, extremities) in 60% of patients; this end point was not achieved in any of the patients treated with excimer laser monotherapy (P<.002).[15] In another double-blind study, this same end point was achieved in 50% of patients treated with tacrolimus 0.1% ointment plus excimer laser, compared with 19% of patients treated with placebo plus excimer laser.[16] Less encouraging results were reported in 2 other double-blind studies. In 1 study, tacrolimus plus narrow-band UVB was equal to placebo plus narrow-band UVB[17]; another study showed tacrolimus 0.1% ointment was superior to clobetasol 0.05%, as measured by computerized morphometric analysis of lesions, but no significant difference when measured by clinical evaluation.[18] One observer-blinded study comparing once or twice daily topical tacrolimus showed favorable results for facial lesions.[19]

One open study of 110 patients showed that greater than 75% repigmentation occurred in the face of 40% of patients, 23% in the limbs, 21.5% in the trunk, but only 1% of the hands/feet, and none in the genitals.[20] In another open study of 9 patients, partial repigmentation occurred in all lesions treated with tacrolimus and excimer laser, and none of the sites treated only with tacrolimus.[21] Five other open studies showed favorable results when tacrolimus was used alone, especially in facial lesions.[22–26] Two retrospective reviews also showed favorable results when tacrolimus was used alone.[27,28]

Pimecrolimus

A double-blind study showed that pimecrolimus plus narrow-band UVB was superior to placebo plus narrow-band UVB in repigmentation of facial lesions (P<.05).[29] Several others have shown mixed results. One study showed pimecrolimus was superior to placebo in vitiligo,[30] but another showed no difference.[31] One study showed pimecrolimus was less effective than clobetasol propionate 0.05% ointment.[32]

Three open studies have shown favorable results with pimecrolimus 1% cream in vitiligo.[33–35] Another open study showed that it was as effective as clobetasol propionate 0.05% cream.[36] A retrospective study of 8 patients with facial vitiligo showed pimecrolimus resulted in mean improvement of surface area of 72.5%.[37] Case reports of 3 patients with facial vitiligo showed favorable results.[38–40]

In 1 open study comparing narrow-band UVB, tacrolimus, and pimecrolimus, no statistically significant differences in repigmentation for any anatomic site were recorded with the 3 treatments.[41]

One study showed that pimecrolimus 1% cream combined with microdermabrasion was superior to pimecrolimus alone and placebo in nonsegmental childhood vitiligo.[42] A single-blinded study showed that pimecrolimus 1% cream plus excimer laser was superior to excimer laser alone in childhood vitiligo.[43]

Summary

Double-blind studies have shown that tacrolimus 0.1% ointment is superior to placebo when combined with excimer laser, especially for UV-resistant areas, and that when used alone, it is almost as effective as clobetasol 0.05%. Open studies have shown it can be effective, especially for facial lesions. Double-blind studies have shown that pimecrolimus 1% cream is superior to placebo when combined with narrow-band UVB, especially for facial lesions. However, double-blind and open studies have shown conflicting results when pimecrolimus is compared with clobetasol propionate. Similarly, double-blind studies showed conflicting results when it is compared with placebo. Additional studies would be helpful in clarifying the role of pimecrolimus in vitiligo.

PSORIASIS

Tacrolimus

One double-blind study of 167 patients showed that tacrolimus 0.1% ointment, when applied twice a day to facial or intertriginous psoriasis, was superior to placebo (P = .004), with improvement as early as day 8.[44] Two other double-blind studies also showed tacrolimus is superior to vehicle,[45,46] and 1 other double-blind study of facial/genital-femoral psoriasis showed tacrolimus 0.03% ointment was superior to calcitriol,[47] which is a natural, bioactive 1,25-dihydroxyvitamin D_3, available as an ointment in Europe. Seven open studies showed favorable results with tacrolimus, especially for facial/inverse/genital psoriasis.[48–54]

Pimecrolimus

Investigators have assessed pimecrolimus in several double-blind studies of inverse psoriasis. One double-blind study showed pimecrolimus is superior to vehicle for inverse psoriasis.[55] Another showed that pimecrolimus is superior to vehicle for inverse psoriasis, but inferior to calcipotriol and clobetasol.[56] Another showed that pimecrolimus is superior to calcipotriol, but inferior to betamethasone valerate 0.1%.[57] One open study showed pimecrolimus 1% cream resulted in significant improvement in all clinical parameters in facial psoriasis lesions.[58]

Summary

Based on double-blind and open studies, tacrolimus 0.1% ointment is effective in psoriasis, especially for facial, inverse, and genital psoriasis. Similarly, 1 double-blind study showed that pimecrolimus 1% cream is superior to vehicle, especially for inverse psoriasis. Further studies are required to determine if pimecrolimus is more or less effective compared with potent corticosteroids and calcipotriol. Considering the high risk for the development of cutaneous atrophy when potent corticosteroids are applied to intertriginous skin, it seems reasonable to initiate therapy with TCI first.

CONTACT DERMATITIS

For nickel-induced allergic contact dermatitis, double-blind studies showed that tacrolimus is superior to placebo[59–61]; pimecrolimus 0.6% cream has been shown to be effective in 1 open study.[62] In 1 double-blind study of contact dermatitis, there was no difference among tacrolimus 0.1% cream, pimecrolimus 1% cream, clobetasol propionate 0.05% ointment, triamcinolone acetonide 0.1% ointment, and placebo, but there was a clear trend in favor of active drug treatment.[63]

Additional studies and case reports have shown positive results for tacrolimus[60,64,65] and pimecrolimus[66] for the management of allergic contact dermatitis. Pimecrolimus has also been effective in irritant contact dermatitis of the skin[67] and lips,[68] and in the cutaneous reaction to jelly fish sting.[69]

SEBORRHEIC DERMATITIS

Two open studies showed favorable results with tacrolimus 0.1%.[70,71] In 1 double-blind study, pimecrolimus 1% cream was superior to vehicle[72]; in another study, it was equal to 1% hydrocortisone acetate cream.[73] In 1 open study, it was equal to ketoconazole 2% cream[74]; another open study showed that pimecrolimus was more effective than topical metronidazole and topical methylprednisolone.[75] Thus, multiple approaches to seborrhea exist, including the use of TCI and antifungal agents instead of topical corticosteroids.

ROSACEA

Two open studies showed that tacrolimus 0.1% ointment can be effective for rosacea.[76,77] One double-blind and 1 open study showed that pimecrolimus 1% cream is not more effective than vehicle.[78,79] One open study showed that pimecrolimus is not more efficacious than metronidazole cream.[80] Two open studies showed that pimecrolimus 1% cream can be effective in steroid-induced rosacea.[81,82] Because there is a paucity of evidence in this regard, TCI should be reserved for otherwise recalcitrant rosacea.

CUTANEOUS LUPUS ERYTHEMATOSUS

In 1 double-blind study, tacrolimus 0.1% ointment was equal to clobetasol propionate 0.05% ointment in facial lupus erythematosus (LE), especially malar rash, and lesions of discoid LE and subacute cutaneous LE.[83] In open studies and case reports, treatment with tacrolimus also led to favorable results.[84–91] A double-blind study showed that pimecrolimus 1% cream was comparable with betamethasone valerate 0.1% cream in discoid lupus.[92] Pimecrolimus 1% cream was effective in cutaneous LE in open studies and case reports.[93–95] More investigation, especially placebo- or vehicle-controlled studies, is required before TCI can be unequivocally recommended for cutaneous LE.

PERIORAL DERMATITIS

Two double-blind studies[96,97] showed pimecrolimus 1% cream was superior to vehicle. Additional work is needed in this area.

CUTANEOUS CROHN DISEASE

One double-blind study showed that tacrolimus 0.1% ointment is superior to placebo in perianal or anal ulcerative Crohn disease, but is unlikely to be effective if there are fistulae.[98] In 1 open study, tacrolimus 0.5% ointment was effective in oral and perineal Crohn disease.[99] In 1 patient treated with tacrolimus 0.05% in Orabase for orofacial Crohn disease, systemic absorption with a blood level of 9 μg/mL was documented.[100]

LICHEN SCLEROSUS

Tacrolimus

In 1 open study of 84 patients (49 women, 32 men, 3 girls) with lichen sclerosus (79 with anogenital lichen sclerosus, 5 with extragenital lichen sclerosus) treated with tacrolimus 0.1% twice a day for 16 weeks, clearance of active lichen sclerosus was reached in 43% of patients at 24 weeks.[101] Favorable results were also seen in smaller open studies in patients with vulvar lichen sclerosus[102,103] and lichen sclerosus of the penis.[104] Several case reports have also shown favorable results in vulvar lichen sclerosus,[105–108] anogenital lichen sclerosus,[109] and extragenital lichen sclerosus[110] including lichen sclerosus of the lip.[111]

Pimecrolimus

Several open studies[112–114] and 1 case report[115] showed favorable results of topical pimecrolimus in vulvar lichen sclerosus. One male patient with extragenital lichen sclerosus did not respond to pimecrolimus cream.[116]

Summary

Potent topical corticosteroids remain the treatment of choice for lichen sclerosus. Nonetheless, response is unpredictable, and TCI offer a viable alternative therapeutic intervention. Lichen sclerosus may be associated with the development of squamous cell carcinoma and, therefore, before TCI therapy is started, the clinician should perform a careful examination to exclude the presence of neoplasia in this situation.

MORPHEA/SCLERODERMA

A double-blind study showed that tacrolimus 0.1% ointment was more effective than petrolatum in morphea.[117] An open study showed favorable results in localized scleroderma.[118] Additional research is necessary.

NETHERTON SYNDROME

In 1 study, 3 patients with Netherton syndrome treated with 0.1% tacrolimus had very high blood tacrolimus levels, up to 37.2 μg/L, but none showed signs or symptoms of toxic effects of tacrolimus.[119] Tacrolimus should be used with extreme caution, if at all, in patients with Netherton syndrome.

TACROLIMUS: LACK OF EFFICACY

One open study[120] and 3 case reports[121–123] showed that tacrolimus 0.1% ointment is not effective in alopecia areata. One double-blind study of 22 patients with hemodialysis-related pruritus showed that tacrolimus was not more effective than vehicle.[124] Additional studies and case reports showed that tacrolimus was not effective in frontal fibrosing alopecia,[125] factitial panniculitis,[126] and UV-induced erythema.[127]

PIMECROLIMUS: LACK OF EFFICACY

Studies have shown lack of efficacy of pimecrolimus in alopecia areata[128] and acne vulgaris.[129] One prospective study of cetuximab-induced papulopustular eruption[130] showed pimecrolimus did not result in clinically meaningful benefit, but 1 case report[131] did show efficacy.

OTHER DISORDERS

Investigators have shown that tacrolimus and pimecrolimus can be effective in many other disorders, sometimes as adjunctive therapy.

Tacrolimus

One review[132] cited reports of favorable results with tacrolimus for the following: balanitis xerotica obliterans, lichen striatus, pyostomatitis vegetans, acrodermatitis continua suppurativa, Sjogren syndrome, Zoon balanitis, ichthyosis linearis circumflexa, lichen nitidus, intertrigo, itch of primary biliary cirrhosis, uremic pruritus, pemphigus folicacious, chronic actinic dermatitis, cutaneous sarcoid, granuloma annulare, lichen amyloidosis, idiopathic annular erythema, epidermolysis bullosa pruriginosa, exfoliative cheilitis, eosinophilic pustular folliculitis, reticular erythematosus, erosive pustular dermatosis of the leg and scalp, necrobiosis lipoidica, pityriasis lichenoides, paraneoplastic pemphigus, skin lesions of dermatomyositis, Hailey-Hailey disease (1 other report documented complete failure of topical tacrolimus), scleroderma, morphea, and vasculitic leg ulcer of rheumatoid arthritis.

In addition, a small number of studies and case reports have shown that tacrolimus can be effective in the following: granuloma faciale,[133] chronic paronychia,[134] lichen planus pigmentosus,[135] pityriasis alba,[136] annular lichenoid dermatitis of youth,[137] genital pruritus,[138] chronic otitis externa,[139] incontinentia pigmenti,[140] plasma cell cheilitis,[141] granulomatous cheilitis,[142] inflammatory linear verrucous epidermal nevus,[143] jogger's nipples,[144] juvenile plantar dermatosis,[145] lower extremity ulcer,[146] localized lichen myxedematosus of discrete type,[147] lichen simplex chronicus,[148] lichenoid tattoo reaction,[149] linear IgA bullous disease,[150] mycosis fungoides,[151] necrolytic acral erythema,[152] plasma cell vulvitis,[153] stasis dermatitis,[154] and cheilitis glandularis.[155]

Pimecrolimus

One review[156] cited reports that pimecrolimus can be effective in Behcet disease, acne keloidalis nuchae, vulvar lichen simplex chronicus, vulvar pruritus,, graft versus host disease, lichen striatus, annular elastolytic giant cell granuloma, balanitis circinata, lichen aureus, granuloma annulare, lichen myxedematosus, nodular scabies, Fox-Fordyce disease, cutaneous plasmacytosis, granuloma faciale, chronic actinic dermatitis, telangiectasia macularis eruptiva perstans, erythema annulare centrifugum, lymphocytic infiltration of Jessner, and eosinophilic pustular folliculitis.

Additional reports indicate pimecrolimus can also be effective in vulvar lichen simplex chronicus,[157] frontal fibrosing alopecia,[158] dyshydrosis eczema,[159] eruptive pseudo-angiomatosis,[160] follicular mucinosis,[161] pityriasis rubra pilari,[162] pyoderma gangrenosum,[163] reticular erythematous mucinosus,[164] Zoon balanitis,[165] and pityriasis alba.[166]

Summary

Topical tacrolimus and pimecrolimus have been assessed in the treatment of many disorders other than atopic dermatitis. Double-blind and open studies have shown favorable results with topical tacrolimus and pimecrolimus in oral lichen planus. In 1 study of oral lichen planus, blood tacrolimus was detected in 54% of patients, but there were no signs of systemic toxicity. Double-blind and open studies of vitiligo have shown favorable results with tacrolimus in combination with excimer laser, especially for lesions over bony prominences and on extremities. Similarly, double-blind studies of vitiligo have shown favorable results when pimecrolimus is combined with narrow-band UVB, especially for facial lesions. Double-blind and open studies of psoriasis have shown favorable results for tacrolimus and pimecrolimus, especially for inverse psoriasis. Topical calcineurin inhibitors have been effective in many other cutaneous disorders, and further studies would help clarify their roles.

REFERENCES

1. Corrocher G, Di Lorenzo G, Martinelli N, et al. Comparative effect of tacrolimus 0.1% ointment and clobetasol 0.05% ointment in patients with oral lichen planus. J Clin Periodontol 2008;35(3): 244–9.
2. Radfar L, Wild RC, Suresh L. A comparative treatment study of topical tacrolimus and clobetasol in oral lichen planus. Oral Surg Oral Med Oral Pathol Oral Radiol Endod 2008;105(2):187–93.
3. Hodgson TA, Sahni N, Kaliakatsou F, et al. Long-term efficacy and safety of topical tacrolimus in the management of ulcerative/erosive oral lichen planus. Eur J Dermatol 2003;13(5):466–70.
4. Vente C, Reich K, Rupprecht R, et al. Erosive mucosal lichen planus: response to topical treatment with tacrolimus. Br J Dermatol 1999;140(2):338–42.
5. Morrison L, Kratochvil FJ 3rd, Gorman A. An open trial of topical tacrolimus for erosive oral lichen planus. J Am Acad Dermatol 2002;47(4):617–20.
6. Olivier V, Lacour JP, Mousnier A, et al. Treatment of chronic erosive oral lichen planus with low concentrations of topical tacrolimus: an open prospective study. Arch Dermatol 2002;138(10):1335–8.
7. Kaliakatsou F, Hodgson TA, Lewsey JD, et al. Management of recalcitrant ulcerative oral lichen planus with topical tacrolimus. J Am Acad Dermatol 2002;46(1):35–41.
8. Laeijendecker R, Tank B, Dekker SK, et al. A comparison of treatment of oral lichen planus with topical tacrolimus and triamcinolone acetonide ointment. Acta Derm Venereol 2006;86(3):227–9.
9. Thomson MA, Hamburger J, Stewart DG, et al. Treatment of erosive oral lichen planus with topical tacrolimus. J Dermatolog Treat 2004;15(5):308–14.
10. Rozycki TW, Rogers RS 3rd, Pittelkow MR, et al. Topical tacrolimus in the treatment of symptomatic oral lichen planus: a series of 13 patients. J Am Acad Dermatol 2002;46(1):27–34.
11. Byrd JA, Davis MD, Bruce AJ, et al. Response of oral lichen planus to topical tacrolimus in 37 patients. Arch Dermatol 2004;140(12):1508–12.
12. Volz T, Caroli U, Ludtke H, et al. Pimecrolimus cream 1% in erosive oral lichen planus–a prospective randomized double-blind vehicle-controlled study. Br J Dermatol 2008;159(4):936–41.
13. Passeron T, Lacour JP, Fontas E, et al. Treatment of oral erosive lichen planus with 1% pimecrolimus cream: a double-blind, randomized, prospective trial with measurement of pimecrolimus levels in the blood. Arch Dermatol 2007;143(4):472–6.
14. Gorouhi F, Solhpour A, Beitollahi JM, et al. Randomized trial of pimecrolimus cream versus triamcinolone acetonide paste in the treatment of oral lichen planus. J Am Acad Dermatol 2007; 57(5):806–13.

15. Passeron T, Ostovari N, Zakaria W, et al. Topical tacrolimus and the 308-nm excimer laser: a synergistic combination for the treatment of vitiligo. Arch Dermatol 2004;140(9):1065–9.
16. Kawalek AZ, Spencer JM, Phelps RG. Combined excimer laser and topical tacrolimus for the treatment of vitiligo: a pilot study. Dermatol Surg 2004; 30(2 Pt 1):130–5.
17. Mehrabi D, Pandya AG. A randomized, placebo-controlled, double-blind trial comparing narrowband UV-B Plus 0.1% tacrolimus ointment with narrowband UV-B plus placebo in the treatment of generalized vitiligo. Arch Dermatol 2006; 142(7):927–9.
18. Lepe V, Moncada B, Castanedo-Cazares JP, et al. A double-blind randomized trial of 0.1% tacrolimus vs 0.05% clobetasol for the treatment of childhood vitiligo. Arch Dermatol 2003;139(5):581–5.
19. Radakovic S, Breier-Maly J, Konschitzky R, et al. Response of vitiligo to once- vs. twice-daily topical tacrolimus: a controlled prospective, randomized, observer-blinded trial. J Eur Acad Dermatol Venereol 2009;23(8):951–3.
20. Fai D, Cassano N, Vena GA. Narrow-band UVB phototherapy combined with tacrolimus ointment in vitiligo: a review of 110 patients. J Eur Acad Dermatol Venereol 2007;21(7):916–20.
21. Ostovari N, Passeron T, Lacour JP, et al. Lack of efficacy of tacrolimus in the treatment of vitiligo in the absence of UV-B exposure. Arch Dermatol 2006;142(2):252–3.
22. Xu AZ, Wei DM, Huang XD, et al. Efficacy and safety of tacrolimus cream 0.1% in the treatment of vitiligo. Int J Dermatol 2009;48(1):86–90.
23. Grimes PE, Morris R, Avaniss-Aghajani E, et al. Topical tacrolimus therapy for vitiligo: therapeutic responses and skin messenger RNA expression of proinflammatory cytokines. J Am Acad Dermatol 2004;51(1):52–61.
24. Hartmann A, Brocker EB, Hamm H. Occlusive treatment enhances efficacy of tacrolimus 0.1% ointment in adult patients with vitiligo: results of a placebo-controlled 12-month prospective study. Acta Derm Venereol 2008;88(5):474–9.
25. Tanghetti EA. Tacrolimus ointment 0.1% produces repigmentation in patients with vitiligo: results of a prospective patient series. Cutis 2003;71(2):158–62.
26. Kanwar AJ, Dogra S, Parsad D. Topical tacrolimus for treatment of childhood vitiligo in Asians. Clin Exp Dermatol 2004;29(6):589–92.
27. Silverberg NB, Lin P, Travis L, et al. Tacrolimus ointment promotes repigmentation of vitiligo in children: a review of 57 cases. J Am Acad Dermatol 2004;51(5):760–6.
28. Choi CW, Chang SE, Bak H, et al. Topical immunomodulators are effective for treatment of vitiligo. J Dermatol 2008;35(8):503–7.
29. Esfandiarpour I, Ekhlasi A, Farajzadeh S, et al. The efficacy of pimecrolimus 1% cream plus narrowband ultraviolet B in the treatment of vitiligo: a double-blind, placebo-controlled clinical trial. J Dermatolog Treat 2009;20(1):14–8.
30. Atwa M. Efficacy and safety of pimecrolimus (ASM 981) 1% in the treatment of vitiligo. J Am Acad Dermatol 2005;52(3 Suppl 1):P168.
31. Dawid M, Veensalu M, Grassberger M, et al. Efficacy and safety of pimecrolimus cream 1% in adult patients with vitiligo: results of a randomized, double-blind, vehicle-controlled study. J Dtsch Dermatol Ges 2006;4(11):942–6.
32. Seckin D, Eryilmaz A, Baba M. A double-blind randomized trial of 1% pimecrolimus versus 0.05% clobetasol propionate for the treatment of vitiligo. J Am Acad Dermatol 2007;56(2 (Suppl 2)):AB170.
33. Boone B, Ongenae K, Van Geel N, et al. Topical pimecrolimus in the treatment of vitiligo. Eur J Dermatol 2007;17(1):55–61.
34. Sendur N, Karaman G, Sanic N, et al. Topical pimecrolimus: a new horizon for vitiligo treatment? J Dermatolog Treat 2006;17(6):338–42.
35. Seirafi H, Farnaghi F, Firooz A, et al. Pimecrolimus cream in repigmentation of vitiligo. Dermatology 2007;214(3):253–9.
36. Coskun B, Saral Y, Turgut D. Topical 0.05% clobetasol propionate versus 1% pimecrolimus ointment in vitiligo. Eur J Dermatol 2005;15(2):88–91.
37. Mayoral FA, Vega JM, Stavisky H, et al. Retrospective analysis of pimecrolimus cream 1% for treatment of facial vitiligo. J Drugs Dermatol 2007; 6(5):517–21.
38. Bilac DB, Ermertcan AT, Sahin MT, et al. Two therapeutic challenges: facial vitiligo successfully treated with 1% pimecrolimus cream and 0.005% calcipotriol cream. J Eur Acad Dermatol Venereol 2009;23(1):72–3.
39. Mayoral FA, Gonzalez C, Shah NS, et al. Repigmentation of vitiligo with pimecrolimus cream: a case report. Dermatology 2003;207(3):322–3.
40. Souza Leite RM, Craveiro Leite AA. Two therapeutic challenges: periocular and genital vitiligo in children successfully treated with pimecrolimus cream. Int J Dermatol 2007;46:986–9.
41. Stinco G, Piccirillo F, Forcione M, et al. An open randomized study to compare narrow band UVB, topical pimecrolimus and topical tacrolimus in the treatment of vitiligo. Eur J Dermatol 2009;19(6): 588–93.
42. Farajzadeh S, Daraei Z, Esfandiarpour I, et al. The efficacy of pimecrolimus 1% cream combined with microdermabrasion in the treatment of nonsegmental childhood vitiligo: a randomized placebo-controlled study. Pediatr Dermatol 2009;26(3):286–91.
43. Hui-Lan Y, Xiao-Yan H, Jian-Yong F, et al. Combination of 308-nm excimer laser with topical

pimecrolimus for the treatment of childhood vitiligo. Pediatr Dermatol 2009;26(3):354–6.
44. Lebwohl M, Freeman AK, Chapman MS, et al. Tacrolimus ointment is effective for facial and intertriginous psoriasis. J Am Acad Dermatol 2004;51(5):723–30.
45. Carroll CL, Clarke J, Camacho F, et al. Topical tacrolimus ointment combined with 6% salicylic acid gel for plaque psoriasis treatment. Arch Dermatol 2005;141(1):43–6.
46. Remitz A, Reitamo S, Erkko P, et al. Tacrolimus ointment improves psoriasis in a microplaque assay. Br J Dermatol 1999;141(1):103–7.
47. Liao YH, Chiu HC, Tseng YS, et al. Comparison of cutaneous tolerance and efficacy of calcitriol 3 microg g(-1) ointment and tacrolimus 0.3 mg g(-1) ointment in chronic plaque psoriasis involving facial or genitofemoral areas: a double-blind, randomized controlled trial. Br J Dermatol 2007;157(5):1005–12.
48. Clayton TH, Harrison PV, Nicholls R, et al. Topical tacrolimus for facial psoriasis. Br J Dermatol 2003;149(2):419–20.
49. Yamamoto T, Nishioka K. Topical tacrolimus: an effective therapy for facial psoriasis. Eur J Dermatol 2003;13(5):471–3.
50. Rallis E, Nasiopoulou A, Kouskoukis C, et al. Successful treatment of genital and facial psoriasis with tacrolimus ointment 0.1%. Drugs Exp Clin Res 2005;31(4):141–5.
51. Martin ES, Herrera RM, Umbert AE, et al. Topical tacrolimus for the treatment of psoriasis on the face, genitalia, intertriginous areas and corporal plaques. J Drugs Dermatol 2006;5(4):334–6.
52. Brune A, Miller DW, Lin P, et al. Tacrolimus ointment is effective for psoriasis on the face and intertriginous areas in pediatric patients. Pediatr Dermatol 2007;24(1):76–80.
53. Freeman AK, Linowski GJ, Brady C, et al. Tacrolimus ointment for the treatment of psoriasis on the face and intertriginous areas. J Am Acad Dermatol 2003;48(4):564–8.
54. Bissonnette R, Nigen S, Bolduc C. Efficacy and tolerability of topical tacrolimus ointment for the treatment of male genital psoriasis. J Cutan Med Surg 2008;12(5):230–4.
55. Gribetz C, Ling M, Lebwohl M, et al. Pimecrolimus cream 1% in the treatment of intertriginous psoriasis: a double-blind, randomized study. J Am Acad Dermatol 2004;51(5):731–8.
56. Mrowietz U, Wustlich S, Hoexter G, et al. An experimental ointment formulation of pimecrolimus is effective in psoriasis without occlusion. Acta Derm Venereol 2003;83(5):351–3.
57. Kreuter A, Sommer A, Hyun J, et al. 1% pimecrolimus, 0.005% calcipotriol, and 0.1% betamethasone in the treatment of intertriginous psoriasis: a double-blind, randomized controlled study. Arch Dermatol 2006;142(9):1138–43.
58. Jacobi A, Braeutigam M, Mahler V, et al. Pimecrolimus 1% cream in the treatment of facial psoriasis: a 16-week open-label study. Dermatology 2008;216(2):133–6.
59. Belsito D, Wilson DC, Warshaw E, et al. A prospective randomized clinical trial of 0.1% tacrolimus ointment in a model of chronic allergic contact dermatitis. J Am Acad Dermatol 2006;55(1):40–6.
60. Saripalli YV, Gadzia JE, Belsito DV. Tacrolimus ointment 0.1% in the treatment of nickel-induced allergic contact dermatitis. J Am Acad Dermatol 2003;49(3):477–82.
61. Pacor ML, Di Lorenzo G, Martinelli N, et al. Tacrolimus ointment in nickel sulphate-induced steroid-resistant allergic contact dermatitis. Allergy Asthma Proc 2006;27(6):527–31.
62. Queille-Roussel C, Graeber M, Thurston M, et al. SDZ ASM 981 is the first non-steroid that suppresses established nickel contact dermatitis elicited by allergen challenge. Contact Dermatitis 2000;42(6):349–50.
63. Bhardwaj SS, Jaimes JP, Liu A, et al. A double-blind randomized placebo-controlled pilot study comparing topical immunomodulating agents and corticosteroids for treatment of experimentally induced nickel contact dermatitis. Dermatitis 2007;18(1):26–31.
64. Katsarou A, Armenaka M, Vosynioti V, et al. Tacrolimus ointment 0.1% in the treatment of allergic contact eyelid dermatitis. J Eur Acad Dermatol Venereol 2009;23(4):382–7.
65. Nakada T, Iijima M, Maibach HI. Eyeglass frame allergic contact dermatitis: does tacrolimus prevent recurrences? Contact Dermatitis 2005;53(4):219–21.
66. Weissenbacher S, Traidl-Hoffmann C, Eyerich K, et al. Modulation of atopy patch test and skin prick test by pretreatment with 1% pimecrolimus cream. Int Arch Allergy Immunol 2006;140(3):239–44.
67. Mensing CO, Mensing CH, Mensing H. Treatment with pimecrolimus cream 1% clears irritant dermatitis of the periocular region, face and neck. Int J Dermatol 2008;47(9):960–4.
68. Erkek E, Kazkayasi M, Bozdogan O. Acute actinic cheilitis-like chemical irritant reaction following accidental contact with ethylene glycol-favorable response to topical 1% pimecrolimus cream: a case report. Cutan Ocul Toxicol 2008;27(2):91–5.
69. Di Costanzo L, Balato N, Zagaria O, et al. Successful management of a delayed and persistent cutaneous reaction to jellyfish with pimecrolimus. J Dermatolog Treat 2009;20(3):179–80.
70. Meshkinpour A, Sun J, Weinstein G. An open pilot study using tacrolimus ointment in the treatment

of seborrheic dermatitis. J Am Acad Dermatol 2003;49(1):145–7.
71. Braza TJ, DiCarlo JB, Soon SL, et al. Tacrolimus 0.1% ointment for seborrhoeic dermatitis: an open-label pilot study. Br J Dermatol 2003;148(6):1242–4.
72. Warshaw EM, Wohlhuter RJ, Liu A, et al. Results of a randomized, double-blind, vehicle-controlled efficacy trial of pimecrolimus cream 1% for the treatment of moderate to severe facial seborrheic dermatitis. J Am Acad Dermatol 2007;57(2):257–64.
73. Firooz A, Solhpour A, Gorouchi F, et al. Pimecrolimus cream, 1%, vs hydrocortisone acetate cream, 1%, in the treatment of facial seborrheic dermatitis: a randomized, investigator-blind, clinical trial. Arch Dermatol 2006;142(8):1066–7.
74. Koc E, Arca E, Kose O, et al. An open, randomized, prospective, comparative study of topical pimecrolimus 1% cream and topical ketoconazole 2% cream in the treatment of seborrheic dermatitis. J Dermatolog Treat 2009;20(1):4–9.
75. Cicek D, Kandi B, Bakar S, et al. Pimecrolimus 1% cream, methylprednisolone aceponate 0.1% cream and metronidazole 0.75% gel in the treatment of seborrhoeic dermatitis: a randomized clinical study. J Dermatolog Treat 2009;20(6):344–9.
76. Bamford JT, Elliott BA, Haller IV. Tacrolimus effect on rosacea. J Am Acad Dermatol 2004;50(1):107–8.
77. Garg G, Thami GP. Clinical efficacy of tacrolimus in rosacea. J Eur Acad Dermatol Venereol 2009; 23(2):239–40.
78. Weissenbacher S, Merkl J, Hildebrandt B, et al. Pimecrolimus cream 1% for papulopustular rosacea: a randomized vehicle-controlled double-blind trial. Br J Dermatol 2007;156(4):728–32.
79. Karabulut AA, Izol Serel B, Eksioglu HM. A randomized, single-blind, placebo-controlled, split-face study with pimecrolimus cream 1% for papulopustular rosacea. J Eur Acad Dermatol Venereol 2008; 22(6):729–34.
80. Koca R, Altinyazar HC, Ankarali H, et al. A comparison of metronidazole 1% cream and pimecrolimus 1% cream in the treatment of patients with papulopustular rosacea: a randomized open-label clinical trial. Clin Exp Dermatol July 6, 2009. [Epub ahead of print].
81. Lee DH, Li K, Suh DH. Pimecrolimus 1% cream for the treatment of steroid-induced rosacea: an 8-week split-face clinical trial. Br J Dermatol 2008;158(5):1069–76.
82. Chu CY. An open-label pilot study to evaluate the safety and efficacy of topically applied pimecrolimus cream for the treatment of steroid-induced rosacea-like eruption. J Eur Acad Dermatol Venereol 2007;21(4):484–90.
83. Tzung TY, Liu YS, Chang HW. Tacrolimus vs. clobetasol propionate in the treatment of facial cutaneous lupus erythematosus: a randomized, double-blind, bilateral comparison study. Br J Dermatol 2007;156(1):191–2.
84. Yoshimasu T, Ohtani T, Sakamoto T, et al. Topical FK506 (tacrolimus) therapy for facial erythematous lesions of cutaneous lupus erythematosus and dermatomyositis. Eur J Dermatol 2002;12(1):50–2.
85. Walker SL, Kirby B, Chalmers RJ. The effect of topical tacrolimus on severe recalcitrant chronic discoid lupus erythematosus. Br J Dermatol 2002; 147(2):405–6.
86. Bohm M, Gaubitz M, Luger TA, et al. Topical tacrolimus as a therapeutic adjunct in patients with cutaneous lupus erythematosus. A report of three cases. Dermatology 2003;207(4):381–5.
87. Kanekura T, Yoshii N, Terasaki K, et al. Efficacy of topical tacrolimus for treating the malar rash of systemic lupus erythematosus. Br J Dermatol 2003;148(2):353–6.
88. Lampropoulos CE, Sangle S, Harrison P, et al. Topical tacrolimus therapy of resistant cutaneous lesions in lupus erythematosus: a possible alternative. Rheumatology (Oxford) 2004;43(11):1383–5.
89. Druke A, Gambichler T, Altmeyer P, et al. 0.1% Tacrolimus ointment in a patient with subacute cutaneous lupus erythematosus. J Dermatolog Treat 2004;15(1):63–4.
90. Sugano M, Shintani Y, Kobayashi K, et al. Successful treatment with topical tacrolimus in four cases of discoid lupus erythematosus. J Dermatol 2006; 33(12):887–91.
91. Heffernan MP, Nelson MM, Smith DI, et al. 0.1% tacrolimus ointment in the treatment of discoid lupus erythematosus. Arch Dermatol 2005;141(9):1170–1.
92. Barikbin B, Givrad S, Yousefi M, et al. Pimecrolimus 1% cream versus betamethasone 17-valerate 0.1% cream in the treatment of facial discoid lupus erythematosus: a double-blind, randomized pilot study. Clin Exp Dermatol 2009;34(7):776–80.
93. Tlacuilo-Parra A, Guevara-Gutierrez E, Gutierrez-Murillo F, et al. Pimecrolimus 1% cream for the treatment of discoid lupus erythematosus. Rheumatology (Oxford) 2005;44(12):1564–8.
94. Kreuter A, Gambichler T, Breuckmann F, et al. Pimecrolimus 1% cream for cutaneous lupus erythematosus. J Am Acad Dermatol 2004;51(3):407–10.
95. Zabawski E. Treatment of cutaneous lupus with Elidel. Dermatol Online J 2002;8(2):25.
96. Schwarz T, Kreiselmaier I, Bieber T, et al. A randomized, double-blind, vehicle-controlled study of 1% pimecrolimus cream in adult patients with perioral dermatitis. J Am Acad Dermatol 2008; 59(1):34–40.
97. Oppel T, Pavicic T, Kamann S, et al. Pimecrolimus cream (1%) efficacy in perioral dermatitis - results of a randomized, double-blind, vehicle-controlled study in 40 patients. J Eur Acad Dermatol Venereol 2007;21(9):1175–80.

98. Hart AL, Plamondon S, Kamm MA. Topical tacrolimus in the treatment of perianal Crohn's disease: exploratory randomized controlled trial. Inflamm Bowel Dis 2007;13(3):245–53.
99. Casson DH, Eltumi M, Tomlin S, et al. Topical tacrolimus may be effective in the treatment of oral and perineal Crohn's disease. Gut 2000;47(3): 436–40.
100. Russell RK, Richardson N, Wilson DC. Systemic absorption with complications during topical tacrolimus treatment for orofacial Crohn disease. J Pediatr Gastroenterol Nutr 2001;32(2):207–8.
101. Hengge UR, Krause W, Hofmann H, et al. Multicentre, phase II trial on the safety and efficacy of topical tacrolimus ointment for the treatment of lichen sclerosus. Br J Dermatol 2006;155(5): 1021–8.
102. Virgili A, Lauriola MM, Mantovani L, et al. Vulvar lichen sclerosus: 11 women treated with tacrolimus 0.1% ointment. Acta Derm Venereol 2007; 87(1):69–72.
103. Luesley DM, Downey GP. Topical tacrolimus in the management of lichen sclerosus. BJOG 2006; 113(7):832–4.
104. Ebert AK, Rosch WH, Vogt T. Safety and tolerability of adjuvant topical tacrolimus treatment in boys with lichen sclerosus: a prospective phase 2 study. Eur Urol 2008;54(4):932–7.
105. Assmann T, Becker-Wegerich P, Grewe M, et al. Tacrolimus ointment for the treatment of vulvar lichen sclerosus. J Am Acad Dermatol 2003; 48(6):935–7.
106. Matsumoto Y, Yamamoto T, Isobe T, et al. Successful treatment of vulvar lichen sclerosus in a child with low-concentration topical tacrolimus ointment. J Dermatol 2007;34(2):114–6.
107. Kunstfeld R, Kirnbauer R, Stingl G, et al. Successful treatment of vulvar lichen sclerosus with topical tacrolimus. Arch Dermatol 2003;139(7):850–2.
108. Ginarte M, Toribio J. Vulvar lichen sclerosus successfully treated with topical tacrolimus. Eur J Obstet Gynecol Reprod Biol 2005;123(1):123–4.
109. Bohm M, Frieling U, Luger TA, et al. Successful treatment of anogenital lichen sclerosus with topical tacrolimus. Arch Dermatol 2003;139(7):922–4.
110. Valdivielso-Ramos M, Bueno C, Hernanz JM. Significant improvement in extensive lichen sclerosus with tacrolimus ointment and PUVA. Am J Clin Dermatol 2008;9(3):175–9.
111. Wakamatsu J, Yamamoto T, Uchida H, et al. Lichen sclerosus et atrophicus of the lip: successful treatment with topical tacrolimus. J Eur Acad Dermatol Venereol 2008;22(6):760–2.
112. Goldstein AT, Marinoff SC, Christopher K. Pimecrolimus for the treatment of vulvar lichen sclerosus: a report of 4 cases. J Reprod Med 2004;49(10): 778–80.
113. Nissi R, Eriksen H, Risteli J, et al. Pimecrolimus cream 1% in the treatment of lichen sclerosus. Gynecol Obstet Invest 2007;63(3):151–4.
114. Oskay T, Sezer HK, Genc C, et al. Pimecrolimus 1% cream in the treatment of vulvar lichen sclerosus in postmenopausal women. Int J Dermatol 2007; 46(5):527–32.
115. Goldstein AT, Marinoff SC, Christopher K. Pimecrolimus for the treatment of vulvar lichen sclerosus in a premenarchal girl. J Pediatr Adolesc Gynecol 2004;17(1):35–7.
116. Arican O, Ciralik H, Sasmaz S. Unsuccessful treatment of extragenital lichen sclerosus with topical 1% pimecrolimus cream. J Dermatol 2004;31(12):1014–7.
117. Kroft EB, Groeneveld TJ, Seyger MM, et al. Efficacy of topical tacrolimus 0.1% in active plaque morphea: randomized, double-blind, emollient-controlled pilot study. Am J Clin Dermatol 2009;10(3):181–7.
118. Stefanaki C, Stefanaki K, Kontochristopoulos G, et al. Topical tacrolimus 0.1% ointment in the treatment of localized scleroderma. An open label clinical and histological study. J Dermatol 2008;35(11): 712–8.
119. Allen A, Siegfried E, Silverman R, et al. Significant absorption of topical tacrolimus in 3 patients with Netherton syndrome. Arch Dermatol 2001;137(6): 747–50.
120. Price VH, Willey A, Chen BK. Topical tacrolimus in alopecia areata. J Am Acad Dermatol 2005;52(1): 138–9.
121. Feldmann KA, Kunte C, Wollenberg A, et al. Is topical tacrolimus effective in alopecia areata universalis? Br J Dermatol 2002;147(5):1031–2.
122. Park SW, Kim JW, Wang HY. Topical tacrolimus (FK506): treatment failure in four cases of alopecia universalis. Acta Derm Venereol 2002; 82(5):387–8.
123. Thiers BH. Topical tacrolimus: treatment failure in a patient with alopecia areata. Arch Dermatol 2000;136(1):124.
124. Duque MI, Yosipovitch G, Fleischer AB Jr, et al. Lack of efficacy of tacrolimus ointment 0.1% for treatment of hemodialysis-related pruritus: a randomized, double-blind, vehicle-controlled study. J Am Acad Dermatol 2005;52(3 Pt 1):519–21.
125. Clark-Loeser L, Latkowski JA. Frontal fibrosing alopecia. Dermatol Online J 2005;11(4):6.
126. Oh CC, McKenna DB, McLaren KM, et al. Factitious panniculitis masquerading as pyoderma gangrenosum. Clin Exp Dermatol 2005;30(3):253–5.
127. Gambichler T, Tomi NS, Moussa G, et al. Topical tacrolimus neither prevents nor abolishes ultraviolet-induced erythema. J Am Acad Dermatol 2006;55(5):882–5.
128. Rigopoulos D, Gregoriou S, Korfitis C, et al. Lack of response of alopecia areata to pimecrolimus cream. Clin Exp Dermatol 2007;32(4):456–7.

129. Tan JK, Morneau K, Fung K. Randomized controlled trial of pimecrolimus 1% cream for treatment of facial acne vulgaris. J Am Acad Dermatol 2005;52(4):738–9.
130. Scope A, Lieb JA, Dusza SW, et al. A prospective randomized trial of topical pimecrolimus for cetuximab-associated acnelike eruption. J Am Acad Dermatol 2009;61(4):614–20.
131. Eiling E, Brandt M, Schwarz T, et al. Pimecrolimus: a novel treatment for cetuximab-induced papulopustular eruption. Arch Dermatol 2008;144(9):1236–8.
132. Lin A. Topical calcineurin inhibitors. In: Wolverton S, editor. Comprehensive dermatologic drug therapy. 2nd edition. Philadelphia: Saunders-Elsevier; 2007. p. 671–91.
133. Patterson C, Coutts I. Granuloma faciale successfully treated with topical tacrolimus. Australas J Dermatol 2009;50(3):217–9.
134. Rigopoulos D, Gregoriou S, Belyayeva E, et al. Efficacy and safety of tacrolimus ointment 0.1% vs. betamethasone 17-valerate 0.1% in the treatment of chronic paronychia: an unblinded randomized study. Br J Dermatol 2009;160(4):858–60.
135. Al-Mutairi N, El-Khalawany M. Clinicopathological characteristics of lichen planus pigmentosus and its response to tacrolimus ointment: an open label, non-randomized, prospective study. J Eur Acad Dermatol Venereol October 15, 2009. DOI:10.1111/j.1468-3083.2009.03460.x.
136. Rigopoulos D, Gregoriou S, Charissi C, et al. Tacrolimus ointment 0.1% in pityriasis alba: an open-label, randomized, placebo-controlled study. Br J Dermatol 2006;155(1):152–5.
137. Kleikamp S, Kutzner H, Frosch PJ. Annular lichenoid dermatitis of youth–a further case in a 12-year-old girl. J Dtsch Dermatol Ges 2008; 6(8):653–6.
138. Weisshaar E. Successful treatment of genital pruritus using topical immunomodulators as a single therapy in multi-morbid patients. Acta Derm Venereol 2008;88(2):195–6.
139. Caffier PP, Harth W, Mayelzadeh B, et al. Tacrolimus: a new option in therapy-resistant chronic external otitis. Laryngoscope 2007;117(6): 1046–52.
140. Jessup CJ, Morgan SC, Cohen LM, et al. Incontinentia pigmenti: treatment of IP with topical tacrolimus. J Drugs Dermatol 2009;8(10):944–6.
141. Jin SP, Cho KH, Huh CH. Plasma cell cheilitis, successfully treated with topical 0.03% tacrolimus ointment. J Dermatolog Treat 2009;1–3. DOI:10.1080/09546630903200620.
142. Kovich OI, Cohen DE. Granulomatous cheilitis. Dermatol Online J 2004;10(3):10.
143. Mutasim DF. Successful treatment of inflammatory linear verrucous epidermal nevus with tacrolimus and fluocinonide. J Cutan Med Surg 2006;10(1):45–7.
144. Tomi NS, Altmeyer P, Kreuter A. Tacrolimus ointment for 'jogger's nipples'. Clin Exp Dermatol 2007;32(1):106–7.
145. Shipley DR, Kennedy CT. Juvenile plantar dermatosis responding to topical tacrolimus ointment. Clin Exp Dermatol 2006;31(3):453–4.
146. Miller S. The effect of tacrolimus on lower extremity ulcers: a case study and review of the literature. Ostomy Wound Manage 2008;54(4):36–42.
147. Rongioletti F, Zaccaria E, Cozzani E, et al. Treatment of localized lichen myxedematosus of discrete type with tacrolimus ointment. J Am Acad Dermatol 2008; 58(3):530–2.
148. Aschoff R, Wozel G. Topical tacrolimus for the treatment of lichen simplex chronicus. J Dermatolog Treat 2007;18(2):115–7.
149. Campbell FA, Gupta G. Lichenoid tattoo reaction responding to topical tacrolimus ointment. Clin Exp Dermatol 2006;31(2):293–4.
150. Dauendorffer JN, Mahe E, Saiag P. Tacrolimus ointment, an interesting adjunctive therapy for childhood linear IgA bullous dermatosis. J Eur Acad Dermatol Venereol 2008;22(3):364–5.
151. Rallis E, Economidi A, Verros C, et al. Successful treatment of patch type mycosis fungoides with tacrolimus ointment 0.1%. J Drugs Dermatol 2006;5(9):906–7.
152. Manzur A, Siddiqui AH. Necrolytic acral erythema: successful treatment with topical tacrolimus ointment. Int J Dermatol 2008;47(10):1073–5.
153. Virgili A, Mantovani L, Lauriola MM, et al. Tacrolimus 0.1% ointment: is it really effective in plasma cell vulvitis? Report of four cases. Dermatology 2008;216(3):243–6.
154. Dissemond J, Knab J, Lehnen M, et al. Successful treatment of stasis dermatitis with topical tacrolimus. Vasa 2004;33(4):260–2.
155. Erkek E, Sahin S, Kilic R, et al. A case of cheilitis glandularis superimposed on oral lichen planus: successful palliative treatment with topical tacrolimus and pimecrolimus. J Eur Acad Dermatol Venereol 2007;21(7):999–1000.
156. Day I, Lin AN. Use of pimecrolimus cream in disorders other than atopic dermatitis. J Cutan Med Surg 2008;12(1):17–26.
157. Kelekci HK, Uncu HG, Yilmaz B, et al. Pimecrolimus 1% cream for pruritus in postmenopausal diabetic women with vulvar lichen simplex chronicus: a prospective non-controlled case series. J Dermatolog Treat 2008;19(5):274–8.
158. Katoulis A, Georgala S, Bozi E, et al. Frontal fibrosing alopecia: treatment with oral dutasteride and topical pimecrolimus. J Eur Acad Dermatol Venereol 2009; 23(5):580–2.
159. Schurmeyer-Horst F, Luger TA, Bohm M. Long-term efficacy of occlusive therapy with topical pimecrolimus in severe dyshidrosiform hand and foot eczema. Dermatology 2007;214(1):99–100.

160. Tan C, Zhu WY, Min ZS. A case of recurrent eruptive pseudo-angiomatosis that responded well to pimecrolimus 1% cream. Dermatology 2009;218(2):181–3.
161. Gorpelioglu C, Sarifakioglu E, Bayrak R. A case of follicular mucinosis treated successfully with pimecrolimus. Clin Exp Dermatol 2009;34(1):86–7.
162. Gregoriou S, Argyriou G, Christofidou E, et al. Treatment of pityriasis rubra pilaris with pimecrolimus cream 1%. J Drugs Dermatol 2007;6(3):340–2.
163. Bellini V, Simonetti S, Lisi P. Successful treatment of severe pyoderma gangrenosum with pimecrolimus cream 1%. J Eur Acad Dermatol Venereol 2008; 22(1):113–5.
164. Mansouri P, Farshi S, Nahavandi A, et al. Pimecrolimus 1 percent cream and pulsed dye laser in treatment of a patient with reticular erythematous mucinosis syndrome. Dermatol Online J 2007; 13(2):22.
165. Bardazzi F, Antonucci A, Savoia F, et al. Two cases of Zoon's balanitis treated with pimecrolimus 1% cream. Int J Dermatol 2008;47(2): 198–201.
166. Fujita WH, McCormick CL, Parneix-Spake A. An exploratory study to evaluate the efficacy of pimecrolimus cream 1% for the treatment of pityriasis alba. Int J Dermatol 2007;46(7):700–5.

Innovative Uses of Rituximab in Dermatology

David R. Carr, MD[a], Michael P. Heffernan, MD[b,*]

KEYWORDS

• Biologics • Rituximab • Dermatology

Rituximab (Rituxan, Genentech, San Francisco, CA, USA and MabThera, Roche, Basel, Switzerland) is a chimeric murine-human monoclonal antibody (IgG1 k) directed against CD20 that induces depletion of B cells in vivo.[1] CD20 is a transmembrane protein found on pre-B–cell and mature lymphocytes. Rituximab was initially developed for treatment of lymphoma, and is currently approved for CD20+ B-cell lymphoma and rheumatoid arthritis unresponsive to other therapies.[2]

Although the US Food and Drug Administration (FDA)-approved indications are limited, numerous off-label uses have evolved. Aside from dermatologic indications, there are reports of efficacy in rheumatology, solid organ transplantation, renal disease, neuromuscular disorders, and endocrine disorders.[3]

Rituximab's site of action is at the CD20 receptor. CD20 is a B-cell specific antigen expressed on the surface of B lymphocytes throughout differentiation from the pre-B–cell to the mature B-cell–stage, but not on plasma cells or stem cells.[1,4] Because plasma cells and hematopoietic precursors are spared, immunoglobulin levels do not fall dramatically and B cells typically begin to return to the circulation within 6 months of therapy.[5,6] Rituximab's cytotoxicity in vitro is mediated by three mechanisms including antibody-dependent cellular cytotoxicity, complement-mediated lysis, and direct disruption of signaling pathways and triggering of apoptosis. The contribution of each mechanism in vivo remains unclear, and different mechanisms may predominate in the treatment of different diseases.[7–9] Additionally, studies in low-grade lymphomas and systemic lupus erythematosus (SLE) have shown that polymorphisms of FcγRIII (receptor for IgG1 found on natural killers cells and macrophages) effect the elimination of B lymphocytes with rituximab therapy. Anolik and colleagues[10] found that subjects with the high affinity FcγRIIIa-158V phenotype had a higher degree of B-cell depletion than those homozygous for FcγRIIIa-158F.

The initial approved dosing regimen was 4 weekly infusions of 375 mg/m^2. This dosage was rather arbitrarily based on two phase I studies looking at single 10 to 500mg/m^2 infusions and 4 weekly infusions of 125 to 500 mg/m^2.[6,11] The results did not show a dose-dependent increase in efficacy or increase in side effects. Alternatively, two 1000 mg intravenous infusions separated by 2 weeks are used for the standard dosage in patients with rheumatoid arthritis. To date, there is no consensus on the most efficacious dosing regimen, and further studies comparing various regimens are necessary.

The incidence of serious adverse effects with rituximab is low. Infusion reactions are the most common adverse event. In most cases these are mild and occur only with the first infusion.[5,12]

This article is completely self-generated and has not received any outside funding.
This article only reflects the views of its authors.
Dr Heffernan has been a paid investigator, lecturer or consultant for Abbott, Amgen, Biogen-IDEC, Centocor, and Genentech.
Contents of this article were presented, in part, at the 64th Annual Meeting of the American Academy of Dermatology, March, 2006.
[a] Department of Dermatology, Wright State University, One Elizabeth Place, Suite 200, Dayton, OH 45408, USA
[b] Central Dermatology, 1034 South Brentwood Avenue, Suite 600, St Louis, MO 63117, USA
* Corresponding author.
E-mail address: Heffernan@centralderm.com

Dermatol Clin 28 (2010) 547–557
doi:10.1016/j.det.2010.03.002
0733-8635/10/$ – see front matter © 2010 Elsevier Inc. All rights reserved.

Patients are often premedicated with acetaminophen and diphenhydramine to prevent or blunt infusion reactions. In a recent study of rituximab for the treatment of rheumatoid arthritis (RA), infections occurred in 35% of subjects in the rituximab group as compared with 28% of the placebo group. Serious infections occurred in 2% of the rituximab group as compared with 1% of the placebo group.[13] Human anti-chimeric antibodies (HACAs) develop in less than 1% of patients treated for lymphoma, though the incidence may be higher in patients treated for autoimmune disease.[14] In a study of rituximab for SLE, 6 of 18 subjects developed detectable HACAs; however, no subjects had adverse events related to this development.[15] HACAs also developed in 2 of 11 subjects in a recent study of rituximab for pemphigus vulgaris. In this report, there was an association between an increase in HACA levels and increased disease activity.[16]

There have also been three cases of rapid onset cutaneous squamous cell carcinoma and two cases of rapid onset Merkel cell carcinoma.[17] Late onset neutropenia has been reported in patients with lymphoma,[18] pemphigus,[19] and vasculitis[20] treated with rituximab.

Recent reports describe two cases of progressive multifocal leukoencephalopathy (PML) in patients with SLE and one patient with rheumatoid arthritis treated with rituximab.[21,22] A review of case reports from the US FDA, the manufacturer, and a literature review from 1997 to 2008 revealed 59 cases of PML in patients who were HIV-negative and treated with rituximab. Of these, 52 had lymphoproliferative disorders, three had RA, two had SLE, and one subject each of idiopathic autoimmune pancytopenia and immune thrombocytopenia.[18] The median time to diagnosis of PML was 5.5 months after the last rituximab dose and the median time to death after PML diagnosis was 2 months with a fatality rate of 90%. The two subjects with SLE had previously been treated with corticosteroids and alkylating agents; whereas, two of the subjects with RA had other risk factors for PML, including chemotherapy and radiation therapy, or long-standing lymphopenia. The most recent report of PML in RA (October 2009) was in a patient who had been treated with leflunomide, hydroxychloroquine, and prednisone. This report was the first of PML in a patient with RA who had not received antecedent therapy with a tumor necrosis factor-alpha antagonist.

OFF-LABEL USES OF RITUXIMAB

Rituximab results in the depletion of normal and malignant B cells, leading to investigation of its use in autoimmune disorders, including SLE, RA, autoimmune thrombocytopenia and hemolytic anemia, and autoimmune neuropathies.[23,24] It has shown promise in the treatment of RA[13,25] and SLE.[23] Although there have been no randomized, controlled trials of rituximab in dermatologic disease, case reports describe its use in pemphigus vulgaris; pemphigus foliaceus; paraneoplastic pemphigus; epidermolysis bullosa acquisita; bullous pemphigoid; mucous membrane pemphigoid; cutaneous B-cell lymphoma; dermatomyositis; cutaneous lupus erythematosus; graft versus host disease (GVHD); Wegener's granulomatosis (WG); microscopic polyangiitis; cryoglobulinemic vasculitis; and Churg-Strauss syndrome.

Pemphigus Vulgaris, Pemphigus Foliaceus, and Paraneoplastic Pemphigus

Rituximab treatment of pemphigus vulgaris (PV) was first attempted based on the success in other autoimmune disorders and the hypothesis that depletion of B cells would result in a decrease in production of the disease-causing autoantibodies.[26] The correlation of decreases in PV autoantibody levels with clinical improvement in most of the patients in which these levels were reported would seem to support this theory.[26–29] This suggests that most PV autoantibodies are produced by CD20+ B-cell clones susceptible to rituximab.[27,29] Alternatively, it has been suggested that although plasma cells and memory B cells may produce PV autoantibodies, plasma cells, which are CD20- and thus resistant to the effects of rituximab, may predominantly produce the less pathogenic IgG1 desmoglein 3 antibodies, whereas the memory B cells produce the IgG4 antibodies responsible for disease. This suggestion might explain the clinical improvement in the face of persistently elevated PV antibody titers observed in one patient and the improvement preceding decreased titers in a second patient.[30,31] Furthermore, in patients with SLE, clinical improvement after rituximab is regularly correlated with B-cell depletion, but not to any decrease in other serologic markers or autoantibody levels. It is postulated that disruption of antibody-independent activities of B cells, including presentation of autoantigens, co-stimulation of T cells, and regulation of leukocytes and dendritic cells, are central to rituximab's effect on the disease.[23] Thus, the critical effects of rituximab in PV may expand beyond decreasing autoantibody production to inhibiting B-cell dependent activation of T cells.

Recent work showed decreased titers of antidesmoglein-1 and antidesmoglein-3 antibodies in response to rituximab treatment. No changes in the titers of antibodies to pneumococcal capsule polysaccharide and tetanus toxoid were noted in one study group[32]; and an increase in anti-varicella zoster virus-IgG and anti-Epstein-Barr virus-IgG titers were seen in a separate group of subjects with PV treated with rituximab. This finding suggests that rituximab may preferentially decrease the numbers of autoreactive (short-lived) plasma cells, while not affecting or increasing the antibody release from pathogen-specific (long-lived) plasma cells.[33]

Over time, the B-cell population re-emerges, though these cells have the phenotype of naïve B cells (not primed B lymphocytes).[31] The repopulation with naïve cells may explain the long-lasting effect of rituximab in many cases.

The successful use of rituximab in over 130 individual cases of treatment resistant pemphigus vulgaris and pemphigus foliaceus have been reported.[26–31,34–46] The majority of cases used a protocol previously described for patients with lymphoma of 375 mg/m^2 intravenously for four weekly dosages. Ahmed and colleagues described nine subjects with PV who received two cycles of 375mg/m^2 of rituximab intravenously for three weekly dosages followed by intravenous immunoglobulin (IVIG) 2g/kg intravenously in the fourth week; then subjects received four monthly infusions of intravenous rituximab and IVIG. Because of rituximab's slower onset of action (generally 2 to 3 weeks), it has also been combined with immunoadsorption, which has a quick onset of action.[47,48] Finally, several series describe chronic infusions every 4 to 12 weeks after an induction of four weekly infusions.[49,50] B-cell depletion following treatment was seen in all cases in which it was measured. In most cases, improvement was noted within the first 2 to 6 weeks. However, there are several reports of a delayed response, where improvement was not noted for 6 to 12 months.[40,45,51]

A recent literature review of rituximab in patients with pemphigus[46] noted in PV a 40% complete remission (clinical remission with no further therapy necessary); 37% clinical remission (clinical remission, but further immunosuppression required); and a 21% partial remission. In pemphigus foliaceus, 40% experienced a complete remission, 45% clinical remission, and 10% partial remission. The relapse rates for PV and pemphigus foliaceus were 13% and 18%, respectively.

Rituximab was well tolerated in most of the PV and PF cases reported, consistent with the observations made in lymphoma and other autoimmune disorders. However, nine serious infections were reported; including three bacterial pneumonias, a relapse of septic arthritis of the hip,[27] four instances of sepsis,[26] two *Pneumocystis carinii* pneumonias,[39] cytomegalovirus gastritis, and pyelonephritis. These events may indicate that close surveillance of patients with pemphigus undergoing rituximab treatment is warranted until the incidence and characterization of infectious complications in this patient population is better understood.

Multiple case reports suggest rituximab's efficacy is less impressive in paraneoplastic pemphigus (PNP). Four case reports describe significant improvement in oral and cutaneous lesions after rituximab[52–55]; however, one report describes only partial improvement[56] and five additional reports describe less successful results, especially with regard to mucosal lesions.[57–61] The mechanism of action in PNP is likely similar to that in PV. In addition, most of the treated patients experienced at least partial remission of the underlying neoplasm and this may have contributed to the observed improvement.

Epidermolysis Bullosa Acquisita

There are seven reports of patients with refractory epidermolysis bullosa acquisita (EBA), treated with rituximab. Four patients achieved complete remission,[62–65] two had a partial response,[65,66] and one patient died of *Pseudomonas* pneumonia 1 week after the patient's first rituximab infusion.[67] Clinical response was seen after 8 weeks to 5 months. In one patient, IgG immunoblot reactivity to type VII collagen was undetectable 12 weeks after rituximab was initiated.[62] Complete remission was achieved 11 weeks after the first infusion and was maintained for over 1 year of follow-up allowing for tapering and discontinuation of the patient's prednisolone and colchicine. Another patient, who had clinical remission 5 months after rituximab, subsequently developed small mechanical blisters and was treated with continued mycophenolate mofetil (MMF) and a decreased dose of prednisolone. IgG immunoblot testing to type VII collagen was 1:10 1 year after treatment (from a height of 1:3200 before beginning rituximab).[63] Two patients were treated with a combination of immunoadsorption and rituximab; one had complete remission, the other only had a partial response.[65] The mechanism of action of rituximab in EBA is likely similar to that in PV.

Bullous Pemphigoid

Eight cases of recalcitrant bullous pemphigoid (BP) treated with rituximab have been reported. The efficacy appears to be quite high, though use of multiple disparate dosing regimens along with only several case reports makes interpretation of efficacy difficult. Of the eight subjects, six had documented clinical remission, one had a partial response, and one died 6 weeks after starting rituximab therapy from nosocomial bacterial pneumonia. Two of those responding also had chronic lymphocytic leukemia (under complete remission).[68] These subjects were treated with the more standard four weekly infusions of 375 mg/m^2, but they subsequently received a rituximab dose of 375 mg/m^2 every 2 months without recurrence of bullae (3 years of follow-up reported). One of the two subjects reported by Schmidt and colleagues[45] (the second died 6 weeks after starting rituximab) was a 2-year-old child who achieved clinical remission after rituximab therapy (24 months of follow-up reported). The subject received four weekly doses of 375mg/m^2 intravenously and had a decrease in BP 180 autoantibody levels from 3538 units/mL to 77 units/mL. A second pediatric subject had complete clinical remission after two courses of rituximab (the dose during the second course was decreased to 187.5 mg/m^2), though there was only 20 weeks of follow-up.[69] Reguiai and colleagues[70] reported a subject who had complete clinical and immunologic response after two courses of rituximab (2.5 years of follow-up reported). The one subject with bullous pemphigoid reported with a partial response only received two doses of rituximab (375 mg/m^2) 4 weeks apart.[71] Notably, in the face of continued clinical disease the subject had undetectable B-cell levels within 3 weeks (persisting for at least 28 weeks) and eventual negative anti-basement membrane zone antibody titers. The mechanism of action is likely similar to that in PV.

Mucous Membrane Pemphigoid

There are three cases of successful use of rituximab in refractory mucous membrane pemphigoid.[72–74] One subject received four weekly infusions of rituximab (375 mg/m^2) and was able to stop oral steroids within 6 months, without recurrence of disease at 12 months after rituximab therapy.[72] Another subject received two infusions of 862.5 mg and remission was maintained at 12 months while the subject continued on prednisolone 10 mg daily and MMF 1 g twice a day (onset of improvement not discussed).[74]

Primary Cutaneous B-cell Lymphoma

Based on its successful use in nodal B-cell lymphoma, rituximab has been employed in the treatment of primary cutaneous B-cell lymphoma (PCBCL). Approximately 60 individual cases of PCBCL treated with systemic rituximab have been reported in the literature. The cases represent a variety of histologic subtypes, including primary cutaneous follicle center lymphoma (PCFCL); primary cutaneous marginal zone lymphoma (PCMZL); primary cutaneous diffuse large B-cell lymphoma-leg type (PCLBCL-LT); diffuse large B cell lymphoma; and mantle cell lymphoma.

Intravenous and intralesional administrations have been used. Intralesional injection allows for considerably smaller doses of rituximab compared with intravenous administration, with single doses of less than 10% of the recommend dose for systemic therapy.[75] However, case reports to date suggest an increase in recurrence rate with intralesional therapy.[75–77] Additionally, one subject treated with intralesional rituximab achieved clearance of one untreated lesion, suggesting a systemic therapeutic effect of locally injected rituximab. This is further supported by the fact that local administration of rituximab also causes depletion of B lymphocytes in the peripheral blood.[75,77]

Primary Cutaneous Marginal Zone Lymphoma

Five reports describe the use of intravenous rituximab in 13 subjects with PCMZL (375 mg/m^2 weekly for 4 to 8 weeks, 12/13 had multifocal disease).[75,76,78] Overall, complete remission was seen in seven (54%), partial remission in four (31%), stable disease in one (8%), and progressive disease in one (8%). Intralesional rituximab (5–30 mg once or three times per week) was reported in 10 subjects (all subjects with less than four lesions clinically), with eight (80%) achieving complete remission and the other two subjects (20%) achieving partial remission.[77,79–81] The relapse rates were four out of seven (57%) and five out of eight (62%) for intravenous and intralesional subjects, respectively.

Primary Cutaneous Follicle Center Lymphoma

Use of intravenous rituximab has been reported in 49 subjects with PCFCL (375 mg/m^2 weekly for 1 to 9 weeks). Overall, complete remission was seen in 40 (82%), partial remission in eight (16%), and progressive disease in one (2%). Intralesional rituximab (10–30 mg two to three times per week; though treatment duration varied from 2 weeks to 6 months) was reported in 12 subjects, with 10 (83%) achieving complete remission and two (17%) achieving partial remission. The relapse rates were 12 out of 40 (30%) and 2 out of 12 (17%) for intravenous and intralesional subjects, respectively.

Primary Cutaneous Diffuse Large B-Cell Lymphoma-Leg Type

Eight reports describe the single-agent use of intravenous rituximab in 13 subjects with PCLBCL-LT (375 mg/m^2 weekly for 4 to 8 weeks).[82–89] Overall, complete remission was seen in five (38%). None of the five subjects with complete remission relapsed, though the average duration of follow-up was short at 7 months. Because of the more aggressive clinical course of PCLBCL-LT, current recommendations are for systemic chemotherapy with or without the addition of rituximab (though single agent rituximab may be a consideration in patients who cannot tolerate other therapies). A recent review of 60 cases of PCLBCL-LT noted a complete remission in 11 out of 12 (92%) subjects treated with various combinations of anthracycline-containing chemotherapies and rituximab, whereas those treated with other therapies had a complete remission of 62%.[90] The authors suggest a short-term advantage to anthracycline-containing chemotherapies and rituximab (follow-up was short, with a mean of 19 months).

Dermatomyositis

There are two pilot studies describing the use of intravenous rituximab in 15 subjects with dermatomyositis (DM).[91,92] In one study, seven subjects received four weekly infusions at a dosage of 100 mg/m^2 (three subjects) or 375 mg/m^2 (three subjects).[91] In the second study, eight subjects received two infusions of 1 g given two weeks apart.[92] Subjects were allowed to continue on a stable regimen of concomitant immunosuppressive medications during the trials. In the first study, all subjects had significant improvement in cutaneous and muscle disease (from 36%–113% improvement in strength scores over baseline testing).[91] In the second study, three out of eight (38%) achieved partial remission (>50% improvement in muscle strength), although there was no change in cutaneous disease in any of the subjects.[92] The authors postulate that the less dramatic results than the previously described open-label study may have been caused by a study population with milder disease or the different dosing regimens used.

The proposed mechanism of rituximab in DM is not well elucidated, and there are still many uncertainties regarding the role of B cells in this disease.[93] The current model for the pathogenesis of DM holds that autoantibodies bind to an antigen on the endothelial cell wall of endomysial capillaries, leading to the activation of complement C3 and the deposition of C5b-9 membrane attack complex. This action is followed by endothelial cell swelling, necrosis, perivascular inflammation, movement of activated T cells into perimysial and endomysial spaces, and finally muscle ischemia.[93,94] Immunopathologic studies also provide support for the role of microvascular injury in skin disease.[95] Rituximab may act by decreasing B-cell production of one of the defined autoantibodies or of an as yet unidentified autoantibody to an endothelial cell autoantigen. Alternatively, it may act through dysregulation of the B cell/T cell interaction and disrupt the expansion of autoreactive T-cell populations as previously suggested in SLE.[23]

Cutaneous Lupus Erythematosus

There have been two cases of refractory subacute cutaneous lupus erythematosus treated with rituximab. One subject responded within 8 weeks of rituximab therapy (four weekly dosages of 375 mg/m^2). There was disease recurrence at 11 months, at which time rituximab was reintroduced as a maintenance regimen of 375 mg/m^2 every 8 weeks for 2 years without recurrence.[96] The second subject received two 1 g dosages 1 week apart. The subject had a partial response and remained under good control with an eventual discontinuation of oral corticosteroids.[97] The follow-up time was short at 6 months.

Graft Versus Host Disease (Acute and Chronic)

The use of rituximab in the treatment of chronic GVHD has been reported in several case series and small clinical trials.[98–105] The largest series is a phase I/II trial featuring 21 subjects with steroid-refractory disease.[98] Cutaneous findings included sclerodermoid and lichenoid changes. Subjects were treated with one, two, or three cycles of four weekly infusions of rituximab at a dosage of 375 mg/m^2. Subjects were allowed to continue on stable dosages of other immunosuppressive medications throughout the trial. The overall clinical response rate was 70%, including two complete responses. Cutaneous and musculoskeletal manifestations of GVHD were more amenable to treatment with rituximab than mucous membrane and hepatic manifestations. The overall response rate in all reported cases was between 43% and 80%; most responses were partial (rare cases of complete response).[106] Currently, there is a phase I/II trial looking at rituximab as a prophylactic treatment for chronic GVHD. Experimental evidence has indicated that T cells and NK cells play a central role in the pathogenesis of chronic GVHD.[107] Evidence for the involvement of B cells has also been accumulating. In one mouse model of chronic GVHD, an expansion of host B cells directed by CD4+ T cells is a critical step in the development of disease.[101] Subjects with chronic GVHD develop autoantibodies similar to those seen in patients with autoimmune disease.[99,107,108] Antibodies to Y chromosome-encoded minor histocompatibility antigens are generated after sex-mismatched transplantation and the presence of these antibodies has been correlated to the occurrence of GVHD.[109,110] In the phase I/II trial discussed previously, there were four male recipients of female grafts. All four of these subjects had autoantibodies before treatment that became undetectable after rituximab, which correlated with their clinical response.[98]

In mice, rates of acute GVHD were decreased with B-cell depletion.[111] Kamble and colleagues[112] reported three cases of rituximab therapy inducing complete remission in acute GVHD. The subjects received between two and four weekly dosages (dosage not reported) and response times were between 15 and 37 days. One of the subjects did go on to develop residual, limited chronic GVHD and died of sepsis 160 days after transplantation (102 days after initiating rituximab). Additionally, rituximab given as part of a conditioning regimen shortly before or after transplantation resulted in lower acute GVHD rates,[101,113–116] whereas post-transplant rituximab did not reduce acute GVHD rates in one series of subjects receiving allogenic stem cell transplantations.[117] The authors of a recent review suggest that the timing of rituximab administration is likely a relevant factor.[106] The role of B cells in acute GVHD is unknown, but their implication is questioned by the efficacy of rituximab in acute GVHD and the increasing research implicating B cells in the pathogenesis of chronic GVHD.

Vasculitis

Rituximab for antineutrophil cytoplasmic antibody-associated vasculitis (AAV) (Wegener's vasculitis and microscopic polyangiitis) has been reported in multiple case reports,[118–122] case series,[123–127] prospective open label trials,[128–131] and recently in a retrospective multicenter study.[20] The results of the multicenter study mirrored the cumulative results of the case reports and series. Most subjects (n = 65) received two infusions of 1 g given 2 weeks apart (n = 32) or four infusions of 375mg/m^2 given at 1-week intervals (n = 26). Overall, 49 out of 65 (75%) had complete remission, 15 out of 65 (23%) had partial remission, and 1 out of 65 (2%) had no response to rituximab.[20] Aries and colleagues[129] reported on eight subjects, of which six did not respond to rituximab. These subjects had prominent granulomatous disease and B-cell depletion was not associated with decreasing antineutrophil cytoplasmic autoantibody (ANCA) titres. Omdal and colleagues[123] reported two subjects with prominent granulomatous disease who did not achieve remission. Conversely, most subjects with vasculitis-prominent disease responded well. This finding suggests rituximab may be effective for AAV vasculitis, whereas the utility for granulomas in WG remains unclear.

A primary effect of rituximab is to deplete the B-cell population. This depletion would decrease the production of ANCA, an important player in the pathogenesis of AAV.[132,133] ANCA titres, though, do not correlate well with disease activity and patients may relapse without detectable ANCA levels. Therefore, the exact role of B cells (and rituximab) in AAV is indeterminate.

In addition to ANCA associated vasculitis, case reports show rituximab may also be efficacious in cryoglobulinemic vasculitis, Churg-Strauss syndrome, and Henoch-Schönlein purpura.

SUMMARY

Rituximab's efficacy has been shown in a variety of dermatologic diseases. As case reports and randomized trials explore the utility of rituximab, the indications for rituximab will continue to be delineated.

REFERENCES

1. Reff ME, Carner K, Chambers KS, et al. Depletion of B cells in vivo by a chimeric mouse human monoclonal antibody to CD20. Blood 1994;83(2):435–45.
2. Grillo-Lopez AJ. Rituximab: an insider's historical perspective. Semin Oncol 2000;27(6 Suppl. 12): 9–16.
3. McDonald V, Leandro M. Rituximab in non-haematological disorders of adults and its mode of action. Br J Haematol 2009;146:233–46.
4. Stashenko P, Nadler LM, Hardy R, et al. Characterization of a human B lymphocyte-specific antigen. J Immunol 1980;125(4):1678–85.
5. Maloney DG, Grillo-Lopez AJ, White CA, et al. IDEC-C2B8 (Rituximab) anti-CD20 monoclonal antibody therapy in patients with relapsed low-grade non-Hodgkin's lymphoma. Blood 1997; 90(6):2188–95.
6. Maloney DG, Liles TM, Czerwinski DK, et al. Phase I clinical trial using escalating single-dose infusion of chimeric anti-CD20 monoclonal antibody (IDEC-C2B8) in patients with recurrent B-cell lymphoma. Blood 1994;84(8):2457–66.

7. Johnson PW, Glennie MJ. Rituximab: mechanisms and applications. Br J Cancer 2001; 85(11):1619–23.
8. Olszewski AJ, Grossbard ML. Empowering targeted therapy: lessons from rituximab. Sci STKE 2004;2004(241):pe30.
9. Cartron G, Watier H, Golay J, et al. From the bench to the bedside: ways to improve rituximab efficacy. Blood 2004;104:2635–42.
10. Anolik JH, Campbell D, Felger RE, et al. The relationship of FcgammaRIIIa genotype to degree of B cell depletion by rituximab in the treatment of systemic lupus erythematosus. Arthritis Rheum 2003;48:455–9.
11. Maloney DG, Grillo-Lopez AJ, Bodkin DJ, et al. IDEC-C2B8: results of a phase I multiple-dose trial in patients with relapsed non-Hodgkin's lymphoma. J Clin Oncol 1997;15:3266–74.
12. Hainsworth JD. Safety of rituximab in the treatment of B cell malignancies: implications for rheumatoid arthritis. Arthritis Res Ther 2003;5(Suppl 4):S12–6.
13. Emery P, Fleischmann R, Filipowicz-Sosnowska A, et al. The efficacy and safety of rituximab in patients with active rheumatoid arthritis despite methotrexate treatment: results of a phase IIB randomized, double-blind, placebo-controlled, dose-ranging trial. Arthritis Rheum 2006;54(5): 1390–400.
14. McLaughlin P, Grillo-Lopez AJ, Link BK, et al. Rituximab chimeric anti-CD20 monoclonal antibody therapy for relapsed indolent lymphoma: half of patients respond to a four-dose treatment program. J Clin Oncol 1998;16(8):2825–33.
15. Looney RJ, Anolik JH, Campbell D, et al. B cell depletion as a novel treatment for systemic lupus erythematosus: a phase I/II dose-escalation trial of rituximab. Arthritis Rheum 2004;50(8):2580–9.
16. Schmidt E, Hennig K, Mengede C, et al. Immunogenicity of rituximab in patients with severe pemphigus. Clin Immunol 2009;132:334–41.
17. Fogarty GB, Bayne M, Bedford P, et al. Three cases of activation of cutaneous squamous cell carcinoma during treatment with prolonged administration of rituximab. Clin Oncol 2006;18(2):155–6.
18. Tesfa D, Gelius T, Sander B, et al. Late-onset neutropenia associated with rituximab therapy: evidence for a maturation arrest at the (pro)myelocyte stage of granulopoiesis. Med Oncol 2008; 25:374–9.
19. Rios-Fernandez R, Gutierrez-Salmeron MT, Callejas-Rubio JL, et al. Late-onset neutropenia following rituximab treatment in patients with autoimmune diseases. Br J Dermatol 2007;157:1271–3.
20. Jones RB, Ferraro AJ, Chaudhry AN, et al. A multicenter survey of rituximab therapy for refractory antineutrophil cytoplasmic antibody-associated vasculitis. Arthritis Rheum 2009;60(7):2156–68.
21. Food and Drug Administration. FDA warns of safety concern regarding Rituxan in new patient population. [online] 2006. Available at: http://www.fda.gov/bbs/topics/NEWS/2006/NEW01532.html. Accessed February 20, 2007.
22. Carson KR, Evens AM, Richey EA, et al. Progressive multifocal leukoencephalopathy after rituximab therapy in HIV-negative patients: a report of 57 cases from the research on adverse drug events and reports project. Blood 2009;113(20): 4834–40.
23. Looney RJ, Anolik J, Sanz I. B cells as therapeutic targets for rheumatic diseases. Curr Opin Rheumatol 2004;16(3):180–5.
24. Silverman GJ, Weisman S. Rituximab therapy and autoimmune disorders: prospects for anti-B cell therapy. Arthritis Rheum 2003;48(6):1484–92.
25. Edwards JC, Szczepanski L, Szechinski J, et al. Efficacy of B-cell-targeted therapy with rituximab in patients with rheumatoid arthritis. N Engl J Med 2004;350(25):2572–81.
26. Salopek TG, Logsetty S, Tredget EE. Anti-CD20 chimeric monoclonal antibody (rituximab) for the treatment of recalcitrant, life-threatening pemphigus vulgaris with implications in the pathogenesis of the disorder. J Am Acad Dermatol 2002;47(5): 785–8.
27. Dupuy A, Viguier M, Bedane C, et al. Treatment of refractory pemphigus vulgaris with rituximab (anti-CD20 monoclonal antibody). Arch Dermatol 2004; 140(1):91–6.
28. Goebeler M, Herzog S, Brocker EB, et al. Rapid response of treatment-resistant pemphigus foliaceus to the anti-CD20 antibody rituximab. Br J Dermatol 2003;149(4):899–901.
29. Herrmann G, Hunzelmann N, Engert A. Treatment of pemphigus vulgaris with anti-CD20 monoclonal antibody (rituximab). Br J Dermatol 2003;148(3):602–3.
30. Cooper HL, Healy E, Theaker JM, et al. Treatment of resistant pemphigus vulgaris with an anti-CD20 monoclonal antibody (Rituximab). Clin Exp Dermatol 2003;28(4):366–8.
31. Espana A, Fernandez-Galar M, Lloret P, et al. Long-term complete remission of severe pemphigus vulgaris with monoclonal anti-CD20 antibody therapy and immunophenotype correlations. J Am Acad Dermatol 2004;50(6):974–6.
32. Mouquet H, Musett P, Gougeon ML, et al. B-cell depletion immunotherapy in pemphigus: effects on cellular and humoral immune responses. J Invest Dermatol 2008;128:2859–69.
33. Nagel A, Podstawa E, Eickmann M, et al. Rituximab mediates a strong elevation of B-cell-activating factor associated with increased pathogen-specific IgG but not autoantibodies in pemphigus vulgaris. J Invest Dermatol 2009;129:2202–10.

34. Virgolini L, Marzocchi V. Anti-CD20 monoclonal antibody (rituximab) in the treatment of autoimmune diseases. Successful result in refractory Pemphigus vulgaris: report of a case. Haematologica 2003;88(7):ELT24.
35. Arin MJ, Engert A, Krieg T, et al. Anti-CD20 monoclonal antibody (rituximab) in the treatment of pemphigus. Br J Dermatol 2005;153(3):620–5.
36. Belgi AS, Azeez M, Hoyle C, et al. Response of pemphigus vulgaris to anti-CD20 antibody therapy (rituximab) may be delayed. Clin Exp Dermatol 2006;31(1):143.
37. Esposito M, Capriotti E, Giunta A, et al. Long-lasting remission of pemphigus vulgaris treated with rituximab. Acta Derm Venereol 2006;86(1): 87–9.
38. Kong HH, Prose NS, Ware RE, et al. Successful treatment of refractory childhood pemphigus vulgaris with anti-CD20 monoclonal antibody (rituximab). Pediatr Dermatol 2005;22(5):461–4.
39. Morrison LH. Therapy of refractory pemphigus vulgaris with monoclonal anti-CD20 antibody (rituximab). J Am Acad Dermatol 2004;51(5):817–9.
40. Niedermeier A, Worl P, Barth S, et al. Delayed response of oral pemphigus vulgaris to rituximab treatment. Eur J Dermatol 2006;16(3):266–70.
41. Schmidt E, Herzog S, Brocker EB, et al. Long-standing remission of recalcitrant juvenile pemphigus vulgaris after adjuvant therapy with rituximab. Br J Dermatol 2005;153(2):449–51.
42. Wenzel J, Bauer R, Bieber T, et al. Successful rituximab treatment of severe pemphigus vulgaris resistant to multiple immunosuppressants. Acta Derm Venereol 2005;85(2):185–6.
43. Ahmed AR, Spigelman Z, Cavacini LA, et al. Treatment of pemphigus vulgaris with rituximab and intravenous immune globulin. N Engl J Med 2006; 355:17772–9.
44. Borel C, Launay F, Garrouste C, et al. [Rituximab induced remission of pemphigus vulgaris: 2 cases]. Rev Med Interne 2007. DOI:10.1016/j.revmed.2006.11.012 [in French].
45. Schmidt E, Seitz CS, Benoit S, et al. Rituximab in autoimmune bullous diseases: mixed responses and adverse effects. Br J Dermatol 2007;156: 352–6.
46. Schmidt E, Goebeler M, Zillikens D. Rituximab in severe pemphigus. Ann N Y Acad Sci 2009;1173: 683–91.
47. Schmidt E, Klinker E, Opitz A, et al. Protein A immunoadsorption: a novel and effective adjuvant treatment of severe pemphigus. Br J Dermatol 2003; 148:1222–9.
48. Shimanovich I, Nitschke M, Rose C, et al. Treatment of severe pemphigus with protein A immunoadsorption, rituximab and intravenous immunoglobulins. Br J Dermatol 2008;158:382–8.
49. Schmidt E, Goebeler M. Use of CD-20-directed therapy in autoimmune skin diseases. Exp Rev Dermatol 2008;3:259–78.
50. Schmidt E, Brocker EB, Goebler M. Rituximab in treatment-resistant autoimmune blistering skin disorders. Clin Rev Allergy Immunol 2008;34: 56–64.
51. Joly P, Mouquet H, Roujeau JC, et al. A single cycle of rituximab for the treatment of severe pemphigus. N Engl J Med 2007;357:545–52.
52. Ahmed AR, Avram MM, Duncan LM. Case records of the Massachusetts general hospital. Weekly clinicopathological exercises. Case 23–2003. A 79-year-old woman with gastric lymphoma and erosive mucosal and cutaneous lesions. N Engl J Med 2003;349(4):382–91.
53. Borradori L, Lombardi T, Samson J, et al. Anti-CD20 monoclonal antibody (rituximab) for refractory erosive stomatitis secondary to CD20(+) follicular lymphoma-associated paraneoplastic pemphigus. Arch Dermatol 2001;137(3):269–72.
54. Heizmann M, Itin P, Wernli M, et al. Successful treatment of paraneoplastic pemphigus in follicular NHL with rituximab: report of a case and review of treatment for paraneoplastic pemphigus in NHL and CLL. Am J Hematol 2001;66(2):142–4.
55. Quian SX, Li JY, Hong M, et al. Nonhematological autoimmunity (glomerulosclerosis, paraneoplastic pemphigus and paraneoplastic neurological syndrome) in a patient with chronic lymphocytic leukemia: diagnosis, prognosis and management. Leuk Res 2009;33:500–9.
56. Barnadas M, Roe E, Brunet S, et al. Therapy of paraneoplastic pemphigus with Rituximab: a case report and review of literature. J Eur Acad Dermatol Venereol 2006;20(1):69–74.
57. Van Rossum MM, Verhaegen NT, Jonkman MF, et al. Follicular non-Hodgkin's lymphoma with refractory paraneoplastic pemphigus: case report with review of novel treatment modalities. Leuk Lymphoma 2004;45(11):2327–32.
58. Schadlow MB, Anhalt GJ, Sinha AA. Using rituximab (anti-CD20 antibody) in a patient with paraneoplastic pemphigus. J Drugs Dermatol 2003; 2(5):564–7.
59. Hoque SR, Black MM, Cliff S. Paraneoplastic pemphigus associated with CD20-positive follicular non-Hodgkin's lymphoma treated with rituximab: a third case resistant to rituximab therapy. Clin Exp Dermatol 2007;32:172–5.
60. Meijs M, Mekkes J, van Noesel C, et al. Paraneoplastic pemphigus associated with follicular dendritic cell sarcoma without Castleman's disease; treatment with rituximab. Int J Dermatol 2008;47:632–4.
61. Schierl M, Foedinger D, Geissler K, et al. Paraneoplastic pemphigus despite treatment with

rituximab, fludarabine, and cyclophosphamide in chronic lymphocytic leukemia. Eur J Dermatol 2008;18(6):717–8.
62. Schmidt E, Benoit S, Brocker EB, et al. Successful adjuvant treatment of recalcitrant epidermolysis bullosa acquisita with anti-CD20 antibody rituximab. Arch Dermatol 2006;142(2):147–50.
63. Crichlow SM, Mortimer NJ, Harman KE. A successful therapeutic trial of rituximab in the treatment of a patient with recalcitrant, high-titre epidermolysis bullosa acquisita. Br J Dermatol 2007;156:194–6.
64. Wallet-Faber N, Franck N, Batteux F, et al. Epidermolysis bullosa acquisita following bullous pemphigoid, successfully treated with the anti-CD20 monoclonal antibody rituximab. Dermatology 2007;215(3):252–5.
65. Niedermeier A, Eming R, Pfutze M, et al. Clinical response of severe mechanobullous epidermolysis bullosa acquisita to combined treatment with immunoadsorption and rituximab (anti-CD20 monoclonal antibodies). Arch Dermatol 2007;143: 192–8.
66. Sadler, Schafleitner B, Lanschuetzer C, et al. Treatment-resistant classical epidermolysis bullosa acquisita responding to rituximab. Br J Dermatol 2007;157:417–8.
67. Mercader P, Rodenas JM, Pena A, et al. Fatal Pseudomona pneumonia following rituximab therapy in a patient with epidermolysis bullosa acquisita. J Eur Acad Dermatol Venereol 2007;21:1141–2.
68. Saouki Z, Papadopoulos A, Kaiafa G, et al. A new approach on bullous pemphigoid therapy. Ann Oncol 2008;19(4):825–6.
69. Schulze J, Bader P, Henke U, et al. Severe bullous pemphigoid in an infant – successful treatment with rituximab. Pediatr Dermatol 2008;25(4):462–5.
70. Reguiai Z, Tchen T, Perceau G, et al. Efficacy of rituximab in a case of refractory bullous pemphigoid. Ann Dermatol Venereol 2009;136(5):431–4.
71. Chee R, Nagendran V, Bansal A, et al. B-cell targeted therapy alone may not be effective in bullous pemphigoid. Clin Exp Dermatol 2006;32:111–2.
72. Schumann T, Schmidt E, Booken N, et al. Successful treatment of mucous membrane pemphigoid with the anti-CD-20 antibody rituximab. Acta Derm Venereol 2009;89:101–2.
73. Taverna JA, Lerner A, Bhawan J, et al. Successful adjuvant treatment of recalcitrant mucous membrane pemphigoid with anti-CD20 antibody rituximab. J Drugs Dermatol 2007;6(7):731–2.
74. Ross AH, Jaycock P, Cook SD, et al. The use of rituximab in refractory mucous membrane pemphigoid with severe ocular involvement. Br J Ophthalmol 2009;93(4):421–2.
75. Senff NJ, Noordijk EM, Kim YH, et al. European organization for research and treatment of cancer and international society for cutaneous lymphoma consensus recommendations for the management of cutaneous B-cell lymphomas. Blood 2008;112: 1600–9.
76. Morales AV, Advani R, Horwitz SM, et al. Indolent primary cutaneous B-cell lymphoma: experience using systemic rituximab. J Am Acad Dermatol 2008;59:953–7.
77. Kyrtsonis MC, Siakantaris MP, Kalpadakis C, et al. Favorable outcome of primary cutaneous marginal zone lymphoma treated with intralesional rituximab. Eur J Haematol 2006;77:300–3.
78. Valencak J, Weihsengruber F, Rappersberger K, et al. Rituximab monotherapy for primary cutaneous B-cell lymphoma: response and follow-up in 16 patients. Ann Oncol 2009;20:326–30.
79. Fink-Puches R, Wolf IH, Zalaudek I, et al. Treatment of primary cutaneous B-cell lymphoma with rituximab. J Am Acad Dermatol 2005; 52(5):847–53.
80. Kerl K, Prins C, Saurat JH, et al. Intralesional and intravenous treatment of cutaneous B-cell lymphomas with the monoclonal anti-CD20 antibody rituximab: report and follow-up of eight cases. Br J Dermatol 2006;155:1197–200.
81. Lozzi GP, Coletti G, Peris K. Persistent CD20-negative primary cutaneous marginal zone lymphoma after treatment with intralesional rituximab therapy. J Am Acad Dermatol 2008;59(5):S110–2.
82. Gellrich S, Muche JM, Wilks A, et al. Systemic eight-cycle anti-CD20 monoclonal antibody (rituximab) therapy in primary cutaneous B-cell lymphomas–an applicational observation. Br J Dermatol 2005; 153(1):167–73.
83. Heinzerling LM, Urbanek M, Funk JO, et al. Reduction of tumor burden and stabilization of disease by systemic therapy with anti-CD20 antibody (rituximab) in patients with primary cutaneous B-cell lymphoma. Cancer 2000;89(8): 1835–44.
84. Lacouture ME, Baron JM, Jani AB, et al. Treatment of radiation-relapsing primary cutaneous B-cell lymphoma. Cancer 2000;89:1835–44.
85. Aboulafia DM. Primary cutaneous large B-cell lymphoma of the legs: a distinct clinical pathologic entity treated with CD20 monoclonal antibody (rituximab). Am J Clin Oncol 2001; 24:237–40.
86. Bonnekoh B, Schulz M, Franke I, et al. Complete remission of a primary cutaneous B-cell lymphoma of the lower leg by first-line monotherapy with the CD20-antibody rituximab. J Cancer Res Clin Oncol 2002;128:161–6.
87. Garbea A, Dippel E, Hildenbrand R, et al. Cutaneous large B-cell lymphoma of the leg masquerading as a chronic venous ulcer. Br J Dermatol 2002;146:144–7.

88. Zinzani PL, Stefoni V, Alinari L, et al. Rituximab in heavily pretreated cutaneous B-cell lymphoma. Leuk Lymphoma 2003;44:1637–8.
89. Sabroe RA, Child FJ, Woolford AJ, et al. Rituximab in cutaneous B-cell lymphoma: a report of two cases. Br J Dermatol 2000;143:157–61.
90. Grange F, Beylot-Barry M, Courville P, et al. Primary cutaneous diffuse large B-cell lymphoma, leg type. Arch Dermatol 2007;143(9):1144–50.
91. Levine TD. Rituximab in the treatment of dermatomyositis: an open-label pilot study. Arthritis Rheum 2005;52(2):601–7.
92. Chung L, Genovese MC, Fiorentino DF. A pilot trial of rituximab in the treatment of patients with dermatomyositis. Arch Dermatol 2007;143:763–7.
93. Greenberg SA, Amato AA. Uncertainties in the pathogenesis of adult dermatomyositis. Curr Opin Neurol 2004;17(3):359–64.
94. Dalakas MC, Hohlfeld R. Polymyositis and dermatomyositis. Lancet 2003;362(9388):971–82.
95. Santmyire-Rosenberger B, Dugan EM. Skin involvement in dermatomyositis. Curr Opin Rheumatol 2003;15(6):714–22.
96. Kieu V, O'Brien T, Yap LM, et al. Refractory subacute cutaneous lupus erythematosus successfully treated with rituximab. Australas J Dermatol 2009; 50:202–6.
97. Uthman I, Taher A, Abbas O, et al. Successful treatment of refractory skin manifestations of systemic lupus erythematosus with rituximab: report of a case. Dermatology 2008;216(3):257–9.
98. Cutler C, Miklos D, Kim HT, et al. Rituximab for steroid-refractory chronic graft-vs.-host disease. Blood 2006;108(2):756–62.
99. Canninga-van Dijk MR, van der Straaten HM, Fijnheer R, et al. Anti-CD20 monoclonal antibody treatment in 6 patients with therapy-refractory chronic graft-versus-host disease. Blood 2004; 104(8):2603–6.
100. Okamoto M, Okano A, Akamatsu S, et al. Rituximab is effective for steroid-refractory sclerodermatous chronic graft-versus-host disease. Leukemia 2006;20(1):172–3.
101. Ratanatharathorn V, Ayash L, Reynolds C, et al. Treatment of chronic graft-versus-host disease with anti-CD20 chimeric monoclonal antibody. Biol Blood Marrow Transplant 2003;9(8):505–11.
102. Carella AM, Biasco S, Nati S, et al. Rituximab is effective for extensive steroid-refractory chronic graft-vs-host-disease. Leuk Lymphoma 2007; 48(3):623–4.
103. Zaja F, Bacigalupo A, Patriarca F, et al. Treatment of refractory chronic GVHD with rituximab: a GITMO study. Bone Marrow Transplant 2007;40(3):273–7.
104. Mohty M, Marchetti N, El-Cheikh J, et al. Rituximab as salvage therapy for refractory chronic GVHD. Bone Marrow Transplant 2008;41(10):909–11.
105. Teshima T, Nagafuji K, Henzan H, et al. Rituximab for the treatment of corticosteroid-refractory chronic graft-versus-host disease. Int J Hematol 2009;90(2):253–60.
106. Shimabukuro-Vornhagen A, Hallek MJ, Storb RF, et al. The role of B cells in the pathogenesis of graft-versus-host disease. Blood 2009;114(24): 4919–27.
107. Gilliam AC. Update on graft versus host disease. J Invest Dermatol 2004;123(2):251–7.
108. Rouquette-Gally AM, Boyeldieu D, Prost AC, et al. Autoimmunity after allogeneic bone marrow transplantation. A study of 53 long-term-surviving patients. Transplantation 1988;46(2):238–40.
109. Miklos DB, Kim HT, Miller KH, et al. Antibody responses to H-Y minor histocompatibility antigens correlate with chronic graft-versus-host disease and disease remission. Blood 2005;105(7):2973–8.
110. Miklos DB, Kim HT, Zorn E, et al. Antibody response to DBY minor histocompatibility antigen is induced after allogeneic stem cell transplantation and in healthy female donors. Blood 2004; 103(1):353–9.
111. Schultz KR, Paquet J, Bader S, et al. Requirement for B cells in T cell priming to minor histocompatibility antigens and development of graft-versus-host disease. Bone Marrow Transplant 1995; 16(2):289–95.
112. Kamble R, Oholendt M, Carrum G. Rituximab responsive refractory acute graft-versus-host disease. Biol Blood Marrow Transplant 2006;12:1201–2.
113. Kebriaei P, Saliba RM, Ma C, et al. Allogeneic hematopoietic stem cell transplantation after rituximab-containing myeloablative preparative regimen for acute lymphoblastic leukemia. Bone Marrow Transplant 2006;38(3):203–9.
114. Shimoni A, Hardan I, Avigdor A, et al. Rituximab reduces relapse risk after allogeneic and autologous stem cell transplantation in patients with high-risk aggressive non-Hodgkin's lymphoma. Br J Haematol 2003;122(3):457–64.
115. Christopeit M, Schuette V, Behre G. Rituximab reduces the incidence of acute graft versus host disease and delays CD3+CD4+ Lymphocyte recovery. Blood 2007;110(11):5005.
116. Khouri IF, McLaughlin P, Saliba RM, et al. Eight-year experience with allogeneic stem cell transplantation for relapsed follicular lymphoma after nonmyeloablative conditioning with fludarabine, cyclophosphamide, and rituximab. Blood 2008; 111(12):5530–6.
117. Glass B, Hasenkamp J, Gorlitz A, et al. Rituximab for graft-versus-host-disease-prophylaxis after allogeneic stem cell transplantation given as treatment of high risk relapse of aggressive lymphoma: results of a randomized phase II Study. Blood 2008;112(11):1974.

118. Cheung CM, Murray PI, Savage CO. Successful treatment of Wegener's granulomatosis associated scleritis with rituximab. Br J Ophthalmol 2005;89:1542.
119. Bachmeyer C, Cadranel JF, Demontis R. Rituximab is an alternative in a case of contra-indication of cyclophosphamide in Wegener's granulomatosis. Nephrol Dial Transplant 2005;20:1274.
120. Ferraro AJ, Day CJ, Drayson MT, et al. Effective therapeutic use of rituximab in refractory Wegener's granulomatosis. Nephrol Dial Transplant 2005;20:622–5.
121. Kallenback M, Duan H, Ring T. Rituximab induced remission in a patient with Wegener's granulomatosis. Nephron Clin Pract 2005;99:c92–6.
122. Specks U, Freeze FC, McDonald TJ, et al. Response of Wegener's granulomatosis to anti-CD20 chimeric monoclonal antibody therapy. Arthiritis Rheum 2001;44:2836–40.
123. Omdal R, Wildhagen K, Hansen T, et al. Anti-CD20 therapy of treatment-resistant Wegener's granulomatosis: favourable but temporary response. Scand J Rheumatol 2005;34:229–32.
124. Eriksson P. Nine patients with anti-neutrophil cytoplasmic antibody-positive vasculitis successfully treated with rituximab. J Intern Med 2005;257: 540–8.
125. Keogh KA, Wylam ME, Stone JH, et al. Induction of remission by B-lymphocyte depletion in eleven patients with refractory antineutrophil cytoplasmic antibody-associated vasculitis. Arthritis Rheum 2005;52:262–8.
126. Tamura N, Matsudaira R, Hirashima M, et al. Two cases of refractory Wegener's granulomatosis successfully treated with rituximab. Intern Med 2007;46:409–14.
127. Brihaye B, Aouba A, Pagnoux C, et al. Adjunction of rituximab to steroids and immunosuppressants for refractory/relapsing Wegener's granulomatosis: a study on 8 patients. Clin Exp Rheumatol 2007; 25(Suppl 44):S23–7.
128. Keogh KA, Ytterberg SR, Fervenza FC, et al. Rituximab for refractory Wegener's granulomatosis: report of a prospective, open-label trial. Am J Respir Crit Care Med 2006;173:180–7.
129. Aries PM, Hellmich B, Reinhold-Keller E, et al. High dose intravenous azathioprine pulse treatment in refractory Wegener's granulomatosis. Rheumatology 2004;43:1307–8.
130. Stasi R, Stipa E, Del Poeta G, et al. Lon-term observation of patients with anti-neutrophil cytoplasmic antibody-associated vasculitis treated with rituximab. Rheumatology 2006;45(11):1432–6.
131. Smith KG, Jones RB, Burns SM, et al. Long-term comparison of rituximab treatment for refractory systemic lupus erythematosus and vasculitis. Arthritis Rheum 2006;54(9):2970–82.
132. Sneller MC. Rituximab and Wegener's granulomatosis: are B-cells a target in vasculitis treatment. Arthritis Rheum 2005;52:1–5.
133. Wong C. Rituximab in refractory antineutrophil cytoplasmic antibody-associated vasculitis: what is the current evidence? Nephrol Dial Transplant 2007;22:32–6.

Innovative Uses of Tumor Necrosis Factor α Inhibitors

Joni Mazza, MA[a,b], Anthony Rossi, MD[a,c], Jeffrey M. Weinberg, MD[a,d,e,*]

KEYWORDS

• Biologic • Etanrcept • Infliximab • Adalimumab
• Skin • Off-label

Tumor necrosis factor α (TNF-α) is an inflammatory cytokine that is released by a variety of cell types, including immune effector cells, such as macrophages, monocytes, lymphocytes, and neutrophils, as well as tissue-specific cells, including keratinocytes and dendritic cells. TNF-α has been shown to promote inflammation via the activation and induction of cytokines interleukin 1 (IL-1), IL-6, and IL-8 and by the upregulation of adhesion molecules on endothelial cells leading to increased leukocyte extravasation.[1–4] Theoretically, the blockade of TNF should have widespread potential in the treatment of numerous inflammatory diseases. Currently, 3 TNF-α inhibitors available in the United States are approved for psoriasis and psoriatic arthritis: infliximab, etanercept, and adalimumab. Numerous case reports and case series have been published in recent years reporting the off-label uses of these drugs in various inflammatory skin diseases. This review summarizes the most recent reports on 20 such conditions.

INFLIXIMAB (REMICADE)

Inflizimab is a chimeric IgG_1 monoclonal antibody against TNF-α that is comprised of the human constant (Fc) region of human IgG and the murine variable (Fab) region that binds to soluble and membrane-bound TNF-α, therefore preventing binding of TNF-α to its receptor. In addition, it also fixes complement and causes apoptosis of cells with cell surface TNF.[5] It is currently approved by the US Food and Drug Administration for the treatment of psoriasis, psoriatic arthritis, Crohn disease and associated fistulas, rheumatoid arthritis (RA), ulcerative colitis, and ankylosing spondylitis. It is contraindicated in patients with a murine protein sensitivity and should be avoided in patients with known or recent malignancies as well as congestive heart failure and multiple sclerosis.[6] The most common side effect is infusion-related reactions, which occur in 16% of patients and have been linked to the presence of antichimeric antibodies. Symptoms include fever, chills, urticaria, chest pain, hypotension, hypertension, and shortness of breath. This infusion reaction risk can be decreased through the concomitant use of methotrexate, azathioprine, or corticosteroids, preventing the formation of antichimeric antibodies.[7] Infections such as pneumonia and sepsis as well as opportunistic infections such as histoplasmosis have been reported, and because of the ability of the drug to inhibit granuloma

[a] Department of Dermatology, St Luke's-Roosevelt Hospital Center and Beth Israel Medical Center, New York, NY, USA
[b] Weill Cornell Medical College, New York, NY, USA
[c] Department of Dermatology, St Luke's-Roosevelt Hospital Center, 1090 Amsterdam Avenue, Suite 11D, New York, NY 10025, USA
[d] Columbia University, New York, NY, USA
[e] Clinical Research Center, Department of Dermatology, St Luke's-Roosevelt Hospital Center, 1090 Amsterdam Avenue, Suite 11D, New York, NY 10025, USA
* Corresponding author. Department of Dermatology, St Luke's-Roosevelt Hospital Center, 1090 Amsterdam Avenue, Suite 11D, New York, NY 10025.
E-mail address: jmw27@columbia.edu

Dermatol Clin 28 (2010) 559–575
doi:10.1016/j.det.2010.03.009
0733-8635/10/$ – see front matter © 2010 Elsevier Inc. All rights reserved.

formation, mycobacterial infection or reactivation is of concern. Therefore a baseline purified protein derivative (PPD) is necessary, and many physicians opt to obtain a chest radiograph before imitation of treatment.[8] There has been a proven increased risk of lymphoproliferative diseases and malignancies as well as onset or flares of multiple sclerosis.[9] Clinical systemic lupus erythematosus (SLE)-like syndromes have been reported with the formation of antinuclear and antinuclear-DNA antibodies. This process has been shown to be reversible on cessation of the agent. Dermatologic conditions such as the paradoxic new onset of psoriasis, cutaneous small vessel vasculitis, and interstitial granulomatous dermatitis have all been reported.[10] Infliximab is pregnancy category B.

ETANERCEPT (ENBREL)

Etanercept is a receptor fusion protein consisting of the extracellular domain of the TNF-α receptor fused with the Fc portion of human IgG, which binds to and inhibits soluble and, to a lesser degree, cell membrane-bound TNF-α. It has 2 p75-binding sites, which confers it a higher affinity for TNF-α compared with the natural receptor.[11] It does not fix complement, cause antibody-dependent cytotoxicity, or trigger T-cell apoptosis compared with infliximab.[12] Etanercept is given as a self-administered subcutaneous injection at a dosage of 25 mg twice weekly for RA, ankylosing spondylitis, and psoriatic arthritis or 50 mg twice weekly for 3 months with a subsequent decrease to 50 mg weekly for psoriasis.[13,14] Entanercept is contraindicated in patients with sepsis or with known hypersensitivity to the medication and should be avoided in patients with a history of an active infection, malignancy, multiple sclerosis, and unstable cardiac disease. Injection site reactions were the most common adverse events in initial clinical trials and occurred in up to 40% of patients. In trials there was an increased rate of upper respiratory infections. Also, there is a debate on the oncogenic potential of etanercept with regard to lymphoma occurrence; some reports show a 3-fold increase. There is an increase in antinuclear antibody formation, with a small series of patients developing signs and symptoms of SLE; this is readily reversible.[15] The rate of development of antietanercept antibodies has been less than 10% and has not been observed to lead to decreased efficacy. Etanercept is pregnancy category B, with no evidence of harm to the fetus in animal studies. However, the drug has not been specifically studied in pregnant women nor is it known if it is secreted in breast milk. Salmon and Alpert[16] have suggested that etanerept and other TNF antagonists be avoided in the first trimester.

ADALIMUMAB (HUMIRA)

Adalimumab is a human recombinant IgG_1 monoclonal antibody against human TNF-α. It binds to soluble and membrane-bound TNF-α, with apoptosis of cells with membrane-bound TNF occurring.[17] Like infliximab, it fixes complement and causes lysis of cells expressing membrane-bound TNF-α. It was initially approved for the treatment of RA and then for psoriatic arthritis, ankylosing spondylitis, and Crohn disease, and is administered as a 40-mg dose subcutaneously or intravenously every other week or weekly. An initial loading dose of 80 mg is used to increase rapidity of response onset. It is contraindicated in patients with known sensitivity reactions and should be avoided in patients with active infections or malignancies as well as multiple sclerosis or congestive heart failure.[18] Live vaccines should be avoided. Mycobacterial infections are a concern and therefore all patients need a baseline PPD. Injection site reactions are the most common adverse event and occur in 20% of patients in clinical trials. In clinical trials for RA, antiadalimumab antibodies were seen in 12% of patients receiving adalimumab as monotherapy and 1% of patients receiving concomitant methotrexate. Antinuclear antibodies seem to be increased in patients being treated with adalimumab, with some patients experiencing SLE-like symptoms. New onset psoriasis as well as cutaneous small vessel vasculitis have been known to complicate therapy.[19] Adalimumab is pregnancy category B and its lactation profile is unknown.[20]

OFF-LABEL USES OF TNF-α ANTAGONISTS

Sarcoidosis

Sarcoidosis is a multiorgan system idiopathic granulomatous disease that affects the lungs, skin, bone, and other organs. TNF-α is believed to play a key role in the pathogenesis of sarcoidosis. In pulmonary sarcoidosis, increased production of TNF-α by alveolar macrophages is seen and TNF-α plays an essential role in the process of granuloma formation. Genetic polymorphisms in the TNF-α promoter are also associated with specific clinical subtypes of sarcoidosis. More than 35 cases of sarcoidosis, including cutaneous, pulmonary, hepatic, and gastrointestinal types, have been reported to be treated with infliximab.[21] Meyerle and Shorr[22] reported the use of infliximab for sarcoidosis. A typical dosing regimen was intravenous infliximab at a dose of 3 to 5 mg/kg as an induction at baseline, week 2, and week 6, followed by maintenance therapy every 4 to 8 weeks thereafter. An improvement was often noted after the second or third infusion and many patients were able to significantly reduce their concomitant corticosteroid requirements.[22]

Using etancercept in the treatment of pulmonary sarcoidosis, Utz and colleagues[23] reported 5 of 17 treatment successes, not as promising as infliximab. Khanna and colleagues[24] reported a patient with lupus pernio and arthritis who was treated with etanercept, 25 mg twice weekly, with improvement in her skin and joint disease within 2 months. The patient's concomitant prednisone and hydroxychloroquine were discontinued by 3 months. Complete remission was reported to be maintained for 18 months on a regimen of etanercept, 25 mg twice weekly, and methotrexate, 5 mg once weekly.

Phillips and colleagues[25] reported the successful treatment of cutaneous sarcoidosis with adalimumab at 40 mg weekly added to the initial treatment of hydroxychloroquine and prednisone. Remission was seen by 9 weeks. Heffernan and Smith[26] reported a case of recalcitrant cutaneous sarcoidosis that showed extensive improvement after adding adalimumab 40 mg once weekly to hydroxychloroquine and pentoxifylline, with results seen at 5 weeks and continued improvement at 10 weeks.

GRANULOMA ANNULARE

Granuloma annulare (GA) is a relatively common skin disease that affects the dermis and subcutaneous tissue. Although most cases resolve spontaneously and without epidermal sequelae, the disease process often results in loss of elastic tissue and leaves behind atrophic lesions. The cause of GA is unknown but it has been speculated to occur after certain inciting factors, such as trauma, insect bites, sun exposure, or psoralen and ultraviolet A therapy. It is postulated that a delayed type hypersensitivity reaction to an unknown antigen is the inciting event, with a subsequent Th1, interferon γ (IFN-γ) producing, lymphocyte reaction causing matrix degradation. Multiple different clinical subtypes of GA exist and they include localized, generalized, patch-type or macular, subcutaneous, perforating, GA in human immunodeficiency virus (HIV) disease, as well as GA associated with malignant disease. Spontaneous resolution of GA occurs within 2 years in 50% of cases, but there is a 40% recurrence rate. Often patients report resolution status following lesional skin biopsy, and because most lesions are asymptomatic no treatment is required. However, generalized cases represent a therapeutic hurdle.[27] The use of TNF-α antagonists has been reported in the literature, although no randomized, double-blinded, placebo-controlled studies have been performed. One case study reports the use of infliximab for the treatment of generalized GA recalcitrant to previous treatments. The patient received infliximab 5 mg/kg intravenously at 0, 2, and 6 weeks and then every 4 weeks thereafter for 4 additional months. A significant improvement was noted by week 2, and by week 6 most lesions had resolved. The patient remained disease free at 1 year.[28] There has also been a case report of the successful use of etanercept for the treatment of generalized GA.[29] The dosing regime was 50 mg biweekly, for a total of 12 months. By 12 weeks of treatment, the patient had cleared mostly all lesions, with only erythema remaining. The patient was still disease free 12 weeks after discontinuing treatment.

NECROBIOSIS LIPOIDICA DIABETICORUM

Necrobiosis lipodica diabeticorum (NLD) is characterized by firm depressed yellowish waxy lesions that start as erythematous papules then later develop into sclerodermalike lesions. Sixty percent of patients with NLD have diabetes mellitus, and 20% have glucose intolerance or a family history of diabetes.[30] It is postulated that immunologically mediated vascular disease is the primary cause of the altered collagen found in NLD and that the microangiopathic vessel changes seen in diabetic patients could also contribute to the collagen degeneration and dermal inflammation.[31] There have been no double-blind placebo-controlled studies to assess treatment efficacy in NLD; first-line therapy includes topical corticosteroids. There have been a few case reports of NLD treated with TNF-α antagonists. Because TNF-α is important in granuloma formation, these antagonists are believed to act in blocking this formation. Cummins and colleagues[32] published a case report of a patient with generalized NLD that was recalcitrant to prednisone and dapsone. The patient was then treated with surgical split thickness autografting followed by prednisone 0.5 mg/kg/d and etanercept at 25 mg twice weekly that was commenced 6 days after surgery. The etanercept was continued for 16 months and the prednisone for 12 months. The patient's lesions cleared and remained disease free at 2 years of follow-up. Another patient with refractory NLD with a single plaque on her shin was treated with intralesional etanercept at 25 mg weekly. The injections were dermal spaced at 1 cm each on the surface of the lesion. At 1 month an initial improvement was noted, with continuing resolution during the next 8 months.[33] A third case report described a patient with an isolated ulcerated lesion of NLD that was unresponsive to multiple treatments. The patient was treated with an infliximab infusion at 5 mg/kg. By the second infusion improvement of the lesion was noted; however, the patient developed military tuberculosis. This case serves to reinforce the importance of pretreatment screening for tuberculosis exposure. Although infliximab was discontinued, this patient's NLD continued to improve thereafter.[34]

PYODERMA GANGRENOSUM

Pyoderma gangrenosum (PG) is an uncommon and recurrent ulcerative disease that is neither infectious nor gangrenous. There are 4 clinical forms: ulcerative, bullous, pustular, and superficial. Initial lesions often start out as a pustule on an erythematous base, or an erythematous nodule or bulla, whereas the classic well-formed lesion is an ulcer with a necrotic undermined border. Histologically, in early PG there is a neutrophilic vascular reaction, which can be folliculocentric, and in untreated lesions a neutrophilic infiltrate often with leukocytoclasia can be seen. Although the disease is idiopathic in nature, it is hypothesized that an underlying immunologic aberration is the cause because of the association of PG with systemic autoimmune processes.[35] Approximately 50% of patients with PG have an associated disease with inflammatory bowel disease, Crohn disease, and ulcerative colitis, being the most commonly associated. It is estimated that between 1.5% and 5% of patients afflicted with inflammatory bowel disease develop PG. Other associated conditions include leukemia, acute and chronic myelogenous leukemia, myeloma, monoclonal gammopathy of the IgA type, polycythemia vera, myeloid metaplasia, chronic active hepatitis, hepatitis C, HIV, SLE, pregnancy, PAPA (pyogenic sterile arthritis, PG, and acne) syndrome, and Takaysu arteritis.[36]

The treatment options for PG are numerous, and the therapeutic approach depends on the number, size, and expansion of lesions, as well as the associated underlying disease. The goal is to reduce the inflammatory process of the wound and to control the underlying disease process. The standard treatment of PG is local or local and combined systemic corticosteroid therapy with or without additional systemic therapy. TNF-α inhibitors have been used with success in PG, especially those associated with inflammatory bowel disease. The published treatment regime for infliximab is 5 mg/kg intravenously at weeks 0, 2, and 6.[37] For adalimumab, it is 80 mg subcutaneously as an initial dose then 40 mg subcutaneously weekly or every other week, and for etanercept the recommended dosing is 50 to 100 mg subcutaneously weekly either in 1 or 2 doses.

The largest case series of patients with PG and inflammatory bowel disease treated with infliximab included 13 patients. In this report, 3 patients had a complete response with infliximab induction alone, whereas 10 patients responded to infliximab induction and maintenance infusion therapy every 4 to 12 weeks. All patients who were also treated with corticosteroids were able to discontinue them after infliximab induction. Eleven patients in this study, however, had to remain on azathioprine and 6-mercaptopurine.[37]

Ljung and colleagues[38] reported a study of 8 patients with PG and associated Crohn disease treated with infliximab; 3 patients experienced completed resolution of the PG and 2 patients experienced partial remission. Many other case reports have been published documenting the treatment of PG with infliximab. Most patients noticed an improvement after the first infusion, with remission occurring within 3 months.[39] A prospective trial of infliximab by Kaufman and colleagues[40] for the use of extraintestinal manifestations of Crohn disease included 4 patients with PG. The mean duration of their PG was 5.5 years. All 4 responded to infliximab, with partial or complete resolution of the PG after 2 or 4 infusions; no adverse events were noted.

McGowan and colleagues[41] published a case report of successful treatment of widespread PG unassociated with inflammatory bowel disease with etancercept. The patient experienced worsening PG while being treated with systemic corticosteroids. She was then started on etanercept 25 mg twice weekly along with prednisone 30 mg orally daily. At 1 month, complete resolution of the PG was noted. However, when the prednisone was tapered to 2.5 mg daily a recurrence was noted. Hydrocortisone intramuscularly was used, and prednisone 60 mg daily was started. Etanercept was increased to 100 mg weekly, which resulted in rapid clearance of the lesions, and the patient remained disease free at 4 months on etancercept and a low concurrent dose of prednisone (5 mg daily).

Hubbard and colleagues[42] reported a more complicated case of PG in a patient with skin ulcerations and abscesses in the spleen and psoas muscle that were believed to be related to the PG. Infliximab was started and the patient was noted to have a rapid improvement of the skin lesions and abscesses. However, the patient suffered an anaphylactoid reaction during the fourth infliximab infusion. Infliximab was discontinued and the PG and abscesses returned. At this time, etanercept was initiated at 25 mg 3 times weekly, although at 3 weeks of treatment no improvement was seen. Etanercept was discontinued and treatment with adalimumab at 40 mg weekly was initiated. On adalimumab the patient experienced rapid resolution of the skin and extracutaneous lesions. Goldenberg and Jorizzo[43] as well as Pastor and colleagues[44] published case reports of the successful use of etanercept for PG.

SWEET SYNDROME

Sweet syndrome, or acute febrile neutrophilic dermatosis, is an uncommon disease with an unknown pathogenesis. A hypersensitivity reaction is proposed suggested by the association with infections, autoimmune diseases, inflammatory bowel diseases, and malignancies. It can also be drug induced or pregnancy related. Up to 50% of patients have idiopathic disease. Initial lesions are tender, erythematous plaques or papules that may enlarge and coalesce. There is associated edema of the lesions and some patients may develop vesiculation and bulla formation. Constitutional signs and symptoms such as fever and malaise are noted. Histologically, a dense perivascular neutrophilic infiltrate with edema is seen, and leukocytoclasia with minimal to no evidence of vasculitis is seen. Sweet syndrome follows a benign course that may last for weeks to months and then involute spontaneously. The most effective therapy is oral prednisone at 0.5 to 1.0 mg/kg/d for 4 to 6 weeks. Increased TNF-α level was reported in lesions of Sweet syndrome, and a study of successful treatment with etanercept of 2 patients with Sweet syndrome with RA has been reported. Etanercept 50 mg twice weekly was used in 1 patient and 25 mg twice weekly in the other patient. Improvement was noted in both patients; however, it is possible that improvement of the patients' underlying RA may have also contributed.[45]

SUBCORNEAL PUSTULAR DERMATOSIS

Subcorneal pustular dermatosis (SPD), or Sneddon-Wilkinson disease, is a chronic sterile subcorneal pustular disease that occurs mainly in middle-aged women. The pustules are superficial and annular or serpiginous in configuration especially on the abdomen, axillae, and groin. Some cases are associated with a monoclonal gammopathy, usually IgA. Histologically, the pustules form below the stratum corneum, with possible spongioform pustules in the upper epidermis. Dapsone, at doses of 50 to 200 mg/d, is effective for most cases. Grob and colleagues[46] reported increased TNF-α levels in the serum and blister fluid of a patient with SPD, and so TNF-α inhibitors are believed to be effective in SPD by disrupting leukocyte adhesion and migration and preventing the accumulation of neutrophils. A report of a dapsone-intolerant patient with SPD was published by Voigtlander and colleagues.[47] This patient was successfully treated with infliximab at 5 mg/kg in addition to acitretin at 0.4 mg/kg/d. Two days after the first infusion of infliximab the patient experienced complete resolution of pustules. The patient had a recurrence of symptoms at 14 days and received a second infusion of infliximab with subsequent resolution. At 6 months the patient remained free of disease on acitretin 0.16 mg/kg/d with the addition of systemic steroids for 1 flare.

VASCULITIS

The vasculitides are a heterogeneous group of disorders similar in their inflammatory destruction of blood vessels. Numerous case reports have been published on the use of TNF antagonists in the treatment of diseases such as Churg-Strauss syndrome, Takayasu arteritis, giant cell arteritis, Kawasaki disease, and leukocytoclastic vasculitis.

The mainstay of treatment of most patients with systemic vasculitis is corticosteroids and concurrent immunosuppressant drugs. As discussed earlier, the anti-TNF agents are particularly useful in the treatment of granulomatous illness, such as sarcoidosis. For this reason, Wegener granulomatosis (WG) has been targeted as a potential indication for TNF blockade. Several open-label trials have shown infliximab to be beneficial in the treatment of WG.[48–52] Josselin and colleagues[53] conducted a long-term follow-up of 15 patients treated with infliximab for several vasculitides, including 10 patients with WG, 1 with microscopic polyangiitis, 3 with RA, and 1 with cryoglobulinemia. By day 45 of treatment, 11 patients had entered remission, and 4 others had some degree of therapeutic response. Despite the continuation of immunosuppression, 10 of the 15 patients ultimately relapsed. Investigators conclude that in treatment-refractory vasculitis, the TNF antagonists may serve as a potential salvage treatment. Etanercept has also been tried but results have been far less promising, pointing to a potential key to understanding the pathogenesis of this illness.[54,55] The risk for using TNF blockers in these patients has largely been related to the increased rates of infection.

BULLOUS PEMPHIGOID AND MUCOUS MEMBRANE PEMPHIGOID

Bullous pemphigoid (BP) is an acute or chronic autoimmune-mediated skin disease characterized by the formation of bullae. In patients with BP, autoantibodies are formed against glycoproteins of the hemidesmosome. Mucous membrane pemphigoid (MMP), also known as cicatricial pemphigoid, shares many common features with BP, but almost always involves the mucosal membranes and is less commonly associated with skin involvement. This disorder carries the risk of serious complications, such as blindness, as a result of scarring of ocular mucous membranes.

Patients with BP have been shown to have increased TNF levels in their serum and in blister fluid, and these levels tend to correlate with severity of disease.[56–59] Patients with ocular MMP were also found to have increased levels of TNF-α in their serum compared with healthy controls.[60] For this reason, TNF antagonists have been used as a potential treatment of this illness.

There has been 1 report of a patient with concurrent BP and psoriasis treated with etanercept after initial treatment with prednisone. This technique allowed the successful tapering of the prednisone without a flare of either illness.[61] Two cases have been reported in which 4 treatment-refractory patients with MMP were treated with 25 mg subcutaneous etanercept twice weekly in addition to their prior regime. Three patients had oral mucosal involvement and 1 had severe, recalcitrant, ocular disease. In all cases, patients achieved clinical remission.[62,63] Recommendations are that this class of drugs may be a useful alternative in patients who may otherwise require, aggressive systemic treatments.

SLE

SLE is a multisystem chronic inflammatory, connective tissue disease that affects the joints, skin, lungs, kidneys, nervous system, and other organs. Immunologic abnormalities, particularly the production of antinuclear antibodies, are the prominent feature of this disease. SLE leads to tissue destruction via activation of the complement cascade and deposition of complement in tissues. TNF, an early proinflammatory cytokine, is implicated as a key player in this disease process. Thus, theoretically, medications aimed at blocking its effects should interrupt the complement cascade and decrease clinical symptoms.[64] However, treatment of patients with SLE with TNF antagonists remains controversial. There have been numerous reported cases of increased production of autoantibodies and several cases of drug-induced lupus secondary to this class of medications. Most cases of increased autoantibody levels have been seen in clinical trials of patients with RA and Crohn disease. However, in many circumstances this potential risk may be outweighed by the beneficial effects of treatment. In a Finnish study of 53 patients treated with TNF antagonists, researchers found a response rate greater than 50% in 74% of patients treated with etanercept and 60% of patients treated with adalimumab. Only 1 patient in this study was noted to show features of drug-induced lupus erythematosus.[65]

Increases in anti–double-stranded DNA (dsDNA) and in anticardiolipin were noted in several patients in a 2004 study on the effect of infliximab in conjunction with azathioprine or methotrexate. However, 6 patients with SLE were noted to have a decrease in symptoms of arthritis and proteinuria. The increases in autoantibody levels were not associated with an increase in disease activity in these patients.[66] Another report described the successful management with etanercept of a patient with subacute cutaneous lupus erythematosis and RA. No increase of autoantibodies was noted in this patient.[67] An additional report described the improvement of a patient with subacute cutaneous lupus erythematosis treated with etanercept; however, no comment was made on autoantibody levels.[68]

Recently, Aringer and colleagues[69] reported on 13 patients with refractory lupus nephritis treated with infliximab. They found that an induction regime of 4 infusions combined with immunosuppressive therapy led to significant improvement in symptoms and may potentially induce long-term remission. However, prolonged use of TNF antagonists may be associated with an increased risk of potentially life-threatening illness, such as *Legionella* pneumonia and cerebral lymphoma. Another study found significant improvement in patients who had infliximab added to standard treatment regimens compared with controls.[70]

In 2008, Costa and colleagues[71] performed a retrospective review of 33 patients who met criteria for drug-induced lupus erythematosis (DILE): 21 caused by infliximab, 10 caused by etanercept, and 2 caused by adalimumab. These investigators found that the patients with DILE secondary to anti-TNF agents differed from patients with classic DILE secondary to traditional agents. In classic DILE there is significantly less cutaneous involvement and the disease is not usually associated with antibodies to dsDNA. In this review, however, 72% of patients with presumed TNF blocker-induced DILE had cutaneous involvement and 90% had positive dsDNA antibodies, suggesting the possibility of a unique reaction. Further complicating this picture is the difficulty in distinguishing a DILE reaction from the underlying rheumatologic disorder.

Based on the reports mentioned earlier, it is possible that although autoantibody levels may increase during treatment with the TNF blockers, this increase does not seem to be related to severity of disease or clinical progression of symptoms, and may be a separate process altogether. Currently, 2 trials are recruiting participants to study the safety profiles of etanercept and infliximab in the treatment of patients with SLE (http://clinicaltrials.gov).[69] Further studies are needed to fully evaluate the efficacy and safety of these drugs in SLE.

SCLERODERMA

Scleroderma is a chronic autoimmune disease characterized by the progressive fibrosis of skin and internal organs, including lungs and gastrointestinal tract. Clinically, these patients display marked variability in the extent and severity of their disease. Although the cause of scleroderma is largely unknown, it is believed to be perpetuated by inflammation following vascular alterations and fibrosis. TNF-α is believed to play a role in increased fibroblast chemotaxis and decreased collagen production.[72] In mouse models of bleomycin-induced scleroderma, etanercept has been shown to lead to a significant reduction in dermal sclerosis, collagen accumulation, and the number of infiltrating myofibroblastic cells.[73]

In 2000, etanercept was studied in a trial of 10 patients with systemic sclerosis. Patients were treated with 25-mg subcutaneous injections twice weekly for 6 months. Four of the 10 patients had improvement of their Rodnan skin score and 3 of 4 patients with digital ulcers reported improvement. Other measures of disease, such as pulmonary function tests, oral aperture, and hand extension, remained stable. One patient had clinical progression of his disease, but no adverse effects were noted.[74]

More recently, in a retrospective analysis of 18 patients at the Johns Hopkins Scleroderma Center treated with etanercept for active inflammatory joint involvement, investigators found that 15 of the 18 patients experienced a significant decrease in signs of inflammation and synovitis. There was no reported worsening of skin involvement during treatment. In addition, they reported no complications, such as opportunistic infections, hospitalizations or death, related to the treatment.[75]

A 2008 study by Denton and colleagues[76] included 16 patients with diffuse cutaneous systemic sclerosis treated with 5 infusions of infliximab 5 mg/kg. After 26 weeks there was no statistically significant change in Rodnan skin score. Nonetheless, clinical stabilization of disease was reported, as well as a decrease in 2 laboratory markers of collagen synthesis. One-third of these patients were reported to have formed anti-infliximab antibodies that resulted in subsequent infusion reactions. A recent case report of a patient with systemic sclerosis, complicated by lung fibrosis and pulmonary hypertension, reported stabilization of lung function and improvement in quality of life during treatment with infliximab 5 mg/kg and methotrexate 10 mg/wk.[77]

There have also been several reports on the adverse effects of TNF antagonists in the treatment of scleroderma. Drug-induced lupus has been reported in association with the use of etanercept and infliximab.[78] Both patients had resolution of clinical symptoms and normalization of autoantibody levels following cessation of treatment. Another report discussed a patient with scleroderma who developed pancytopenia and a fungal infection following treatment with infliximab.[79] These adverse events highlight the potential concern in using TNF blockers and emphasize the need for more research on the safety and efficacy of these drugs in the treatment of scleroderma.

DERMATOMYOSITIS

Dermatomyositis (DM) is a connective tissue disease characterized by inflammation of the muscles and skin. The cause is largely unknown. Regardless of the definite cause, multiple studies have implicated TNF as playing a significant role in the pathogenesis of DM. In addition, there have been reports of successful management of DM with etanercept and infliximab.[80] In a study of 5 children with refractory juvenile DM, all patients showed significant clinical benefit following treatment with infliximab.[81] An open-label trial of anti-TNF-α in combination with methotrexate in treatment-naive patients with DM and polymyositis yielded less promising results. Only 2 patients of 6 reached the primary end point at 26 weeks, with 3 dropping out of the study because of disease progression. Based on previous studies and reports, as well as their own data, investigators concluded that anti-TNF treatment is beneficial in some patients with DM and polymyositis, whether treatment naive or refractory, but that it remains difficult to predict which patients will respond to TNF blockade.[82] Another case report of 2 patients with DM treated with infliximab reported a favorable response to treatment after 3 infusions. One patient was noted to be progressing well, whereas the other succumbed to aspiration pneumonia during the course of a fourth infusion while on concomitant high-dose prednisone treatment.[83]

There has been 1 report of a patient with refractory DM who became septic after her third infusion with infliximab. The patient recovered with antibiotics, but 4 months later was diagnosed with non-Hodgkin lymphoma. Although it is more likely that the lymphoma is the result of the DM or of her long-standing use of immunosuppressives, given the time course, it is not possible to completely rule out infliximab as a potential contributor. For this reason, these investigators suggested using caution when prescribing TNF blockers for patients with syndromes known to have paraneoplastic associations.[84]

BEHÇET DISEASE

Behçet disease is a chronic, multisystemic, inflammatory disease, seen primarily in Middle Eastern and Mediterranean populations. It is characterized by the hallmark of oral aphthae along with any of the following: genital ulcers, skin lesions, eye inflammation, pathergy reaction, neurologic disease, and vascular disease. Most symptoms are believed to be caused by vasculitis, which is unique in its ability to involve blood vessels of all sizes. The pathogenesis of this inflammatory disease is related to aberrant T-cell function with subsequent increase in TNF-α levels. TNF antagonists have been used to treat this disease for many years. In 2001, Goossens and colleagues[85] reported on a patient with severe refractory oral and genital ulcers successfully treated with 2 infusions of 10 mg/kg infliximab. Since that time, many case reports have been published describing the treatment of various Behçet lesions with TNF blockers.

Since the Goossens report in 2001, infliximab has frequently been reported as a successful treatment option.[86,87] Recently, a retrospective clinical chart review was performed comparing the efficacy and safety of infliximab with cyclosporine in refractory uveoretinitis associated with Behçet disease. The investigators concluded that during the initial 6 months of treatment, infliximab was more effective than cyclosporine in reducing acute episodes of uveitis.[88] Infliximab has also been reported as successful in the treatment of refractory entro-Behçet disease, particularly when started early before organ damage occurs.[89]

The use of etanercept in the treatment of Behçet disease was studied in a randomized trial of 40 patients in 2005. Treatment groups were assigned either to etanercept administered as a 25-mg subcutaneous injection twice weekly for 4 weeks or placebo injections on the same schedule. The treatment group was noted to have more patients free of oral ulcers compared with controls (45% vs 5%), and more treatment patients remained free of nodular skin lesions (85% vs 25%). Significantly, this report did not assess the effect of etanercept on the more serious manifestations of this illness such as uveitis.[90]

Adalimumab has also been shown to be effective in patients with Behçet disease.[91–93] In a report of a patient with severe Behçet disease-related uveitis and a hypersensitivity to infliximab, the patient was successfully treated and attained remission when switched to adalimumab. This finding suggests that adalimumab may be a useful alternative in infliximab-sensitive patients.[94]

To date, 3 cases of failure have also been reported: 2 with infliximab and 1 with etanercept. In the case that was refractory to etanercept, the patient was subsequently successfully treated with infliximab.[95,96] TNF antagonists may represent a promising treatment in the management of this disease, and so-called TNF switching may be an appropriate maneuver should 1 agent fail or ultimately lose effectiveness.

GRAFT-VERSUS-HOST DISEASE

TNF-α is an established contributor to graft-versus-host disease (GVHD). Murine bone marrow models have shown that donor- and host-derived TNF-α are key players in the development of GVHD.[97–100] In addition, treatment with anti-TNF antibodies slows the progression of the disease. In humans, higher levels of TNF have been correlated with the development of GVHD.[101] Therefore, experimental and clinical data support the use of TNF antagonists in the treatment of this disease.

Acute GVHD

Despite significant advancements in donor selection and prophylaxis, GVHD still remains a major cause of morbidity and mortality among patients undergoing hematopoietic stem cell transplant. Currently steroid combined with a calcineurin inhibitor is the mainstay of treatment of acute GVHD (aGVHD). However, less than 50% of patients with grade II disease or higher achieve sustainable remission with this therapy.

In 2000, Couriel and colleagues[102] reported on 37 patients with acute GVHD treated with

10-mg/kg weekly infusions of infliximab. Response rates were 75% for skin GVHD, 81% for upper gastrointestinal tract GVHD, 91% for lower gastrointestinal tract GVHD, and 35% for liver GVHD. Despite these promising figures, 22 patients died of GVHD during the course of the study. Subsequent smaller studies of patients with aGVHD treated with infliximab yielded similar results, with significant improvements in symptoms but an overall high mortality. In 2003, Jacobsohn and colleagues[103] reported even less promising results. Of the 11 steroid-refractory patients, only 2 were noted to have a complete response to treatment with infliximab. Another 5 of the 9 remaining patients were reported to have a partial response; all 9 of these patients eventually succumbed to progressive GVHD and infection. However, 2 retrospective studies of steroid-resistant patients treated with infliximab alone reported an overall response rate of 67% and 59%.[104,105] In addition, in a study of 12 adult steroid-resistant patients with matched sibling donor transplants and nonmyeloablative conditioning therapy, infliximab in combination with daclizumab was shown to have survival rates of 73%.[106] Rao and colleagues[107] looked at this same regime in the treatment of 22 children with GVHD and found a 68% survival at 31 months.

These cases were all patients with steroid-refractory disease. To compare the efficacy of steroids alone or steroids plus infliximab, a small trial randomized patients into these groups.[108] The investigators found that response rates were not statistically significant, suggesting that early treatment with infliximab does not provide a benefit to patients who are not resistant to steroids.

Etanercept has also shown promise in the treatment of aGVHD. A case report of an 11-year-old girl reported complete remission of steroid-refractory aGVHD after treatment with etanercept. Etanercept has also been studied in combination with daclizumab; an overall response rate of 67% was obtained. Another study looked at etanercept in combination with tacrolimus and methlyprednisone and found that for the 20 patients in the study with stage II or III aGVHD, 75% of patients attained complete remission after 4 weeks.[109]

Chronic GVHD

In their 2000 study, Couriel and colleagues[102] also reported on 22 patients with chronic GVHD treated with a median of 4 weekly 10-mg/kg infusions in addition to prednisone and other immunosuppressive therapies. These investigators reported a response rate of 57% for skin disease and 92% for gastrointestinal disease, with 11 mortalities. Another study reported a more than 50% alleviation of symptoms in 5 of 8 patients.[110]

Many infections have been reported in the case reports of chronic GVHD treated with TNF blockers. It is not possible to ascertain the degree to which these medications contribute to these infections, because patients are significantly immunosuppressed and being treated with various immunosuppressives. Infliximab has been reported in association with fungal infections and this relationship necessitates further evaluation.[111]

Overall it seems that for patients with steroid-refractory GVHD, TNF antagonists may offer a reasonable alternative treatment option. However, more research is still needed to evaluate the safety and efficacy of TNF antagonists in this setting.

PITYRIASIS RUBRA PILARIS

Pityriasis rubra pilaris (PRP) is a chronic papulosquamous disorder characterized by reddish-orange, scaly plaques, palmoplantar keratoderma, and follicular hyperkeratosis. In some cases, patients progress to erythroderma, with islands of sparing. Although the pathogenesis remains unknown, it is believed to be an immunologic response to an antigenic trigger. Topical steroids, topical retinoids, vitamin D analogs, and methotrexate have all been used as therapeutics, but this rare disorder remains difficult to treat.

A 2003 case report described 3 patients with PRP treated with infliximab infusions of 5 mg/kg administered at monthly intervals. Patients in this series were also being treated with concomitant antibiotics, topical steroids, antihistamines, and UVB. All patients reported marked improvement in symptoms within 2 weeks of the initial infusion.[112] Another report described 2 patients with refractory PRP who showed significant improvement in symptoms after infliximab was added to treatment with acitretin. More recently, 2 case reports have also been published describing the successful treatment of PRP with infliximab in combination with methotrexate[113] and as monotherapy.[114]

Two reports have also been published describing the successful treatment of adult patients with PRP with etanercept, 1 in combination with isoretinoin treatment and 1 without. In the first case, a 55-year-old man with PRP continued to be symptomatic despite the use of calcipotriene ointment, clobestasol cream, acitretin, and UVB therapy. When his regime was modified to include etanercept 50 mg subcutaneously twice a week and acitretin 25 mg each day, he experienced 85% to 90% resolution of plaque lesions after 7 months.[115] In the second report, a 37-year-old man was started on etanercept 50 mg subcutaneously twice a week after he was discontinued on oral retinoids because of increased liver enzymes. After 6 months of treatment and a decrease in dosage to 25 mg twice a week, the patient was noted to be "almost clear."[116] An additional case report describes a 16-year-old girl with treatment-refractory PRP who was successfully treated with etanercept.[117]

Recently, a case report was published describing a 72-year-old man treated for biopsy-proven PRP with adalimumab subcutaneous injections. An initial dose of 80 mg was followed by 40-mg doses weekly for 32 weeks. After 8 weeks of monotherapy with adalimumab, the patient was reported to have dramatic and rapid near resolution of his symptoms.[118]

The clinical and histopathologic similarities between PRP and psoriasis, coupled with the numerous anecdotal reports of clinical improvement with the TNF antagonists, suggest that this class of drugs may play a role in the treatment of this disease. Randomized, controlled trials are needed to further explore this treatment option and to determine an optimum dosing regimen.

SAPHO SYNDROME

SAPHO syndrome is characterized by synovitis, acne, pustulosis, hyperostosis, and osteitis. Although the cause of this syndrome is unknown, high amounts of TNF-α have been seen in the bone biopsies of patients with this syndrome.[119] In addition, several case reports have described the successful treatment of these patients with TNF antagonists, suggesting a possible etiopathogenic association. The authors of 1 report discuss the treatment of 2 patients with infliximab at 5 mg/kg at 0, 2, and 6 weeks, with both requiring a fourth infusion for relapse of symptoms at 8 to 10 weeks after the third dose. The first patient initially presented with severe acne and osteitis of the clavicle. The second patient initially reported painful swelling of the sternum and sternoclavicular joints and a history of palmoplantar pustulosis. At 18 months after treatment, both patients had complete clinical remission.[120]

Another report of 2 patients with SAPHO treated with TNF antagonists also showed promising results. The first presented with diffuse sclerosing osteomyelitis of the mandible. After 8 weeks on eternercept, 25 mg twice weekly, the patient reported significant alleviation of her symptoms and was able to decrease her dose of prednisolone from 20 mg to 7.5 mg daily after 8 weeks. The second patient in this report presented with treatment-refractory bone pain and swelling that achieved complete remission with 4 infusions of infliximab. However, because of dyspnea after infusions, the patient was switched to etanercept 25 mg twice weekly. Both patients in this report remained in remission at 9 months follow-up while continuing on the etanercept treatment.[119]

A 2008 review of the syndrome reported the results of 18 patients with SAPHO treated with TNF blockers, focusing primarily on osteoarticular and skin responses. In this report, 16 patients were treated with infliximab infusion in a dose of 5 mg/kg, and 2 patients received etanercept. All patients were reported to have some initial improvement in symptoms, with many reporting sustained clinical response. There was a favorable cutaneous response in most patients with skin lesions.[121]

Current recommendations for treatment remain conservative, with nonsteroidal antiinflammatory drugs being used as a first-line treatment. However, based on the satisfactory results of the case reports mentioned earlier, TNF antagonists can potentially be useful in patients with refractory disease.

MULTICENTRIC RETICULOHISTIOCYTOSIS

Multicentric reticulohistiocytosis (MR) is a rare disorder characterized by destructive arthritis in association with papulonodular skin lesions composed of a proliferation of histiocytes and multinucleated giant cells. One-quarter of cases are associated with an underlying malignancy. Although the precise pathogenesis remains unknown, TNF-α levels are increased in the blood and tissues of patients with this disorder. There have been several reports on the use of TNF antagonists in its treatment. In most of these cases, the patients had been refractory to several prior immunosuppressive therapies. In these cases, the TNF blocker was added to a regime of other immunosuppressive therapies.

In 2 of the cases of treatment with etanercept, patients experienced a significant improvement in skin and joint symptoms within 4 to 6 weeks, allowing for tapering of more toxic immunosuppressive drugs.[122,123] One patient treated with infliximab was reported as experiencing symptom improvement of skin lesions after the first infusion and improvement of joint symptoms after 3 months.[124] In the case of adalimumab use, the patient had improvement of skin and joint symptoms within 8 weeks.[125]

Other reports have not been so successful. One patient treated with etanercept and intramuscular steroids had no meaningful response to treatment. In a report of infliximab use, 2 patients experienced improvement of their skin lesions, but no substantial improvement of joint symptoms.[126]

A 2008 case report described a 63-year-old man with MR who had previously been refractory to all medications, including treatment with etanercept 50 mg subcutaneous injections weekly for 4 weeks. The patient was then tried on infliximab 5 mg/kg infusions at 0, 2, and 6 weeks and then every 8 weeks in combination with his treatment regime of prednisone and methotrexate. After 3 infusions, the patient was noted to be less fatigued and with resolution of a prominent chest lesion and with no new cutaneous lesions.[127]

These results suggest that TNF blockade monotherapy may not be successful in treating patients with MR. In addition, the 2008 case report highlights the differences in efficacy among various TNF blockers. The different responses to treatment may be explained by the differential binding of the drugs. Infliximab tends to bind TNF quickly and irreversibly compared with etanercept. This difference may have implications for treatment of patients and for further understanding of the pathogenesis of this disease.[127]

TOXIC EPIDERMAL NECROLYSIS

Toxic epidermal necrolysis (TEN) is a life-threatening skin reaction, often to a medication, that results in widespread erythema, necrosis, and bullous detachment of the epidermis and mucous membranes. Overproduction of TNF-α has been shown to play a role in the pathogenesis of this disease. Several studies have reported an increase in TNF-α in blister fluid from patients with TEN compared with similar lesions in patients with burns.[128–130] This proinflammatory cytokine may function indirectly to recruit T cells and macrophages and directly through the assistance in keratinocyte apoptosis.[131,132] It has been suggested that the increase in TNF-α is a keratinocyte defensive measure designed to counteract T-cell invasion.

Currently, no 1 specific treatment has been shown to be effective. Most recently, intravenous immunoglobulin has been used to halt progression of this illness, although efficacy has not been proved. To date, there have been 5 reported cases of patients with TEN treated with TNF antagonists. The first report discussed 3 patients with TEN who displayed significant improvement following single infusions of infliximab (5 mg/kg in 2 patients and 3 mg/kg in 1 patient). In 1 case, improvement was correlated with a decrease in TNF-α expression in the skin and perivascular inflammatory cells.[133] Two patients have been reported as successfully treated for TEN with etanercept. In 2007, a case report described a 59-year-old man treated with etanercept subcutaneous injections after developing TEN secondary to ciprofloxacin. After the first injection, epithelial detachment stopped, and several days after the second injection reepithelialization was complete.[134] The second patient was treated with a combination of 2 25-mg etanercept injections and corticosteroids following TEN induced by phenobarbital. The patient was noted to have complete reepithelialization 20 days after the second injection.[135] TNF-α plays a major role in TEN, and additional research is needed to further elucidate the potential role of TNF antagonists in its treatment. Because the skin is largely denuded in TEN, there is justifiable concern that TNF antagonists might predispose such patients to serious wound infection and/or sepsis.

ERYTHEMA ANNULARE CENTRIFIGUM

Erythema annulare centrifigum (EAC) is a figurate erythema of unknown cause, but believed to be a hypersensitivity reaction. Pathologic evaluation reveals parakeratosis and spongiosis within the epidermis and a lymphohistiocytic perivascular infiltrate with red blood cell extravasation in the dermis. Whereas antihistamines and topical steroids have been largely unsuccessful in treatment, topical calcitriol and tacrolimus have been shown to be somewhat beneficial.

One report has been published describing the successful treatment of a 57-year-old man with refractory EAC with etanercept. The patient was treated with 50-mg doses once per week, and after 4 weeks experienced a 95% clearance of his skin lesions. After 3 months, clearance was noted to be 100%; after 6 months, the patient was discontinued from treatment with the drug. Two months later, the patient relapsed. He was again started on etanercept and displayed similar improvement of symptoms.[136] The authors of this report suggested that perhaps EAC is a T1-mediated disease, with TNF involved in its pathogenesis. Additional studies are necessary to help establish this potential connection and to determine the true effectiveness of TNF blockade in this clinical scenario.

HAILEY-HAILEY DISEASE (BENIGN FAMILIAL PEMPHIGUS)

Hailey-Hailey disease is a genetic condition that causes rashes and blisters to form in skin folds. The disease is caused by a defect in the calcium pump ATP2C1, located on chromosome 3. Numerous therapies have been attempted to treat this condition, including topical steroids for management of symptoms during outbreaks, and antibiotics, antifungals, steroids, dapsone, methotrexate, thalidomide, and cyclosporine to prevent outbreaks. To date, most treatments have been largely unsuccessful for the more chronic and frequently relapsing forms of this disease.

In 2006, Norman and colleagues[68] published a case report of a 47-year-old woman with chronic, treatment-refractory Hailey-Hailey disease who was being treated with weekly subcutaneous injections of etanercept, with doses increasing from 25 mg to 75 mg weekly for 10 months. The patient was noted to improve markedly after 15 months of treatment. However, the patient also lost 22.7 kg (50 lbs) during the course of this treatment, which may also have contributed to symptom and disease amelioration. However, the investigators point out that disease improvement occurred before the weight loss, and suggest the potential role of TNF in the pathogenesis of this illness.

HIDRADENITIS SUPPURATIVA

The TNF antagonist agents have proved to be variably effective in management of this typically refractory, chronic disorder. See the article by Shuja and colleagues elsewhere in this issue for further exploration of this topic.

SUMMARY

The TNF-α antagonists infliximab, etanercept, and adalimumab have been increasingly used in the treatment of many conditions. This class of medications has been markedly successful in several illnesses, particularly when the disease has been refractory to traditional treatments. In addition, the safety profile of the TNF-blocking drugs is believed to be more acceptable compared with chronic administration of immunosuppressants, such as corticosteroids. However, use of the TNF-α antagonists is not without risk. The incidence of tuberculosis is significantly higher in patients treated with TNF blockers, with many cases presenting as disseminated or atypical disease. There have also been reported cases of histoplasmosis, aspergillosis, cryptococcus, and listeriosis, in conjunction with TNF-antagonist use. Moreover, increased rates of lymphoma, demyelinating disease, increased transaminase levels, congestive heart failure, and the development of antinuclear autoantibodies have been seen in association with these medications. There is an omnipresent risk of bacterial superinfection in the types of disorders with which these biologic drugs have been tried. These drugs are also expensive, making them an unrealistic option for many patients. Insurance coverage is uncertain for off-label usage.

Despite the risks and difficulties associated with their use, TNF antagonists remain an important and life-changing treatment for many patients. Based on current data, TNF blockers comprise significant and potentially beneficial therapeutics, particularly as a second-line therapy in treatment-refractory illness. As more is learned about the pathogenesis of these diseases, and the role that the cytokine TNF plays in each, their use and benefits are likely to expand exponentially.

REFERENCES

1. Kupper TS. Immunologic targets in psoriasis. N Engl J Med 2003;349(21):1987–90.
2. Robert C, Kupper TS. Inflammatory skin diseases, T cells, and immune surveillance. N Engl J Med 1999;341(24):1817–28.
3. Wajant H, Pfizenmaier K, Scheurich P. Tumor necrosis factor signaling. Cell Death Differ 2003; 10(1):45–65.
4. Gisondi P, Gubinelli E, Cocuroccia B, et al. Targeting tumor necrosis factor-alpha in the therapy of psoriasis. Curr Drug Targets Inflamm Allergy 2004;3(2):175–83.
5. Chaudhari U, Romano P, Mulcahy LD, et al. Efficacy and safety of infliximab monotherapy for plaque type psoriasis: a randomized trial. Lancet 2001;357:1842–6.
6. Behnam SM, Behnam SE, Koo JY. TNF-alpha inhibitors and congestive heart failure. Skinmed 2005;4:363–8.
7. Baert F, Noman M, Vermeire S, et al. Influence of immunogenicity on the longterm efficacy of infliximab in Crohn's disease. N Engl J Med 2003; 348:601–8.
8. Hanauer SB, Feagan BG, Lichtenstein GR, et al. Maintenance infliximab for Crohn's disease: the ACCENT I randomised trial. Lancet 2002;359: 1541–9.
9. Mohan N, Edwards ET, Cupps TR, et al. Demyelination occurring during anti-tumor necrosis factor alpha therapy for inflammatory arthritides. Arthritis Rheum 2001;44:2862–9.
10. Kary S, Worm M, Audring H, et al. New onset or exacerbation of psoratic skin lesions in patients with definite rheumatoid arthritis receiving tumour necrosis factor alpha antagonists. Ann Rheum Dis 2006;65:405–7.
11. Yamauchi PS, Gindi V, Lowe NJ. The treatment of psoriasis and psoriatic arthritis with etanercept: practical considerations on monotherapy, combination therapy, and safety. Dermatol Clin 2004;22: 449–59, ix.

12. Khanna D, McMahon M, Furst DE. Safety of tumour necrosis factor-alpha antagonists. Drug Saf 2004; 27(5):307–24.
13. Mohler KM, Torrance DS, Smith CA, et al. Soluble tumor necrosis factor (TNF) receptors are effective therapeutic agents in lethal endotoxemia and function simultaneously as both TNF carriers and TNF antagonists. J Immunol 1993;151:1548–61.
14. Bathon JM, Martin RW, Fleischmann RM, et al. A comparison of etanercept and methotrexate in patients with early rheumatoid arthritis. N Engl J Med 2000;343:1586–93.
15. Weinblatt ME, Kremer JM, Bankhurst AD, et al. A trial of etanercept, a recombinant tumor necrosis factor receptor: Fc fusion protein, in patients with rheumatoid arthritis receiving methotrexate. N Engl J Med 1999;340:253–9.
16. Salmon JE, Alpert D. Are we coming to terms with tumor necrosis factor inhibition in pregnancy? Arthritis Rheum 2006;54:2353–5.
17. Mease PJ. Adalimumab: an anti-TNF agent for the treatment of psoriatic arthritis. Expert Opin Biol Ther 2005;5:1491–504.
18. Keystone E, Haraoui B. Adalimumab therapy in rheumatoid arthritis. Rheum Dis Clin North Am 2004;30:349–64, vii.
19. Bongartz T, Sutton AJ, Sweeting MJ, et al. Anti-TNF antibody therapy in rheumatoid arthritis and the risk of serious infections and malignancies; systematic review and meta-analysis of rare harmful effects in randomized controlled trials. JAMA 2006;295:2275–85.
20. Deng A, Harvey V, Sina B, et al. Interstitial granulomatous dermatitis associated with the use of tumor necrosis factor alpha inhibitors. Arch Dermatol 2006;142:198–202.
21. Roberts SD, Wilkes DS, Burgett RA, et al. Refractory sarcoidosis responding to infliximab. Chest 2003;124:2028–31.
22. Meyerle JH, Shorr A. The use of infliximab in cutaneous sarcoidosis. J Drugs Dermatol 2003; 2:413–4.
23. Utz JP, Limper AH, Kalra S, et al. Etanercept for the treatment of stage II and III progressive pulmonary sarcoidosis. Chest 2003;124:177–85.
24. Khanna D, Liebling MR, Louie JS. Etanercept ameliorates sarcoidosis arthritis and skin disease. J Rheumatol 2003;30:1864–7.
25. Philips MA, Lynch J, Azmi FH. Ulcerative cutaneous sarcoidosis responding to adalimumab. J Am Acad Dermatol 2005;53:917.
26. Heffernan MP, Smith DI. Adalimumab for treatment of cutaneous sarcoidosis. Arch Dermatol 2006;142: 17–9.
27. Adams BB. Colocalization of granuloma annulare and mid-dermal elastolysis. J Am Acad Dermatol 2003;48:S25.
28. Hertl MS, Haendle I, Schuler G, et al. Rapid improvement of recalcitrant disseminated granuloma annulare upon treatment with the tumour necrosis factor-alpha inhibitor, infliximab. Br J Dermatol 2005;152:552–5.
29. Shupack J, Siu K. Resolving granuloma annulare with etanercept. Arch Dermatol 2006;142:394–5.
30. Lowitt MH, Dover JS. Necrobiosis lipoidica. J Am Acad Dermatol 1991;25:735.
31. Ullman S, Dahl MV. Necrobiosis lipoidica. An immunofluorescence study. Arch Dermatol 1977; 113:1671–3.
32. Cummins DL, Hiatt KM, Mimouni D, et al. Generalized necrobiosis lipoidica treated with a combination of split-thickness autografting and immunomodulatory therapy. Int J Dermatol 2004;43:852–4.
33. Zeichner JA, Stern DW, Lebwohl M. Treatment of necrobiosis lipoidica with the tumor necrosis factor antagonist etanercept. J Am Acad Dermatol 2006; 54(Suppl):S120–1.
34. Kolde G, Muche JM, Schulze P, et al. Infliximab: a promising new treatment option for ulcerated necrobiosis lipoidica. Dermatology 2003;206:180–1.
35. Wolff K, Stingl G. Pyoderma gangrenosum. In: Freedberg IM, Eisen AZ, Wolff K, et al, editors. Fitzpatrick's dermatology in general medicine. 5th edition. New York: McGraw-Hill Health Professions Division; 1999. p. 1140–8.
36. Crowson AN, Mihm MC Jr, Magro C. Pyoderma gangrenosum: a review. J Cutan Pathol 2003; 30:97.
37. Regueiro M, Valentine J, Plevy S, et al. Infliximab for treatment of pyoderma gangrenosum associated with inflammatory bowel disease. Am J Gastroenterol 2003;98(8):1821–6.
38. Ljung T, Staun M, Grove O, et al. Pyoderma gangrenosum associated with Crohn disease: effect of TNF-alpha blockade with infliximab. Scand J Gastroenterol 2002;37:1108–10.
39. Arnott ID, McDonald D, Williams A, et al. Clinical use of Infliximab in Crohn's disease: the Edinburgh experience. Aliment Pharmacol Ther 2001;15: 1639–46.
40. Kaufman I, Caspi D, Yeshurun D, et al. The effect of infliximab on extraintestinal manifestations of Crohn's disease. Rheumatol Int 2005;25(6):406–10.
41. McGowan JW 4th, Johnson CA, Lynn A. Treatment of pyoderma gangrenosum with etanercept. J Drugs Dermatol 2004;3:441–4.
42. Hubbard VG, Friedmann AC, Goldsmith P. Systemic pyoderma gangrenosum responding to infliximab and adalimumab. Br J Dermatol 2005; 152:1059–61.
43. Goldenberg G, Jorizzo JL. Use of etanercept in treatment of pyoderma gangrenosum in a patient with autoimmune hepatitis. J Dermatolog Treat 2005;16:347–9.

44. Pastor N, Betlloch I, Pascual JC, et al. Pyoderma gangrenosum treated with anti-TNF alpha therapy (etanercept). Clin Exp Dermatol 2006;31:152–3.
45. Yamauchi PS, Turner L, Lowe NJ, et al. Treatment of recurrent Sweet's syndrome with coexisting rheumatoid arthritis with the tumor necrosis factor antagonist etanercept. J Am Acad Dermatol 2006;54(Suppl):S122–6.
46. Grob JJ, Mege JL, Capo C, et al. Role of tumor necrosis factor-alpha in Sneddon-Wilkinson subcorneal pustular dermatosis. A model of neutrophil priming in vivo. J Am Acad Dermatol 1991; 25:944–7.
47. Voigtlander C, Luftl M, Schuler G, et al. Infliximab (antitumor necrosis factor alpha antibody): a novel, highly effective treatment of recalcitrant subcorneal pustular dermatosis (Sneddon-Wilkinson disease). Arch Dermatol 2001;137:1571–4.
48. Bartolucci P, Ramanoelina J, Cohen P, et al. Efficacy of the anti-TNF-alpha antibody infliximab against refractory systemic vasculitides: an open pilot study in 10 patients. Rheumatology (Oxford) 2002;41:1126–32.
49. Booth A, Harper L, Hammad T, et al. Prospective study of TNFalpha blockade with infliximab in anti-neutrophil cytoplasmic antibody-associated systemic vasculitis. J Am Soc Nephrol 2004;15:717–21.
50. Booth AD, Jefferson HJ, Ayliffe W, et al. Safety and efficacy of TNF-alpha blockade in relapsing vasculitis. Ann Rheum Dis 2002;61:559.
51. Gause A, Arbach O, Reinhold-Keller E, et al. Induction of remission with infliximab in active generalized Wegener's granulomatosis is effective but complicated by serious infection [abstract]. Arthritis Rheum 2003;48:s208.
52. Lamprecht P, Voswinkel J, Lilienthal T, et al. Effectiveness of TNF-alpha blockade with infliximab in refractory Wegener's granulomatosis. Rheumatology (Oxford) 2002;41:1303–7.
53. Josselin L, Mahr A, Cohen P, et al. Infliximab efficacy and safety against refractory systemic necrotising vasculitides: long-term follow-up of 15 patients. Ann Rheum Dis 2008;67(9):1343–6.
54. Keystone EC. The utility of tumour necrosis factor blockade in orphan diseases. Ann Rheum Dis 2004;63(Suppl 2):ii79–83, 189.
55. Stone JH, Uhlfelder ML, Hellmann DB, et al. Etanercept combined with conventional treatment in Wegener's granulomatosis: a six-month open-label trial to evaluate safety. Arthritis Rheum 2001;44:1149–54.
56. D'Auria L, Cordiali Fei P, Ameglio F. Cytokines and bullous pemphigoid. Eur Cytokine Netw 1999;10:123–34.
57. D'Auria L, Mussi A, Bonifati C, et al. Increased serum IL-6, TNF-alpha and IL-10 levels in patients with bullous pemphigoid: relationships with disease activity. J Eur Acad Dermatol Venereol 1999;12:11–5.
58. Giacalone B, D'Auria L, Bonifati C, et al. Decreased interleukin-7 and transforming growth factor-beta1 levels in blister fluids as compared to the respective serum levels in patients with bullous pemphigoid. Opposite behavior of TNF-alpha, interleukin-4 and interleukin-10. Exp Dermatol 1998;7:157–61.
59. Rhodes LE, Hashim IA, McLaughlin PJ, et al. Blister fluid cytokines in cutaneous inflammatory bullous disorders. Acta Derm Venereol 1999;79:288–90.
60. Lee SJ, Li Z, Sherman B, et al. Serum levels of tumor necrosis factor-alpha and interleukin-6 in ocular cicatricial pemphigoid. Invest Ophthalmol Vis Sci 1993;34:3522–5.
61. Yamauchi PS, Lowe NJ, Gindi V. Treatment of coexisting bullous pemphigoid and psoriasis with the tumor necrosis factor antagonist etanercept. J Am Acad Dermatol 2006;54(Suppl):S121–2.
62. Sacher C, Rubbert A, Konig C, et al. Treatment of recalcitrant cicatricial pemphigoid with the tumor necrosis factor alpha antagonist etanercept. J Am Acad Dermatol 2002;46:113–5.
63. Canizares MJ, Smith DI, Conners MS, et al. Successful treatment of mucous membrane pemphigoid with etanercept in 3 patients. Arch Dermatol 2006;142:1457–61.
64. Aringer M, Smolen JS. TNF inhibition in SLE: where do we stand? Lupus 2009;18(1):5–8.
65. Levälampi T, Korpela M, Vuolteenaho K, et al. Etanercept and adalimumab treatment in patients with rheumatoid arthritis and spondyloarthropathies in clinical practice: adverse events and other reasons leading to discontinuation of the treatment. Rheumatol Int 2008;28(3):261–9.
66. Aringer M, Graninger WB, Steiner G, et al. Safety and efficacy of tumor necrosis factor alpha blockade in systemic lupus erythematosus: an open-label study. Arthritis Rheum 2004; 50:3161–9. 9–16.
67. Fautrel B, Foltz V, Frances C, et al. Regression of subacute cutaneous lupus erythematosus in a patient with rheumatoid arthritis treated with a biologic tumor necrosis factor alpha-blocking agent: comment on the article by Pisetsky and the letter from Aringer et al. Arthritis Rheum 2002;46:1408–9 [author reply: 1409].
68. Norman R, Greenberg RG, Jackson JM. Case reports of etanercept in inflammatory dermatoses. J Am Acad Dermatol 2006;54(Suppl):S139–42.
69. Aringer M, Houssiau F, Gordon C, et al. Adverse events and efficacy of TNF-{alpha} blockade with infliximab in patients with systemic lupus erythematosus: long-term follow-up of 13 patients. Rheumatology (Oxford) 2009;48(11):1451–4.

70. Uppal SS, Hayat SJ, Raghupathy R. Efficacy and safety of infliximab in active SLE: a pilot study. Lupus 2009;18(8):690–7.
71. Costa MF, Said NR, Zimmermann B. Drug-induced lupus due to anti-tumor necrosis factor alpha agents. Semin Arthritis Rheum 2008; 37(6):381–7.
72. Shi-Wen X, Panesar M, Vancheeswaran R, et al. Expression and shedding of intercellular adhesion molecule 1 and lymphocyte function-associated antigen 3 by normal and scleroderma fibroblasts. Effects of interferon-gamma, tumor necrosis factor alpha, and estrogen. Arthritis Rheum 1994;37(11): 1689–97.
73. Koca SS, Isik A, Ozercan IH, et al. Effectiveness of etanercept in bleomycin-induced experimental scleroderma. Rheumatology (Oxford) 2008;47(2): 172–5.
74. Ellman MH, MacDonald PA, Hayes FA. Etanercept as a treatment for diffuse scleroderma: a pilot study. Arthritis Rheum 2000;43:s392.
75. Lam GK, Hummers LK, Woods A, et al. Efficacy and safety of etanercept in the treatment of scleroderma-associated joint disease. J Rheumatol 2007; 34(7):1636–7.
76. Denton CP, Engelhart M, Tvede N, et al. An open-label pilot study of infliximab therapy in diffuse cutaneous systemic sclerosis. Ann Rheum Dis 2009;68(9):1433–9.
77. Bargagli E, Galeazzi M, Bellisai F, et al. Infliximab treatment in a patient with systemic sclerosis associated with lung fibrosis and pulmonary hypertension. Respiration 2008;75(3):346–9.
78. Christopher-Stine L, Wigley F. Tumor necrosis factor-alpha antagonists induce lupus-like syndrome in patients with scleroderma overlap/ mixed connective tissue disease. J Rheumatol 2003;30:2725–7.
79. Menon Y, Cucurull E, Espinoza LR. Pancytopenia in a patient with scleroderma treated with infliximab. Rheumatology (Oxford) 2003;42:1273–4 [author reply: 1274].
80. Efthimiou P, Schwartzman S, Kagen LJ. Possible role for tumor necrosis factor inhibitors in the treatment of resistant dermatomyositis and polymyositis: a retrospective study of eight patients. Ann Rheum Dis 2006;65(9):1233–6.
81. Riley P, McCann LJ, Maillard SM, et al. Effectiveness of infliximab in the treatment of refractory juvenile dermatomyositis with calcinosis. Rheumatology (Oxford) 2008;47(6):877–80.
82. Hengstman GJ, De Bleecker JL, Feist E, et al. Open-label trial of anti-TNF-alpha in dermato- and polymyositis treated concomitantly with methotrexate. Eur Neurol 2008;59(3–4):159–63.
83. Dold S, Justiniano ME, Marquez J, et al. Treatment of early and refractory dermatomyositis with infliximab: a report of two cases. Clin Rheumatol 2007;26:1186–8.
84. Roddy E, Courtney PA, Morris A. Non-Hodgkin's lymphoma in a patient with refractory dermatomyositis which had been treated with infliximab. Rheumatology (Oxford) 2002;41:1194–5.
85. Goossens PH, Verburg RJ, Breedveld FC. Remission of Behcet's syndrome with tumour necrosis factor alpha blocking therapy. Ann Rheum Dis 2001;60:637.
86. Olivieri I, Padula A, Leccese P, et al. Long-lasting remission of severe Behçet's disease after the end of infliximab therapy. J Rheumatol 2009; 36(4):855.
87. Jalili A, Kinaciyan T, Barisani T, et al. Successful treatment of refractory Behçet's disease with the TNF-alpha blocker infliximab. Iran J Immunol 2009;6(1):55–8.
88. Yamada Y, Sugita S, Tanaka H, et al. Comparison of infliximab versus cyclosporine during the initial 6-month treatment period in Behcet's disease. Br J Ophthalmol 2010;94(3):284–8.
89. Iwata S, Saito K, Yamaoka K, et al. Effects of anti-TNF-alpha antibody infliximab in refractory entero-Behcet's disease. Rheumatology (Oxford) 2009; 48(8):1012–3.
90. Melikoglu M, Kural-Seyahi E, Tascilar K, et al. The unique features of vasculitis in Behçet's syndrome. Clin Rev Allergy Immunol 2008;35(1–2):40–6.
91. Belzunegui J, López L, Paniagua I, et al. Efficacy of infliximab and adalimumab in the treatment of a patient with severe neuro-Behçet's disease. Clin Exp Rheumatol 2008;26(4 Suppl 50):S133–4.
92. Ariyachaipanich A, Berkelhammer C, Nicola H. Intestinal Behçet's disease: maintenance of remission with adalimumab monotherapy. Inflamm Bowel Dis 2009;15(12):1769–71.
93. Yildiz N, Alkan H, Ardic F, et al. Successful treatment with adalimumab in a patient with coexisting Behçet's disease and ankylosing spondylitis. Rheumatol Int 2009. [Epub ahead of print].
94. Takase K, Ohno S, Ideguchi H, et al. Successful switching to adalimumab in an infliximab-allergic patient with severe Behçet disease-related uveitis. Rheumatol Int 2009. [Epub ahead of print].
95. Estrach C, Mpofu S, Moots RJ. Behcet's syndrome: response to infliximab after failure of etanercept. Rheumatology (Oxford) 2002;41:1213–4.
96. Yucel AE, Kart-Koseoglu H, Akova YA, et al. Failure of infliximab treatment and occurrence of erythema nodosum during therapy in two patients with Behcet's disease. Rheumatology (Oxford) 2004;43: 394–6.
97. Cooke KR, Hill GR, Gerbitz A, et al. Tumor necrosis factor-alpha neutralization reduces lung injury after experimental allogeneic bone marrow transplantation. Transplantation 2000;70:272–9.

98. Hattori K, Hirano T, Miyajima H, et al. Differential effects of anti-Fas ligand and anti-tumor necrosis factor alpha antibodies on acute graft-versus-host disease pathologies. Blood 1998;91:4051–5.
99. Schmaltz C, Alpdogan O, Muriglan SJ, et al. Donor T cell-derived TNF is required for graft-versus-host disease and graft-versus-tumor activity after bone marrow transplantation. Blood 2003;101:2440–5.
100. Tsukada N, Kobata T, Aizawa Y, et al. Graft-versus-leukemia effect and graft-versus-host disease can be differentiated by cytotoxic mechanisms in a murine model of allogeneic bone marrow transplantation. Blood 1999;93:2738–47.
101. Holler E, Kolb HJ, Moller A, et al. Increased serum levels of tumor necrosis factor alpha precede major complications of bone marrow transplantation. Blood 1990;75:1011–6.
102. Couriel D, Hicks K, Ipolotti C. Infliximab for the treatment of graft-versus-host disease in allogeneic transplant recipients: an update. Blood 2000;96:400a.
103. Jacobsohn DA, Hallick J, Anders V, et al. Infliximab for steroid-refractory acute GVHD: a case series. Am J Hematol 2003;74:119–24.
104. Couriel D, Saliba R, Hicks K, et al. Tumor necrosis factor-alpha blockade for the treatment of acute GVHD. Blood 2004;104:649–54.
105. Patriarca F, Sperotto A, Damiani D, et al. Infliximab treatment for steroid-refractory acute graft-versus-host disease. Haematologica 2004;89:1352–9.
106. Srinivasan R, Chakrabarti S, Walsh T. Improved survival in steroid refractory acute graft versus host disease after nonmyeloablative allogeneic transplantation using daclizumab-based strategy with comprehensive infection prophylaxis. Br J Haematol 2004;124:777–86.
107. Rao K, Rao A, Karlsson H, et al. Improved survival and preserved antiviral responses after combination therapy with daclizumab and infliximab in steroid-refractory graft-versus-host disease. J Pediatr Hematol Oncol 2009;31(6):456–61.
108. Antin JH, Chen AR, Couriel DR, et al. Novel approaches to the therapy of steroid-resistant acute graft-versus-host disease. Biol Blood Marrow Transplant 2004;10:655–68.
109. Uberti JP, Ayash L, Ratanatharathorn V, et al. Pilot trial on the use of etanercept and methylprednisolone as primary treatment for acute graft-versus-host disease. Biol Blood Marrow Transplant 2005; 11:680–7.
110. Chiang KY, Abhyankar S, Bridges K, et al. Recombinant human tumor necrosis factor receptor fusion protein as complementary treatment for chronic graft-versus-host disease. Transplantation 2002;73:665–7.
111. Marty FM, Lee SJ, Fahey MM, et al. Infliximab use in patients with severe graft-versus-host disease and other emerging risk factors of non-Candida invasive fungal infections in allogeneic hematopoietic stem cell transplant recipients: a cohort study. Blood 2003;102:2768–76.
112. Drosou A, Kirsner RS, Welsh E, et al. Use of infliximab, an anti-tumor necrosis alpha antibody, for inflammatory dermatoses. J Cutan Med Surg 2003;7:382–6.
113. Barth D, Harth W, Treudler R, et al. Successful treatment of pityriasis rubra pilaris (type 1) under combination of infliximab and methotrexate. J Dtsch Dermatol Ges 2009;7(12):1071–3.
114. Müller H, Gattringer C, Zelger B, et al. Infliximab monotherapy as first-line treatment for adult-onset pityriasis rubra pilaris: case report and review of the literature on biologic therapy. J Am Acad Dermatol 2008;59(Suppl 5):S65–70.
115. Davis KF, Wu JJ, Murase JE, et al. Clinical improvement of pityriasis rubra pilaris with combination etanercept and acitretin therapy. Arch Dermatol 2007;143(12):1597–9.
116. Seckin D, Tula E, Ergun T. Successful use of etanercept in type I pityriasis rubra pilaris. Br J Dermatol 2008;158(3):642–4.
117. Cox V, Lesesky EB, Garcia BD, et al. Treatment of juvenile pityriasis rubra pilaris with etanercept. J Am Acad Dermatol 2008;59(5 Suppl):S113–4.
118. Walling HW, Swick BL. Pityriasis rubra pilaris responding rapidly to adalimumab. Arch Dermatol 2009;145(1):99–101.
119. Wagner AD, Andresen J, Jendro MC, et al. Sustained response to tumor necrosis factor alpha-blocking agents in two patients with SAPHO syndrome. Arthritis Rheum 2002;46:1965–8.
120. Olivieri I, Padula A, Ciancio G, et al. Persistent efficacy of tumor necrosis factor alpha blockage therapy in SAPHO syndrome: comment on the article by Wagner et al. Arthritis Rheum 2003; 48(5):1467 [author reply: 1468].
121. Moll C, Hernández MV, Cañete JD, et al. Ilium osteitis as the main manifestation of the SAPHO syndrome: response to infliximab therapy and review of the literature. Semin Arthritis Rheum 2008;37(5):299–306.
122. Kovach BT, Calamia KT, Walsh JS, et al. Treatment of multicentric reticulohistiocytosis with etanercept. Arch Dermatol 2004;140:919–21.
123. Matejicka C, Morgan GJ, Schlegelmilch JG. Multicentric reticulohistiocytosis treated successfully with an anti-tumor necrosis factor agent: comment on the article by Gorman et al. Arthritis Rheum 2003;48:864–6.
124. Lee MW, Lee EY, Jeong YI, et al. Successful treatment of multicentric reticulohistiocytosis with a combination of infliximab, prednisolone and methotrexate. Acta Derm Venereol 2004;84: 478–9.

125. Shannon SE, Schumacher HR, Self S, et al. Multicentric reticulohistiocytosis responding to tumor necrosis factor-alpha inhibition in a renal transplant patient. J Rheumatol 2005;32:565–7.
126. Sellam J, Deslandre CJ, Dubreuil F, et al. Refractory multicentric reticulohistiocytosis treated by infliximab: two cases. Clin Exp Rheumatol 2005;23:97–9.
127. Kalajian AH, Callen JP. Multicentric reticulohistiocytosis successfully treated with infliximab: an illustrative case and evaluation of cytokine expression supporting anti-tumor necrosis factor therapy. Arch Dermatol 2008;144:1360–6.
128. Correia O, Delgado L, Barbosa IL, et al. Increased interleukin 10, tumor necrosis factor alpha, and interleukin 6 levels in blister fluid of toxic epidermal necrolysis. J Am Acad Dermatol 2002;47:58–62.
129. Paquet P, Nikkels A, Arrese JE, et al. Macrophages and tumor necrosis factor alpha in toxic epidermal necrolysis. Arch Dermatol 1994;130(5):605–8.
130. Paquet P, Pierard GE. Soluble fractions of tumor necrosis factor-alpha, interleukin-6 and of their receptors in toxic epidermal necrolysis: a comparison with second-degree burns. Int J Mol Med 1998;1: 459–62.
131. Paquet P, Paquet F, Al Saleh W, et al. Immunoregulatory effector cells in drug-induced toxic epidermal necrolysis. Am J Dermatopathol 2000;22:413–7.
132. Paul C, Wolkenstein P, Adle H, et al. Apoptosis as a mechanism of keratinocyte death in toxic epidermal necrolysis. Br J Dermatol 1996;134: 710–4.
133. Fischer M, Fiedler E, Marsch WC, et al. Antitumour necrosis factor-alpha antibodies (infliximab) in the treatment of a patient with toxic epidermal necrolysis. Br J Dermatol 2002;146:707–9.
134. Famularo G, Di Dona B, Canzona F, et al. Etanercept for toxic epidermal necrolysis. Ann Pharmacother 2007;41:1083–4.
135. Gubinelli E, Canzona F, Tonanzi T, et al. Case report: toxic epidermal necrolysis successfully treated with etanercept. J Dermatol 2009;36:150–3.
136. Minni J, Sarro R. A novel therapeutic approach to erythema annulare centrifugum. J Am Acad Dermatol 2006;54(Suppl):S134–5. 138:916–22.

Innovative Uses of Thalidomide

Meng Chen, BA[a], Sean D. Doherty, MD[b], Sylvia Hsu, MD[c,*]

KEYWORDS

• Thalidomide • Off-label use • Dermatology • Birth defects

Thalidomide is a synthetic glutamic acid derivative first introduced in 1956 in Germany as an over-the-counter sedative marketed as Countergan.[1,2] Initially thought a safe medication, thalidomide was marketed to other industrialized nations by 1958 and was also widely used as an antiemetic by pregnant women.[3–5] Thalidomide was withdrawn from the world market in 1961 due to occurrences of rare congenital abnormalities, such as phocomelia, in infants born to women who ingested thalidomide during pregnancy.[3] It had not been approved in the United States at that time due to concerns of a potential link between thalidomide and peripheral neuropathy.[5,6] In 1965, Dr Jacob Sheskin, an Isreali dermatologist, made a fortuitous discovery when giving thalidomide to his leprosy patients for its sedative properties.[4,7] Patients with erythema nodosum leprosum (ENL) had unexpected improvement of skin lesions soon after initiating therapy. This discovery triggered a renewal of interest and research into thalidomide. In 1998, the drug was approved by the Food and Drug Administration for ENL and, in May 2006, it was approved for treating multiple myeloma.[1,8] Thalidomide's status as an orphan drug has led to its off-label and innovative use in several dermatologic disorders unresponsive to traditional treatments.[3]

PHARMACOLOGY

Thalidomide's structure has a left-sided pthalimide ring and a right-sided glutarimide ring.[4] Thalidomide is given orally, with peak plasma concentrations occurring approximately 2.9 to 5.7 hours after ingestion.[7] The drug is metabolized mainly through spontaneous, nonenzymatic hydrolysis in blood and tissue, although a minute amount is metabolized via the hepatic cytochrome P450 system.[7] Thalidomide distributes extensively in the body and has been found in semen, making it necessary for male patients taking the medication to wear condoms even if they have had a vasectomy; their female partners are also advised to use an additional form of birth control.[9] Mean elimination time is 5 to 7 hours, and less than 1% of the medication is excreted unchanged in urine.[4] Most dosages of thalidomide used in dermatology have been low (range of 25 to 400 mg daily), although higher doses have been administered in select situations. The mechanism of action for thalidomide is still not completely understood, although it has been shown to have sedative, anti-inflammatory, immunomodulatory, and antiangiogenic activity.[3]

OFF-LABEL DERMATOLOGIC USES

Aphthous Stomatitis

Several studies have shown thalidomide to be effective for recurrent aphthous stomatitis. Mascaro and colleagues[10] reported 6 cases of aphthous stomatitis that completely resolved after 7 to 10 days of therapy with thalidomide (100 mg daily). Jenkins and colleagues[11] reported similar results: 15 patients with aphthous stomatitis were treated with thalidomide (400 mg daily tapered to 200 mg daily). Fourteen of the patients

[a] Department of Dermatology, Baylor College of Medicine, BCM Debakey Building M220, One Baylor Plaza, Mail Stop BCM368, Houston, TX 77030, USA
[b] Department of Dermatology, Baylor College of Medicine, 1709 Dryden, Suite 10.50, Houston, TX 77030, USA
[c] Department of Dermatology, Baylor College of Medicine, 6620 Main Street, Suite 1425 Houston, TX 77030, USA
* Corresponding author.
E-mail address: shsu@bcm.edu

Dermatol Clin 28 (2010) 577–586
doi:10.1016/j.det.2010.03.003
0733-8635/10/$ – see front matter © 2010 Elsevier Inc. All rights reserved.

had complete resolution of lesions within 5 to 21 days, and the remaining patient had significant improvement. Unfortunately, most of the treated patients relapsed after therapy was discontinued.

Larger, open-label, noncontrolled studies have also reported successful treatment of severe aphthosis with thalidomide. In a 40-patient trial, severe oral aphthosis was treated with thalidomide at initial dosages of 300 mg daily; mild cases were started on 100 mg daily.[12] In both groups, 75% of patients responded well to therapy. For patients who relapsed after discontinuing therapy, the investigators recommended a dosage of 100 mg daily for 12 days. A controlled, crossover, randomized trial of 73 patients with severe aphthous stomatitis reported 32 patients (44%) with complete remission while on thalidomide (100 mg daily); most other patients in the study experienced dramatic improvement.[13]

A recent open trial of 21 patients compared the efficacy of thalidomide, dapsone, colchicine, and pentoxifylline in treating severe recurrent aphthous stomatitis.[14] Each patient was given 1 of the 4 test drugs for 6 months and switched drugs if toxicity or lack of efficacy occurred. Of the 4 drugs, thalidomide (100 mg daily) was the most effective and well tolerated, resulting in complete remission for 7 of 8 patients. Other studies have shown that thalidomide therapy is also an effective option for recurrent aphthous ulcers in patients with HIV.[15,16] Aphthous ulcers have a variable natural course and many cases resolve spontaneously, making the interpretation of any therapeutic study somewhat difficult. Thalidomide therapy should be considered only for severe, recurrent, and seemingly recalcitrant cases.[17]

Behçet Disease

Behçet disease (BD) is a systemic disorder with various skin lesions, ocular disease (panuveitis), arthritis, intestinal bleeding, and recurrent aphthous orogenital ulcers.[18] After reports of thalidomide's efficacy for aphthous stomatitis, a 1982 open trial treated 22 BD patients with thalidomide (400 mg daily for 5 days and 200 mg daily for the next 15–60 days).[19] Although ocular and arthritic symptoms did not improve, orogenital ulcerations healed quickly. Ulcers recurred after withdrawal of thalidomide, but they were milder and less frequent than before treatment.[19] Other studies have shown similar beneficial effects but have also noted recurrence of disease after treatment ended.[3,20,21]

A randomized, double-blind trial compared thalidomide dosages (100 mg daily and 300 mg daily) to placebo.[18] The results showed thalidomide dosages of 100 mg daily to be similar in efficacy to 300 mg daily, with both dosages demonstrating better efficacy compared with the placebo control. Withdrawal of either treatment dosage led to prompt recurrence. In a study to find an optimal dosage with minimal toxicity, 50 mg daily of thalidomide was concluded as efficacious, and remission was sustained in more than 60% of patients by a dosage of 50 mg every 2 to 3 days.[22] Recent trials treating BD with thalidomide have used dosages ranging from 25 to 200 mg daily with reported high efficacy.[23,24] Like aphthous stomatitis, some orogenital ulcerations of BD resolve without treatment, so thalidomide should be reserved for severe, unresponsive BD cases where orogenital ulcerations are prominent features of the disorder.[3]

Lupus Erythematosus

The first reported successful thalidomide treatment of chronic cutaneous lupus erythematosus (CCLE) was in 1977 in a case series of 20 patients.[25] Since that time, there have been at least 200 reported cases demonstrating thalidomide's efficacy for severe CCLE.[26] One large clinical trial of 60 patients with CCLE reported complete or marked responses in 54 patients (90%), but 71% of patients relapsed after discontinuing treatment.[27] Patients with relapse again responded when therapy was reinitiated.

Subacute cutaneous lupus erythematosus has also shown response to thalidomide therapy.[28–30] Pelle and Werth[31] reviewed 8 separate case series that reported a total of 171 patients with various forms of cutaneous lupus treated with thalidomide. The overall response rate was 85%, with complete resolution in 59%; the response rates for discoid lupus erythematosus and subacute cutaneous lupus erythematosus were comparable at 90.3% and 82.4%, respectively.

Thalidomide has also been used to effectively treat refractory tumid lupus erythematosus,[32] but the drug has not been as successful in treating lupus panniculitis. Coelho and colleagues[33] reported a complete or partial response in 99% of patients with all types of cutaneous lupus treated with thalidomide (100 mg daily tapered to 50 mg daily or less when clinically feasible). Two-thirds of patients with lupus panniculitis, however, had no response to treatment.

Thalidomide has proved effective for treating cutaneous aspects of systemic lupus erythematosus (SLE) as well.[31,33] Stevens and colleagues,[30] however, observed that the drug does not significantly suppress systemic disease in SLE. Dosage for treating lupus erythematosus has varied among studies. Published treatment guidelines recommend starting at 100 to 200 mg daily.[34] This dosage can be tapered as the clinical situation warrants. Because relapse of disease occurs in more than 70% of patients after discontinuing thalidomide, low maintenance dosages (50 mg 3–7 times weekly) may be required to sustain remission.[27,31,33] Although shown effective in various forms of lupus erythematosus, thalidomide is still considered second-line treatment of cutaneous lupus refractory to other therapies.[34]

Prurigo Nodularis

Prurigo nodularis (PN) is a pruritic type of neurodermatitis with skin-colored, erythematous, or hyperpigmented cutaneous nodules.[4] Patients with PN can be difficult to treat, and standard therapies with corticosteroids and antihistamines may be ineffective.[35] The initial report of thalidomide's efficacy in treating PN was in 1965 by Sheskin.[36] A more recent retrospective study presented 12 patients with PN who were given thalidomide for at least 1 month at an initial dosage of 100 mg daily.[32] Response was noted in 8 of 12 patients, ranging from mild to moderate improvement, with complete resolution in 1 patient. In another study, 22 patients with PN were given thalidomide (50 to 300 mg daily) for a mean duration of 1 year.[37] In 20 patients, there was immediate, pronounced alleviation of pruritus along with significant reduction in size and number of lesions after 1 to 2 months. Thirteen patients, however, discontinued treatment due to side effects, 5 of them due to neuropathy.[37] Combination therapy of thalidomide treatment followed by narrowband ultraviolet B phototherapy has also been studied and induced excellent therapeutic response.[38] The mechanism of thalidomide's efficacy for PN is thought to be the drug's direct toxic effect on proliferative neural tissues.[8,39] Although thalidomide is efficacious in treating PN at higher doses, the high rate of peripheral neuropathy seen in these studies makes treatment with thalidomide at high doses less than ideal.

Sarcoidosis

There are several case reports and small, open-label, clinical trials using thalidomide to treat cutaneous sarcoidosis. In a review by Doherty and Rosen,[40] it was reported that thalidomide dosing for sarcoidosis has ranged from 50 mg to more than 400 mg daily, and dosages for long-term maintenance have ranged from 50 mg every 15 days to 100 mg every other day.[41–45] Baughman and colleagues[46] used thalidomide to treat 14 patients with unresponsive chronic cutaneous sarcoidosis for 4 months. All patients experienced subjective improvement, and photographic scoring showed objective improvement in 10 of 12 patients. In another study, 8 patients with cutaneous sarcoidosis were treated with thalidomide for 16 weeks at a dosage of 50 mg daily increased, as needed, to a maximum of 200 mg daily; 6 patients also concomitantly received stable prednisone dosages.[47] After treatment, skin biopsies of all 8 patients showed reductions in granuloma size and epidermal thickness. In a French study of 10 patients given thalidomide for refractory cutaneous sarcoidosis, 3 patients had total regression of skin lesions and 4 had a partial response; 3 patients had no response.[48] The investigators noted relapse of symptoms when the drug was discontinued, but reintroduction of thalidomide was efficacious.

Sarcoidosis involves a Th1-type immune response characterized by increased levels of interferon γ (IFN-γ), interleukin (IL)-2, and IL-12.[49] Also, tumor necrosis factor α (TNF-α) plays a major role by escalating macrophage recruitment into granulomatous lesions.[50] Thalidomide inhibits TNF-α and IFN-γ and has also been shown to induce and enhance IL-4 and IL-5 production, indicating that thalidomide may help modulate a therapeutic switching from disease-inducing predominant Th1 activation—the type principally seen in sarcoidosis—to Th2 activation.[51]

Actinic Prurigo

In the initial 1973 study, 32 of 34 patients with actinic prurigo exhibited clinical improvement after receiving thalidomide (initial dosage of 300 mg daily tapered to 15 mg daily for a mean of 50 days). Patients promptly relapsed, however, on discontinuation of treatment.[52] A 1977 study of 51 patients demonstrated parallel results.[53] In another study of 14 patients with actinic prurigo, 11 patients had lasting improvement with thalidomide (50 to 200 mg daily), but 8 patients required maintenance dosages (50 to 100 mg weekly).[54] As is true of many of the disorders discussed in this article, actinic prurigo also may require ongoing, maintenance drug to prevent relapse of disease.

Graft-versus-host disease

Thalidomide's efficacy for acute and chronic graft-versus-host disease (GVHD) in humans was first reported in 1988, when a patient was successfully treated with thalidomide for acute cutaneous GVHD after allogeneic bone marrow transplant.[55] More recent studies, however, have shown mixed results. Vogelsang and colleagues[56] used thalidomide (200 mg 4 times daily) as salvage therapy for 23 patients with refractory chronic GVHD and 21 patients with high-risk GVHD; complete response was achieved in 14 patients and partial response in 12 patients. The study concluded thalidomide is a safe and effective treatment option for chronic GVHD.

A randomized, placebo-controlled study of 59 patients concluded thalidomide was not effective as a prophylactic agent for preventing GVHD; the thalidomide group developed a higher incidence of GVHD than did the placebo group.[57] In a 2001 randomized trial, when thalidomide was incorporated as initial therapy for GVHD in a regimen of cyclosporine and prednisone, no significant clinical benefit was found.[58] A 2003 study compared thalidomide's effect on 21 acute GVHD patients and 59 chronic GVHD patients.[59] Thalidomide was not effective for acute GVHD but did produce clinical benefit in chronic GVHD, and patients responsive to thalidomide had significantly better survival rates.[59] In the study, thalidomide was added to the regimen after patients had already started a variety of other agents, including corticosteroids, cyclosporine, and azathioprine, making the actual benefit of the thalidomide difficult to ascertain.[59]

In summary, although thalidomide has not been shown clinically beneficial as prophylactic or first-line therapy for GVHD, thalidomide can be an effective salvage treatment of chronic GVHD. Common side effects with thalidomide treatment of GVHD include constipation, sleepiness, and neuropathy.[56] In one case report, pancreatitis resulted from thalidomide usage for a patient with chronic GVHD.[60]

Langerhans Cell Histiocytosis

Since the initial report in 1987, several case studies have reported that thalidomide is effective in treating Langerhans cell histiocytosis.[61] In many instances, however, patients relapsed after cessation of treatment and ultimately required maintenance dosages.[3,62–66] Broekaert and colleagues[65] recommended an initial dosage of 50 to 200 mg daily and a maintenance dosage as low as 25 mg twice weekly, depending on the course of disease. These investigators also concluded that thalidomide is a safe, well-tolerated, and easy-to-administer treatment choice that is rapidly efficacious on mucocutaneous lesions.[65] Thalidomide has not been reported to have effects on visceral manifestations of the disease, however.[3,62–66] A recent article described a phase II trial of 15 patients, in which 7 of 9 patients without organ involvement showed complete or partial response to therapy, but all patients with organ involvement did not respond to therapy.[67] After review of their data and previous reports, the investigators recommended thalidomide for treating patients with refractory skin and bone Langerhans cell histiocytosis but not for treatment of advanced, high-risk disease.[67]

Erythema Multiforme

A 1982 article reported a case of recurrent erythema multiforme (EM) treated with thalidomide (200 mg daily); after a few days, the patient's lesions on the hands, feet, lips, and glans penis healed, and there was no relapse after tapering dosage to 100 mg daily.[68] A recent report noted an excellent response to thalidomide (200 mg daily) for 2 patients with severe, persistent EM.[69] Neither patient relapsed with a maintenance dosage (50 mg daily), although 1 patient developed neuropathy after 2 years on thalidomide.[69] There are several other case reports treating recurrent EM with thalidomide. In a larger retrospective study, 26 patients with EM were given thalidomide (100 mg daily) after other therapies failed.[70] The 20 patients with recurrent disease had reduction in duration of episodes by an average of 11 days, and 6 patients had lesions disappear within 5 to 8 days, which was maintained with low-dose treatment.[70]

Lichen Planus

Treatment of lichen planus (LP) has often been inadequate, especially for widespread cases of LP.[71] Thalidomide has been reported to treat severe, refractory LP at dosage ranges of 25 to 300 mg daily.[3,32] In a retrospective study of 6 patients with severe oral LP, thalidomide was initiated at 50 to 100 mg daily and gradually tapered.[72] Four patients had complete healing and 1 patient had partial healing. Oral erosions rapidly recurred when thalidomide was discontinued, however, and 2 patients had side effects of phlebitis and neuropathy.[72]

In a 2009 report, 8 patients with cutaneous LP were treated with thalidomide (100 mg daily) until they had complete resolution of lesions, although 3 patients withdrew due to neuropathy.[71] For patients finishing the study, there was healing of skin lesions at a mean of 4 weeks and complete remission at a mean of 3 months; no recurrences were noted 6 months after treatment.[71]

Torti and colleagues[73] treated 50 oral LP cases through a therapeutic ladder ranging from topical corticosteroids to oral thalidomide. Among treatments, thalidomide resulted in the highest percentage (80%) of patients with substantial or complete healing, but only 5 of 50 patients were given thalidomide, because it was used only for recalcitrant cases unresponsive to other agents. Thalidomide can be a valuable treatment of LP; however, it is reserved only for severe, unresponsive disease. Dosages of 100 mg daily initially have been effective, and clinical response frequently occurs after 3 to 4 months or more of treatment. Patients must be monitored for adverse effects, especially neuropathy.

There have been a few case reports of successful thalidomide treatment of lichen planopilaris, a follicular type of LP.[32,74,75] In contrast, a case series of 4 patients of lichen planopilaris showed no clinical improvement from thalidomide treatment.[76]

Kaposi Sarcoma

Thalidomide was first noted to have therapeutic effects for Kaposi sarcoma (KS) in 1996, when a 14-year-old girl with HIV and KS given thalidomide for oral ulcers was noted to have improvement in KS lesions.[77] A phase II study ensued; thalidomide (100 mg daily) was given to 17 HIV patients with KS for 8 weeks.[78] There were 6 (35%) partial responses, but 8 patients withdrew from the study (6 due to toxicity).[78] Another phase II trial treated 20 HIV patients who had KS with thalidomide at an initial dosage of 200 mg daily escalated to a maximum of 1000 mg daily.[79] After a median of 6.3 months of therapy, there were 8 (40%) partial responses, with a median dosage of 500 mg daily at time of response.[79]

Two recent articles analyzed thalidomide therapy for non–AIDS-related KS. One was a retrospective study of 11 patients who received thalidomide at a median dosage of 100 mg daily for a median duration of 16 weeks. There were 3 partial responders and 4 had stable disease, but 3 patients discontinued thalidomide due to neuropathy and vertigo.[80] The second study also used thalidomide (100 mg daily) but treated patients for a longer duration of 12 months. Two of 3 patients had complete remission after 12 months and all 3 had partial response after 4 months.[81] Although effective for some cases of KS—HIV-related and non–HIV-related—thalidomide has not materialized as a first-line treatment of this vascular tumor.

Jessner Lymphocytic Infiltrate

In 2 French case series, thalidomide has shown promise for treating Jessner lymphocytic infiltrate. Moulin and colleagues[82] successfully treated 5 patients with thalidomide (100 mg daily). On stopping thalidomide, skin lesions returned in 4 patients, but continuous dosage of 25 to 50 mg daily for more than 2 years resulted in normal skin for 3 patients.[82] The second study was a controlled, randomized, crossover trial of 28 patients. There was complete resolution in 19 (76%) patients treated with thalidomide (100 mg daily) compared with 4 (16%) patients receiving placebo.[83] Six patients responding to thalidomide relapsed after switching to placebo.[83] For Jessner lymphocytic infiltrate, thalidomide (100 mg daily) seems beneficial. Maintenance dosing may be needed, because withdrawal of treatment has uniformly resulted in clinical relapse.

Uremic Pruritus

For uremic patients receiving hemodialysis, pruritus occurs in 80% to 90% of patients at some point.[84] The cause remains unclear, and no standard treatments have yet been established. In a crossover, randomized, double-blind trial, thalidomide (100 mg daily for 7 days) was compared with placebo for treating refractory uremic pruritus in 29 patients. Of 18 patients finishing the study, approximately 55% showed a response to thalidomide whereas none responded to placebo.[85] In responsive patients, there was an average decrease of 78% to 81% in pruritus scoring. Although promising, additional investigation is needed to evaluate thalidomide's efficacy for management of uremic pruritus.

Pyoderma Gangrenosum

Pyoderma gangrenosum (PG) is a noninfectious skin disorder that begins as painful pustules or papulonodules that enlarge and ulcerate.[86] Several case reports have reported thalidomide's effectiveness in PG unresponsive to other treatments. One recent case of PG related to myelodysplastic syndrome had dramatic improvement of massive ulcerovegetative lesions after 4 months of combination therapy with IFN-α2a and thalidomide (200 mg daily).[87] In another recent report, a patient with PG and multiple myeloma had complete healing of PG after receiving dexamethasone and thalidomide (200 mg daily for 5 weeks).[86] Another patient with PG unresponsive to several courses of methylprednisolone had complete response to thalidomide (ranging from 100 mg to 200 mg daily over 10 weeks).[88] In one case, thalidomide (100 mg daily) led to complete healing of PG, but withdrawal of treatment after 2 years due to neuropathy led to prompt relapse.[89] Effective dosages of thalidomide in case reports have ranged from 100 to 400 mg daily, with treatment durations ranging from 5 days to 6 months or more.[90–93] Ehling and colleagues[94] designated thalidomide a third-choice treatment of PG, reserving thalidomide for severe, progressive disease. Controlled clinical trials are needed to further assess thalidomide's efficacy in PG.

Scleromyxedema

Thalidomide has also been used to treat scleromyxedema. Since a report in 2004 of a scleromyxedema case responding well to thalidomide, a handful of new case reports have described remarkable improvement in skin lesions and monoclonal gammopathy after using thalidomide for scleromyxedema.[95–97] In one case series, 200 mg daily given in divided doses was effective.[98] Dosages of 100 mg daily have also been successful.[95–97] Additional studies are required to assess the true efficacy of thalidomide in this setting.

Necrobiosis Lipoidica

A case of necrobiosis lipoidica that was unresponsive to therapy was treated with thalidomide (150 mg daily). Four months after initiation of therapy, there was clinical improvement in all lesions, and thalidomide was tapered to 50 mg daily.[99] After complete resolution at 1 year of therapy, the dosage was further lowered to 50 mg twice weekly with no adverse effects or recurrence after 2 years of therapy.[99] Further studies are needed to confirm thalidomide's efficacy for necrobiosis lipoidica.

TOXIC EPIDERMAL NECROLYSIS–CONTRAINDICATED USE

Toxic epidermal necrolysis (TEN) has been associated with elevated TNF-α activity. Due to its known anti–TNF-α effect, thalidomide was used to treat TEN in a double-blind, randomized, controlled study.[100] Ten of 12 patients receiving thalidomide died, however, compared with only 3 of 10 patients given placebo.[100] Due to excess mortality in the thalidomide group, the study was prematurely discontinued. Based on limited but alarmingly compelling data, TEN should not be treated with thalidomide.

ADVERSE EFFECTS

Teratogenicity

Thalidomide's most severe toxicity is teratogenicity. This agent should never be used by pregnant women or anyone who could become pregnant, because it is labeled pregnancy category X.[8] Severe birth defects can result from only a single dose of thalidomide, with teratogenic risk at its highest during the critical period of 35 to 50 days after the last menstrual period.[101] Birth defects have included phocomelia, amelia, absent or hypoplastic bones, external ear abnormalities, facial palsy, eye defects, and internal organ malformations.[102] Although such teratogenic effects have been among thalidomide's most devastating toxicities, they are also readily prevented by taking precautions and following guidelines for avoiding pregnancy while on thalidomide. Due to teratogenic potential, the manufacturer requires all physicians prescribing thalidomide to follow the System for Thalidomide Education and Prescribing Safety (S.T.E.P.S.).[3] Thalidomide can be prescribed for only 28 days at a time with no refills. Prescriptions are valid for 1 week only, and monthly pregnancy tests are required.[4]

Peripheral Neuropathy

Peripheral neuropathy is another major side effect and can be a highly limiting factor for prescribing thalidomide. In some cases, neuropathy can be slow to resolve or even irreversible.[7] There has been much disagreement over whether or not a direct correlation exists between neuropathy occurrence and daily doses or total cumulative dose.[103] In a review of 65 patients receiving a wide range of thalidomide doses, analysis indicated that there was a significant correlation between neuropathy and cumulative doses for patients receiving more than 20 g of thalidomide.[104] The severity of neuropathy was also dose related for this group. For patients given less than 20 g, neuropathy occurred less often.[104] The lowest effective thalidomide dose should be used whenever possible, and close monitoring of nerve function is essential. Apfel and colleagues[103] suggested that if neuropathy does occur, consideration for discontinuing thalidomide should be done on an individual basis with regards to the severity of the underlying condition being managed and the severity of neuropathy.

Thromboembolic Events

Thromboembolic complications due to thalidomide are mostly associated with thalidomide's use in the cancer setting, especially when given concomitantly with chemotherapeutic agents.[105] It is also an emerging toxicity of thalidomide in the dermatologic setting, however. There are at least 15 cases of thalidomide-related thromboses in the noncancer setting, including among cases of sarcoidosis, lupus erythematosus, and atopic dermatitis.[105] The risk increases when thalidomide is combined with corticosteroids (such as dexamethasone).[105] The mechanism of this complication is not clear and is likely multifactorial. It may be advisable to screen patients for possible thrombotic predisposition before thalidomide treatment.

Fabi and colleagues[105] suggested that warfarin or aspirin (81 mg daily) may be effective as thrombotic prophylaxis, although there is no direct evidence yet for optimal thrombotic prophylaxis in the dermatology setting.

OTHER SIDE EFFECTS

Other common side effects are somnolence, constipation, nonspecific rash, and dizziness.[3] Neutropenia is a rare toxicity that occurs in less than 1% of cases.[4] The incidence is higher in HIV patients, however. Baseline complete blood cell counts with differential should be monitored closely in high risk patients.[4] Uncommon side effects include hypotension, headache, peripheral edema, weight gain, nausea, amenorrhea, pruritus, and mood changes.[3] A rare hypersensitivity reaction has been reported and may present as an erythematous macular rash associated with fever, tachycardia, and hypotension. Therapy should be discontinued if this occurs.[106] Dermatologic side effects have been noted as well, including allergic vasculitis, thrombocytopenic purpura, TEN, and exfoliative reactions.[3,107,108]

SUMMARY

Thalidomide is Food and Drug Administration approved only for ELN and multiple myeloma. There is evidence, however, that thalidomide is effective for treating certain cutaneous conditions. These off-label therapies for thalidomide are not considered first line, but should be considered when the underlying conditions are disabling or disfiguring and recalcitrant to other therapies. Thalidomide has many reported side effects and can lead to birth defects. Anyone using thalidomide should follow the S.T.E.P.S. program and closely monitor for side effects in treated patients.

Side effects may be minimized by using lower doses of thalidomide. Because many of the conditions discussed in this article relapse when treatment is discontinued, all patients should be treated with the lowest dose of medication that effectively controls their disease. This is especially true if a patient requires long-term suppressive therapy. Newer thalidomide analogs, such as lenalidomide, require further study but may have increased efficacy with lower potential for side effects and may replace thalidomide in the future.

REFERENCES

1. Melchert M, List A. The thalidomide saga. Int J Biochem Cell Biol 2007;39(7–8):1489–99.
2. Mellin GW, Katzenstein M. The saga of thalidomide. Neuropathy to embropathy, with case reports of congenital abnormalities. N Engl J Med 1962;267:1184–93.
3. Wu JJ, Huang DB, Pang KR, et al. Thalidomide: dermatological indications, mechanisms of action and side-effects. Br J Dermatol 2005;153(2):254–73.
4. Perri AJ 3rd, Hsu S. A review of thalidomide's history and current dermatological applications. Dermatol Online J 2003;9(3):5.
5. Rosenbach M, Werth VP. Dermatologic therapeutics: thalidomide. A practical guide. Dermatol Ther. 2007;20(4):175–86.
6. Kelsey FO. Thalidomide update: regulatory aspects. Teratology 1988;38:221–6.
7. Stirling DI. Thalidomide and its impact in dermatology. Semin Cutan Med Surgery 1988;17(4):231–42.
8. Radomsky CL, Levine N. Thalidomide. Dermatol Clin 2001;19:87–103.
9. Nasca MR, O'Toole EA, Palicharla P, et al. Thalidomide increases human keratinocyte migration and proliferation. J Invest Dermatol 1999;113(5):720–4.
10. Mascaro JM, Lecha M, Torras H. Thalidomide in the treatment of recurrent, necrotic, and giant mucocutaneous aphthae and apthosis. Arch Dermatol 1979;115:636–7.
11. Jenkins JS, Powell RJ, Allen BR, et al. Thalidomide in severe orogenital ulceration. Lancet 1984;2:1424–6.
12. Grinspan D. Significant response of oral aphthosis to thalidomide treatment. J Am Acad Dermatol 1985;12:85–90.
13. Revuz J, Guillaume JC, Janier M, et al. Crossover study of thalidomide vs placebo in severe recurrent aphthous stomatitis. Arch Dermatol 1990;126:923–7.
14. Mimura MA, Hirota SK, Sugaya NN, et al. Systemic treatment in severe cases of recurrent aphthous stomatitis: an open trial. Clinics (Sao Paulo) 2009;64(3):193–8.
15. Jacobson JM, Greenspan JS, Spritzler J, et al. Thalidomide for the treatment of oral aphthous ulcers in patients with human immunodeficiency virus infection. N Engl J Med 1997;336:1487–93.
16. Shetty K. Thalidomide in the management of recurrent aphthous ulcerations in patients who are HIV-positive: a review and case reports. Spec Care Dentist 2005;25(5):236–41.
17. Bowers PW, Powell RJ. Effect of thalidomide on orogenital ulceration. Br Med J (Clin Res Ed) 1983;287(6395):799–800.
18. Hamuryudan V, Mat C, Saip S, et al. Thalidomide in the treatment of the mucocutaneous lesions of the Behçet syndrome. A randomized, double-blind, placebo-controlled trial. Ann Intern Med 1998;128(6):443–50.
19. Saylan T, Saltik I. Thalidomide in the treatment of Behcet's syndrome. Arch Dermatol 1982;118:536.

20. Hamza MH. Treatment of Behcet's disease with thalidomide. Clin Rheumatol 1986;5:365–71.
21. Gardner-Medwin JM, Smith NJ, Powell RJ. Clinical experience with thalidomide in the management of severe oral and genital ulceration in conditions such as Behcet's disease: use of neurophysiological studies to detect thalidomide neuropathy. Ann Rheum Dis 1994;53:828–32.
22. De Wazières B, Gil H, Magy N, et al. Treatment of recurrent ulceration with low doses of thalidomide. Pilot study in 17 patients. Rev Med Interne 1999; 20(7):567–70.
23. Sharma NL, Sharma VC, Mahajan VK, et al. Thalidomide: an experience in therapeutic outcome and adverse reactions. J Dermatolog Treat 2007;18: 335–40.
24. Yasui K, Uchida N, Akazawa Y, et al. Thalidomide for treatment of intestinal involvement of juvenile-onset Behçet disease. Inflamm Bowel Dis 2008; 14(3):396–400.
25. Barba-Rubio J, Franco-Gonzalez F. Fixed lupus erythematosus (its treatment with thalidomide). Med Cutan Ibero Lat Am 1977;146:878–81.
26. Lyakhovisky A, Baum S, Shpiro D, et al. [Thalidomide therapy for discoid lupus erythematosus]. Harefuah 2006;145(7):489–92 [in Hebrew].
27. Knop J, Bonsmann G, Happle R, et al. Thalidomide in the treatment of sixty cases of chronic discoid lupus erythematosus. Br J Dermatol 1983;108(4):461–6.
28. Ordi-Ros J, Cortes F, Cucurull E, et al. Thalidomide in the treatment of cutaneous lupus refractory to conventional therapy. J Rheumatol 2000; 27:1429–33.
29. Hasper MF. Chronic cutaneous lupus erythematosus. Thalidomide treatment of 11 patients. Arch Dermatol 1983;119:812–5.
30. Stevens RJ, Andujar C, Edwards CJ, et al. Thalidomide in the treatment of the cutaneous manifestations of lupus erythematosus: experience in sixteen consecutive patients. Br J Rheumatol 1997;36:353–9.
31. Pelle MT, Werth VP. Thalidomide in cutaneous lupus erythematosus. Am J Clin Dermatol. 2003; 4(6):379–87.
32. Doherty SD, Hsu S. A case series of 48 patients treated with thalidomide. J Drugs Dermatol 2008; 7(8):769–73.
33. Coelho A, Souto MI, Cardoso CR, et al. Long-term thalidomide use in refractory cutaneous lesions of lupus erythematosus: a 65 series of Brazilian patients. Lupus. 2005;14(6):434–9.
34. Drake LA, Dinehart SM, Farmer ER, et al. Guidelines of care for cutaneous lupus erythematosus. American Academy of Dermatology. J Am Acad Dermatol 1996;34(5 Pt 1):830–6.
35. Alfadley A, Al-Hawsawi K, Thestrup-Pedersen K, et al. Treatment of prurigo nodularis with thalidomide: a case report and review of the literature. Int J Dermatol 2003;42(5):372–5.
36. Sheskin J. Thalidomide in the treatment of lepra reactions. Clin Pharmacol Ther 1965;6:303–6.
37. Jøhnke H, Zachariae H. [Thalidomide treatment of prurigo nodularis]. Ugeskr Laeger 1993;155(38): 3028–30 [in Danish].
38. Ferrándiz C, Carrascosa JM, Just M, et al. Sequential combined therapy with thalidomide and narrow-band (TL01) UVB in the treatment of prurigo nodularis. Dermatology 1997;195(4): 359–61.
39. Grosshans E, Illy G. Thalidomide therapy for inflammatory dermatoses. Int J Dermatol 1984; 23(9):598–602.
40. Doherty CB, Rosen T. Evidence-based therapy for cutaneous sarcoidosis. Drugs 2008;68(10): 1361–83.
41. Barriere H. Cutaneous sarcoidosis. Treatment with thalidomide. Presse Med 1983;12:963.
42. Grasland J, Pouchot D, Chaumaiziere G, et al. Effectiveness of thalidomide treatment during cutaneous sarcoidosis. Rev Med Interne 1998; 19:208–9.
43. Lee JB, Koblenzer PS. Disfiguring cutaneous manifestation of sarcoidosis treated with thalidomide: a case report. J Am Acad Dermatol 1998;39:835–8.
44. Carlesimo M, Giustini S, Rossi A, et al. Treatment of cutaneous and pulmonary sarcoidosis with thalidomide. J Am Acad Dermatol 1995;32:866–9.
45. Rousseau L, Beylot-Barry M, Doutre MS, et al. Cutaneous sarcoidosis successfully treated with low dose of thalidomide. Arch Dermatol 1998;134:1045–6.
46. Baughman RP, Judson MA, Teirstein AS, et al. Thalidomide for chronic sarcoidosis. Chest 2002; 122(1):227–32.
47. Oliver SJ, Kikuchi T, Kreuger JG, et al. Thalidomide induces granuloma differentiation in sarcoid skin lesions associated with disease improvement. Clin Immunol 2002;102:225–36.
48. Estines O, Revuz J, Wolkenstein P, et al. Sarcoidosis: thalidomide treatment in ten patients. Ann Dermatol Venereol 2001;128(5):611–3.
49. Badgwell C, Rosen T. Cutaneous sarcoidosis therapy updated. J Am Acad Dermatol 2007; 56(1):69–83.
50. Moller DR. Involvement of T-cells and alterations in T-cell receptors in sarcoidosis. Semin Respir Infect 1998;13:174–83.
51. McHugh SM, Rifkin IR, Deighton J, et al. The immunosuppressive drug thalidomide induces T helper cell type 2 (Th2) and concomitantly inhibits Th1 cytokine production in mitogen- and antigen-stimulated human peripheral blood mononuclear cell cultures. Clin Exp Immunol 1995;99:160–7.
52. Londoño F. Thalidomide in the treatment of actinic prurigo. Int J Dermatol 1973;12(5):326–8.

53. Calnan CD, Meara RH. Actinic prurigo (Hutchinson's summer prurigo). Clin Exp Dermatol 1977; 2(4):365–72.
54. Lovell CR, Hawk JL, Calnan CD, et al. Thalidomide in actinic prurigo. Br J Dermatol 1983;108(4):467–71.
55. Lim SH, McWhannell A, Vora AJ, et al. Successful treatment with thalidomide of acute graft-versus-host disease after bone-marrow transplantation. Lancet 1988;1(8577):117.
56. Vogelsang GB, Farmer ER, Hess AD, et al. Thalidomide for the treatment of chronic graft-versus-host disease. N Engl J Med 1992;326(16):1055–8.
57. Chao NJ, Parker PM, Niland JC, et al. Paradoxical effect of thalidomide prophylaxis on chronic graft-vs.-host disease. Biol Blood Marrow Transplant 1996;2(2):86–92.
58. Arora M, Wagner JE, Davies SM, et al. Randomized clinical trial of thalidomide, cyclosporine, and prednisone versus cyclosporine and prednisone as initial therapy for chronic graft-versus-host disease. Biol Blood Marrow Transplant 2001;7(5):265–73.
59. Kulkarni S, Powles R, Sirohi B, et al. Thalidomide after allogeneic haematopoietic stem cell transplantation: activity in chronic but not in acute graft-versus-host disease. Bone Marrow Transplant 2003;32(2):165–70.
60. Chung LW, Yeh SP, Hsieh CY, et al. Life-threatening acute pancreatitis due to thalidomide therapy for chronic graft-versus-host disease. Ann Hematol 2008;87(5):421–3.
61. Gnassia AM, Gnassia RT, Bonvalet D. Histiocytose X avec 'granulome eosinophile vulvaire': effet spectaculaire de la thalidomide. Ann Dermatol Venereol 1987;114:1387–9.
62. Thomas L, Ducros B, Secchi T, et al. Successful treatment of adult's Langerhans cell histiocytosis with thalidomide. Report of two cases and literature review. Arch Dermatol 1993;129(10):1261–4.
63. Misery L, Larbre B, Lyonnet S, et al. Remission of Langerhans cell histiocytosis with thalidomide treatment. Clin Exp Dermatol 1993;18(5):487.
64. Padula A, Medeiros LJ, Silva EG, et al. Isolated vulvar Langerhans cell histiocytosis: report of two cases. Int J Gynecol Pathol 2004;23(3):278–83.
65. Broekaert SM, Metzler G, Burgdorf W, et al. Multisystem Langerhans cell histiocytosis: successful treatment with thalidomide. Am J Clin Dermatol 2007;8(5):311–4.
66. Moravvej H, Yousefi M, Barikbin B. An unusual case of adult disseminated cutaneous Langerhans cell histiocytosis. Dermatol Online J 2006;12(6):13.
67. McClain KL, Kozinetz CA. A phase II trial using thalidomide for Langerhans cell histiocytosis. Pediatr Blood Cancer 2007;48(1):44–9.
68. Bahmer FA, Zaun H, Luszpinski P. Thalidomide treatment of recurrent erythema multiforme. Acta Derm Venereol 1982;62(5):449–50.
69. Conejo-Mir JS, del Canto S, Muñoz MA, et al. Thalidomide as elective treatment in persistent erythema multiforme; report of two cases. J Drugs Dermatol 2003;2(1):40–4.
70. Cherouati K, Claudy A, Souteyrand P, et al. Treatment by thalidomide of chronic multiforme erythema: its recurrent and continuous variants. A retrospective study of 26 patients. Ann Dermatol Venereol 1996;123(6-7):375–7.
71. Moura AK, Moure ER, Romiti R. Treatment of cutaneous lichen planus with thalidomide. Clin Exp Dermatol 2009;34(1):101–3.
72. Macario-Barrel A, Balguerie X, Joly P. Treatment of erosive oral lichen planus with thalidomide. Ann Dermatol Venereol 2003;130(12 Pt 1):1109–12.
73. Torti DC, Jorizzo JL, McCarty MA. Oral lichen planus: a case series with emphasis on therapy. Arch Dermatol 2007;143(4):511–5.
74. Boyd AS, King LE Jr. Thalidomide-induced remission of lichen planopilaris. J Am Acad Dermatol 2002;47(6):967–8.
75. George SJ, Hsu S. Lichen planopilaris treated with thalidomide. J Am Acad Dermatol 2001;45(6):965–6.
76. Jouanique C, Reygagne P, Bachelez H, et al. Thalidomide is ineffective in the treatment of lichen planopilaris. J Am Acad Dermatol 2004; 51(3):480–1.
77. Solèr RA, Howard M, Brink NS, et al. Regression of AIDS-related Kaposi's sarcoma during therapy with thalidomide. Clin Infect Dis 1996;23(3):501–3 [discussion: 504–5].
78. Fife K, Howard MR, Gracie F, et al. Activity of thalidomide in AIDS-related Kaposi's sarcoma and correlation with HHV8 titre. Int J STD AIDS 1998;9(12): 751–5.
79. Little RF, Wyvill KM, Pluda JM, et al. Activity of thalidomide in AIDS-related Kaposi's sarcoma. J Clin Oncol 2000;18(13):2593–602.
80. Ben M'barek L, Fardet L, Mebazaa A, et al. A retrospective analysis of thalidomide therapy in non-HIV-related Kaposi's sarcoma. Dermatology 2007; 215(3):202–5.
81. Rubegni P, Sbano P, De Aloe G, et al. Thalidomide in the treatment of Kaposi's sarcoma. Dermatology 2007;215(3):240–4.
82. Moulin G, Bonnet F, Barrut D, et al. Treatment of Jessner-Kanof disease with thalidomide. Ann Dermatol Venereol. 1983;110(8):611–4.
83. Guillaume JC, Moulin G, Dieng MT, et al. Crossover study of thalidomide vs placebo in Jessner's lymphocytic infiltration of the skin. Arch Dermatol 1995;131(9):1032–5.
84. Arndt KA, Bowers KE. Pruritus. In: Manual of dermatologic therapeutics. 6th edition. Philadelphia: Lippincott Williams & Wilkins; 2002. p. 167.
85. Silva SR, Viana PC, Lugon NV, et al. Thalidomide for the treatment of uremic pruritus: a crossover

randomized double-blind trial. Nephron 1994; 67(3):270–3.
86. Verrou E, Kartsios C, Banti A, et al. IgG multiple myeloma presented with ulcerative pyoderma gangrenosum. Leuk Lymphoma 2007;48(7):1420–2.
87. Koca E, Duman AE, Cetiner D, et al. Successful treatment of myelodysplastic syndrome-induced pyoderma gangrenosum. Neth J Med 2006;64(11): 422–4.
88. Federman GL, Federman DG. Recalcitrant pyoderma gangrenosum treated with thalidomide. Mayo Clin Proc 2000;75(8):842–4.
89. Buckley C, Bayoumi AH, Sarkany I. Pyoderma gangrenosum with severe pharyngeal ulceration. J R Soc Med 1990;83(9):590–1.
90. Venencie PY, Saurat JH. Pyoderma gangrenosum in a child: treatment with thalidomide. Ann Pediatr 1982;29:67–9.
91. Hecker MS, Lebwohl MG. Recalcitrant pyoderma gangrenosum: treatment with thalidomide. J Am Acad Dermatol 1998;38:490–501.
92. Farrell AM, Black MM, Bracka A, et al. Pyoderma gangrenosum of the penis. Br J Dermatol 1998; 138(2):337–40.
93. Munro CS, Cox NH. Pyoderma gangrenosum associated with Behçet's syndrome—response to thalidomide. Clin Exp Dermatol 1988;13(6):408–10.
94. Ehling A, Karrer S, Klebl F, et al. Therapeutic management of pyoderma gangrenosum. Arthritis Rheum 2004;50(10):3076–84.
95. Peter LM, Ammoury A, Chiavassa-Gandois H, et al. Scleromyxoedema with associated peripheral neuropathy: successful treatment with thalidomide. Clin Exp Dermatol 2008;33(5):606–10.
96. Amini-Adle M, Thieulent N, Dalle S, et al. Scleromyxedema: successful treatment with thalidomide in two patients. Dermatology 2007;214(1):58–60.
97. Wu MY, Hong JB, Yang CC, et al. Scleromyxedema with myopathy was successfully treated by thalidomide. J Eur Acad Dermatol Venereol 2009;23(2): 189–90.
98. Sansbury JC, Cocuroccia B, Jorizzo JL, et al. Treatment of recalcitrant scleromyxedema with thalidomide in 3 patients. J Am Acad Dermatol 2004; 51(1):126–31.
99. Kukreja T, Petersen J. Thalidomide for the treatment of refractory necrobiosis lipoidica. Arch Dermatol 2006;142(1):20–2.
100. Wolkenstein P, Latarjet J, Roujeau JC, et al. Randomised comparison of thalidomide versus placebo in toxic epidermal necrolysis. Lancet 1998; 352(9140):1586–9.
101. Ghobrial IM, Rajkumar SV. Management of thalidomide toxicity. J Support Oncol 2003;1(3):194–205.
102. Mcbride WG. Thalidomide embryopathy. Teratology 1977;16(1):79–82.
103. Apfel SC, Zochodne DW. Thalidomide neuropathy: too much or too long? Neurology 2004;62(12): 2158–9.
104. Cavaletti G, Beronio A, Reni L, et al. Thalidomide sensory neurotoxicity: a clinical and neurophysiological study. Neurology 2004;62:2291–3.
105. Fabi SG, Hill C, Witherspoon JN, et al. Frequency of thromboembolic events associated with thalidomide in the non-cancer setting: a case report and review of the literature. J Drugs Dermatol 2009; 8(8):765–9.
106. Thalidomide. Warren (NJ): Celgene Corporation; 2003. [package insert].
107. Salafi A, Kharkar RD. Thalidomide and exfoliative dermatitis. Int J Lepr 1988;56:625.
108. Koch HP. Thalidomide and congeners as anti-inflammatory agents. Prog Med Chem 1985;22: 165–242.

Innovative Uses for Zinc in Dermatology

Yoon Soo Bae, MD[a], Nikki D. Hill, BSc[a],
Yuval Bibi, MD, PhD[a,*], Jacob Dreiher, MD, MPH[b,c],
Arnon D. Cohen, MD, MPH, PhD[b,c]

KEYWORDS

• Zinc • Zinc deficiency • Dermatology

In 1869, Raulin[1] described zinc as an essential component for *Aspergillus niger*. Since this observation, zinc was shown to be a cofactor for more than 300 metalloenzymes[2] and 2000 transcription factors.[3,4] Zinc is a vital prosthetic group in zinc/copper superoxide dismutase, thereby affecting cellular reduction/oxidation status. This metal is also putatively involved in gene transcription with factors possessing zinc-finger motifs and participates in histone deacetylase reactions.[5] Overall, zinc has been recognized as crucial for the normal development and physiology of a variety of organisms,[6] including humans.[7] Zinc is found in all types of tissue. The skin contains approximately 6% of total body zinc[8] and is second only to muscle and bone in zinc content. Foods that are rich in zinc include beef, oysters, and liver.[9] Zinc is absorbed in the distal duodenum and proximal jejunum. Absorption of zinc by the intestine is inhibited by phytate, among other molecules.[10] Zinc is primarily excreted through the intestine and to a lesser extent in urine.[11] For more than 3000 years, zinc salts, such as zinc oxide or calamine, have been applied topically to facilitate wound healing. In the past 50 years, progress has been made to associate zinc with numerous skin pathologies. The roles of zinc in dermatology will be discussed later. Refer to **Table 1** for a summary of skin conditions associated with zinc deficiency and the proposed modes of treatment, respectively.

METHODS

In 2005, the authors conducted a PubMed search using zinc and the dermatosis in question as search words. Literature beyond the scope of the authors' initial search was added for background purposes and to compliment their results. The results of this review were previously published.[12] In September 2009, the authors repeated this method searching articles written since 2005, in addition to the previous search.

RESULTS

Dermatologic Diseases Attributed to Systemic Zinc Abnormalities

Three separate major entities involving systemic zinc deficiency have been described to date.

Moderate systemic zinc deficiency

In 1961, Prasad and colleagues[13] described several series of subjects from the Mediterranean suffering from growth retardation, male hypogonadism appearing in adolescence, cell-mediated immune dysfunctions, abnormal neurosensory changes, rough and dry skin, and delayed wound healing.[14] This syndrome was attributed to inadequate dietary zinc intake or disruption of its absorption by other molecules in the intestine (eg, phytate),[15] resulting in moderate zinc deficiency. When treated with dietary zinc supplementation, these subjects greatly improved.[16,17]

[a] Department of Dermatology, Boston University School of Medicine, 609 Albany Street, Boston, MA 02118, USA
[b] Clalit Health Services, Beer-Sheva, Israel
[c] Siaal Research Center for Family Medicine and Primary Care, Faculty of Health Sciences, Ben-Gurion University, Beer-Sheva, Israel
* Corresponding author.
E-mail address: yuvalbn@yahoo.com

Dermatol Clin 28 (2010) 587–597
doi:10.1016/j.det.2010.03.006
0733-8635/10/$ – see front matter © 2010 Elsevier Inc. All rights reserved.

Table 1
Zinc treatment for various dermatopathologies

Disease	Mode	Efficacy	References	Study Design
Acne vulgaris				
...	Systemic	++	Hillstrom et al[28]	Double-blind RCT[a]
...	Systemic	++	Göransson et al[29]	Double-blind RCT
...	Systemic	++	Verma et al[30]	Double-blind RCT
...	Systemic	++	Liden et al[31]	Double-blind RCT
...	Systemic	–	Orris et al[32]	Double-blind RCT
...	Systemic	+	Weimar et al[33]	Double-blind RCT
...	Systemic	++	Dreno et al[35]	Double-blind RCT
...	Systemic	–	Dreno et al[36]	Double-blind RCT
...	Topical	–	Sharquie et al[39] Sharquie et al[115]	Single-blind RCT
...	Systemic	=	Michaelsson et al[26] Michaelsson et al[27] Michaelsson et al[38]	Double-blind RCT
...	Topical	=	Feucht et al[40]	Double-blind RCT
...	Topical	+	Habbema et al[41]	Double-blind RCT
...	Topical	+	Schachner et al[42] Schachner et al[43]	Double-blind Randomized cross-over trial
...	Topical	+	Schachner et al[42] Schachner et al[43]	Double-blind RCT
...	Topical	–	Langner et al[44]	Investigator-Blind RCT
...	Topical	=	Cunliffe et al[46]	Investigator-blind RCT
...	Topical	+	Strauss & Stranieri[48]	Double-blind RCT
...	Topical	=	Bojar et al[50]	Double-blind RCT
...	Topical	+	Pierard-Franchimont et al[55]	Double-blind RCT
Aphthous ulcers/mucositis				
...	Systemic	+	Sharquie et al[39] Sharquie et al[115]	Double-blind RCT
Diaper dermatitis				
...	Topical	–	Arad et al[79]	Observation
...	Topical	–	Wananukul et al[80]	Investigator-blind RCT
Eczema				
...	Topical	+	Faghihi et al[76]	Double-blind RCT
Seborrheic dermatitis and dandruff				
...	Topical	+	Marks et al[71]	Parallel observation
...	Topical	–	Pierard-Franchimont et al[73]	Randomized, parallel observation
...	Topical	+	Shin et al[74]	Randomized
Androgenic alopecia				
...	Topical	+	Berger et al[64]	Investigator-blind RCT
Recalcitrant viral warts				
...	Topical	+	Khattar et al[86]	Double-blind RCT
Leprosy				
...	Topical	–	Reinar et al[116]	RCT
Psoriasis				
...	Topical	=	Housman et al[99]	Double-blind RCT
Rosacea				
...	Systemic	+	Sharquie et al[58] Sharquie et al[63]	Double-blind RCT
Chronic cutaneous ulcers				
...	Topical	+	Brandrup et al[104]	Randomized trial
...	Topical	+	Stromberg et al[105]	Double-blind
...	Topical	=	Agren et al[106]	Single-blind RCT
...	Topical	+	Apelqvist et al[107]	Open RCT

[a] Randomized controlled trial.

Acrodermatitis enteropathica

Acrodermatitis enteropathica, also known as Danbolt-Closs syndrome, is an autosomal recessive condition initially reported by Danbolt and Closs in 1942.[18] Acrodermatitis enteropathica is characterized by gastrointestinal disturbances, eye infections, growth failure, vesiculobullous, and psoriasiform dermatitis. These skin lesions are distributed in the perioral, acral and perineal areas in a symmetric pattern (**Fig. 1**). In 1973, Barnes and Moynahan[19] noted the association between the acrodermatitis enteropathica phenotype and severe zinc deficiency. Consequently, acrodermatitis enteropathica was successfully treated by supplementation of dietary zinc.[19,20] Recently, mutations in the *SLC39A4* gene, encoding a zinc transporter protein (hZIP4) were identified to be responsible for the acrodermatitis enteropathica phenotype[21] by impeding zinc absorption in the intestinal tract. In addition to congenital acrodermatitis enteropathica, an acquired class of syndromes with a similar phenotype was described.[22]

Acute zinc deficiency

With the advances in intensive care made in the latter half of the 20th century, an acute form of zinc deficiency was identified.[23] This condition is associated with parenteral alimentation. The hallmarks of acute zinc deficiency are diarrhea; mental apathy; depression; alopecia; and acute dermatitis (more pronounced in the perioral region). This syndrome is usually reversible with appropriate zinc supplementation. Severe to moderate zinc deficiency is increasingly rare, especially in developed countries; however, one should be alert to the possibility of zinc deficiency as a differential diagnosis, especially in intensive care-associated dermatoses.

The states mentioned earlier are closely linked to systemic zinc depletion. Beyond these conditions, many dermatologic diseases are associated and treated with topical or systemic zinc preparations with varying degrees of success. As a general note, with the exception of systemic zinc deficiency states, this trace element is not currently used as a first-line dermatologic treatment. The following discussion will explore skin conditions for which zinc was postulated to carry a therapeutic effect and the efforts made to investigate the role of zinc in those dermatoses.

Utility of Zinc in General Dermatology

Acneiform dermatoses

Acne vulgaris The initial link between zinc deficiency and acne was made as early as the 1970s by Michaelsson and Fitzherbert[20,24] who reported the improvement of acne upon supplementation of zinc in zinc-deficient patients. Michaelsson first noted the favorable effects of zinc on acne in a patient suffering from acrodermatitis enteropathica. Subsequently, serum levels of zinc surveyed in patients suffering from severe inflammatory acne vulgaris were found to be significantly lower than normal.[25,26] Following these observations, several double-blinded, randomized controlled trials (RCT) reported oral zinc sulfate to be effective in the treatment of severe acne[27–31] and less efficient for the treatment of mild to moderate acne.[32,33] Nausea, vomiting, and diarrhea were noted as side effects with this mode of treatment[33,34] and may have lead to low compliance. Orally administered zinc gluconate was also found to be effective in treating inflammatory acne[35,36] with no additional benefit for an initial loading dose.[37] When compared with systemic tetracycline treatment in a multicenter, double-blinded randomized trial, zinc salts appear to be equal to or less effective than this class of antibiotics[34,36,38] and are not considered first-line treatment for this condition.

Sharquie and colleagues[39] evaluated the effectiveness of 2% tea lotion in comparison with topical 5% zinc sulfate solution in the treatment of acne vulgaris. In a single-blind, randomized study of 47 subjects with mild acne, the 5% zinc

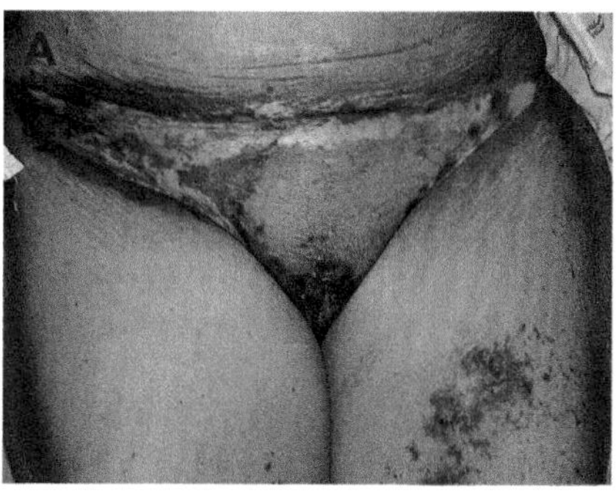

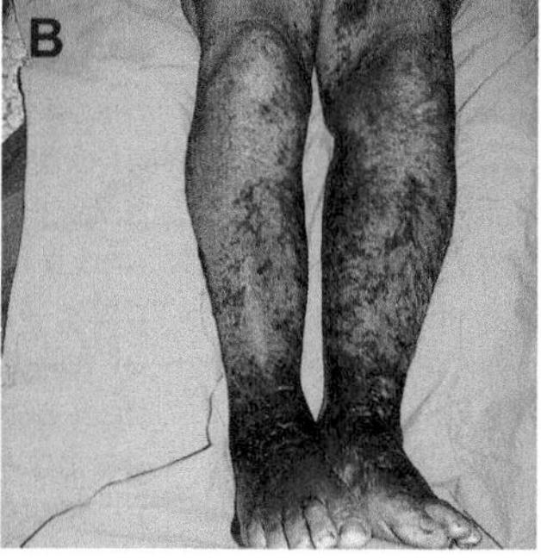

Fig. 1. A female patient suffering from acrodermatitis enteropathica. Note the dermatitic and erosive lesions with postinflammatory hypopigmentation distributed over the pelvic region and the extremities. The erosions are a result of vesiculobullous disease. (*Courtesy of* Dr Dafna Hallel-Halevy, Soroka University Medical Center, Beer Sheva, Israel.)

sulfate solution was shown to be beneficial, but did not reach statistically significance, whereas the tea lotion did. Topically applied preparations containing zinc salts (ie, zinc acetate, zinc octoate) with or without erythromycin were either equal to or superior to a single antibiotic (ie, erythromycin, tetracycline, or clindamycin) in reducing the severity of acne and the number of lesions in some studies.[40–43] However, a study by Langner and colleagues[44] found that the onset of action of clindamycin phosphate plus benzoyl peroxide once daily was quicker than twice daily erythromycin plus zinc acetate and there was no overall difference in efficacy or adverse events. Conversely, topical zinc sulfate was found to be ineffective in the treatment of acne[45] and caused considerable local irritation. The differences between the two salts may be caused by different absorption rates and solubility. A recent study of 24 subjects with mild to moderate acne demonstrated that the systemic absorption of clindamycin in subjects using a combined topical zinc/clindamycin 1% gel was 30% to 50% less than in subjects using a clindamycin lotion alone. No differences in efficacy were noted leading the investigators to believe that this inhibitory effect of systemic absorption may lead to improved compliance. To further improve compliance, it was observed that subjects using zinc in combination with clindamycin once daily or twice daily compared with clindamycin lotion alone led to equivalent efficacy and safety.[46]

From a mechanistic point of view, the role of zinc in the treatment of acne vulgaris is not well understood. Several studies noted a reduction in local skin microbial parameters such as the *Propionibacterium acnes* count and free fatty acids levels.[47–49] Zinc appears to target *P acnes* specifically and does not affect *Staphylococcus* sp.[50] Whether zinc is effective against *Micrococcaceae* has yet to be determined because existing data are controversial.[50,51] A possible mechanism for this antimicrobial effect is inhibition of *P acnes* lipase by zinc.[52] Treatment with zinc gluconate improved polymorphonuclear chemotaxis in subjects suffering from acne.[53] This finding suggests a role for zinc as an inflammation modulating agent in skin. An additional proposed mechanism for the benefit of zinc in the treatment of acne is suppression of sebum delivery, perhaps by anti-androgenic activity.[54,55] Zinc appears to enhance the topical absorption of erythromycin.[56] This observation alludes to a possible benefit in combining erythromycin with zinc salts. In summary, zinc is thought to be linked to acne through direct effects on the microbial-inflammatory equilibrium, and possible facilitation of topical antibiotic absorption in combined zinc preparations. Regardless, these studies provide evidence that zinc may be regarded as a second-line treatment that could be considered especially in patient groups in which first-line treatments for acne may be contraindicated, such as pregnant women, or poorly tolerated, minimizing the concern of side effects.[57]

Rosacea Rosacea is typically treated with topical and systemic therapies, such as antibiotics, metronidazole, retinoids, topical antifungals, azelaic acid, tacrolimus, and others.[58] In a double-blind, placebo-controlled crossover trial, 25 subjects were treated with 100 mg of zinc sulfate three times daily. A statistically significant improvement was demonstrated after 1 month of therapy. Thus, zinc sulfate is thought to have therapeutic and prophylactic effects in rosacea.[58] The mechanisms of action in rosacea are unknown and are postulated to be mediated through effects on oxidative status, antiinflammatory properties, and targeting various organisms implicated in rosacea. Alternatively, zinc may be beneficial in rosacea acting as a modulator of inflammation.

Hidradenitis suppurativa No standard of therapy exists for hidradenitis suppurativa. Many therapies including local antiseptics, antibiotics, long-term antibiotic therapy, isotretinoin, oral contraceptives, anti-androgens, corticosteroids, and surgery have been used.[59] In an investigation of 22 subjects with grade I or II in Hurley's classification, 90 mg of zinc gluconate was administered for 4 months. All subjects were noted to have a clinical response with eight complete remissions and 14 partial remissions. Also, recurrences disappeared when the dose of zinc salts was increased. Thus, this treatment appears to be suppressive rather than curative.[60]

Folliculitis decalvans Folliculitis decalvans is a chronic inflammatory condition of the scalp, commonly leading to scarring alopecia. Care is focused on antibiotic usage in patients with folliculitis decalvans and in severe cases steroids have been effective.[61] Abeck reported three subjects responding to a combination therapy consisting of oral and topical fusidic acid 1000 mg daily for 3 weeks and 1.5% cream for 2 weeks respectively and a 6 month course of oral zinc sulfate 400 mg daily. After 1 year, two subjects had no evidence of folliculitis decalvans, whereas another subject had a recurrence after a 2-month disease-free period when zinc therapy was stopped. Abeck attributes the antiinflammatory effect to zinc sulfate.[61]

Vasculitic conditions

Behcet's disease Behcet's disease (BD) is a vasculitic syndrome presenting as oral aphthous ulcers; genital ulcers; ocular lesions; skin lesions, such as pustules and erythema nodosum; and a positive pathergy test. Conventionally, immunosuppressants and antiinflammatory drugs are used to control the symptoms of BD. Najim and colleagues studied 76 subjects with BD who showed increased levels of serum malondialdehyde and copper while glutathione and zinc levels were decreased (*P*<.05). Furthermore, zinc levels were found to be inversely correlated with the clinical manifestation index and pathergy test positivity grades (*P*<.01). In a randomized, controlled, double-blind cross-over trial of 30 subjects treated with 100 mg zinc sulfate or identical placebo tablet three times daily, a statistically significant difference was observed in the clinical manifestation index.[62,63] In addition, mean serum zinc level in patients with BD was significantly lower than mean serum zinc levels in the control group. The investigators attribute the antioxidant and immunomodulatory effects of zinc sulfate to effectively treating patients with BD.

Conditions affecting hair

Androgenic alopecia Treatment of androgenic alopecia with topical zinc pyrithione resulted in a modest, though sustained increase in hair growth.[64] In a 6-month, randomized, investigator-blinded, parallel-group clinical study, the efficacy of a 1% pyrithione zinc shampoo was compared with that of a 5% minoxidil topical solution, a placebo shampoo, and a combination of 1% pyrithione zinc shampoo and 5% minoxidil topical solution. The 1% pyrithione zinc shampoo group showed a relative increase in hair count that was less than half that for the topical minoxidil. There was no advantage seen in using combined solution, perhaps indicating a joint pathway of action.

Telogen effluvium Zinc serum concentrations and the efficacy of zinc supplementation were tested in women with chronic telogen effluvium, which was traditionally linked with zinc deficiency.[65] Low levels of zinc were detected in only 7% of the women in this study. Moreover, treatment of subjects who were supposedly zinc deficient with the essential amino acid L-lysine resulted in the achievement of normal serum zinc levels with the exception of one subject. Thus, zinc deficiency is most likely not associated with telogen effluvium.

Seborrheic dermatitis and dandruff Seborrheic dermatitis (SD) and dandruff are traditionally treated with topical zinc pyrithione-containing preparations (eg, shampoo). Pyrithione is a zinc ionophore putatively facilitating local absorption of zinc. The stratum corneum of scalp samples taken from subjects with dandruff showed remarkable improvement after treatment with zinc pyrithione.[66] Zinc pyrithione has been proposed to exert its effects through inhibition of keratinocyte proliferation[67]; however, in vivo studies fail to substantiate this claim.[68] It is currently thought that in the case of dandruff and SD, the beneficial effects of zinc pyrithione are caused by direct inhibition of the growth of *Malassezia* sp.[69,70] Clinically, several randomized controlled trials reported significant efficacy for zinc pyrithione in the treatment of dandruff and SD.[71,72] However, in an open, randomized trial, 331 subjects were assigned to using a ketoconazole 2% or a zinc pyrithione 1% shampoo for 4 weeks twice weekly. Ketoconazole treatment resulted in a significantly greater improvement in the total dandruff severity score than zinc pyrithione (*P*<.02). In addition, the recurrence rate of dandruff was significantly lower in the ketoconazole group when compared with zinc pyrithione.[73] Another randomized trial by Shin and colleagues[74] showed subjects using conventional treatment of zinc pyrithione improved continuously even after cessation of treatment, in contrast with betamethasone or tacrolimus therapy, and suggest zinc pyrithione be used in a combination with a topical steroid to improve results.

Dermatitis

Eczema Hand Eczema is usually managed with emollients, barrier creams, corticosteroids, calcineurin inhibitors, immunosuppressants, and antimicrobial agents.[75] The addition of 2.5% zinc sulfate to 0.05% clobetasol cream twice a daily for two weeks was more effective than Clobetasol 0.05% cream alone (*P*<.05) in a study of 47 patients with chronic hand eczema. In addition, the recurrence rate of eczema was significantly lower in the group treated with this combination treatment (*P*<.05).[76] Multiple mechanisms of action of zinc were proposed, including antiinflammatory effects, promotion of wound repair, etc.[76]

Diaper dermatitis Diaper rash is traditionally treated with topical zinc preparations.[77] A recent report shows clinical efficacy for zinc oxide in the reduction of the inflammatory parameters of diaper dermatitis.[78] Arad and colleagues investigated 54 infants with diaper dermatitis and randomly assigned each subject to one of three treatment groups including zinc oxide paste, clobetasone butyrate 0.05%, and aqueous solution of eosin 2%. After 5 days of treatment, the rate of complete healing in the eosin group was significantly higher than that in the zinc oxide paste and corticosteroid groups (P = .048). In addition, partial healing was higher in the eosin group than in the other groups (P = .021).[79] A similar study in Thailand evaluating irritant diaper dermatitis from diarrhea demonstrated transepidermal water loss to be less on the side treated with 5% dexpanthenol and zinc oxide ointment (vs ointment base), but no statistical significance in the severity of the rash.[80]

Infectious disease

Recalcitrant viral warts Al-Gurairi and colleagues[81] reported a cure rate of more than 80% of recalcitrant viral warts with oral zinc sulfate. However, this is a preliminary study, which merits additional research.[82] In a randomized, placebo-controlled, double-blind study, Sadighha treated 13 subjects with oral zinc sulfate (10 mg/kg to a maximum dose of 600 mg/day) for 1 to 2 months, with a 54% response rate within the first month of treatment.[83] Serum zinc levels were also studied in those subjects. The mean value of zinc in the subjects' sera was 53.3 $\pm$ 9.7 μg/dl before the study and 181.5 $\pm$ 22.1 μg/dl in those who responded, whereas the mean level of serum zinc after 1 month of treatment in those who did not respond to treatment reached 69 $\pm$ 10.11 μg/dl. Some of the remaining subjects who had originally not responded within the first month eventually responded and were found to have mean serum zinc levels of 201.3 $\pm$ 22.0 μg/dl, whereas in the rest of the non-responders, the mean serum zinc levels were 69.8 $\pm$ 10.3 μg/dl.[83] After a course of 2 months' treatment with zinc sulfate, the success rate rose to 76.9% (10 subjects). This study demonstrates a dose-dependent response in subjects with recalcitrant warts treated with zinc. Yaghoobi conducted a similar study in 32 subjects with an oral dosage of 10 mg/kg zinc sulfate and found that elevated serum zinc levels corresponded with successful treatment of verrucae.[84]

In a small subject population (n = 10), Sharquie looked into the use of 10% topical zinc sulfate solution three times daily for 4 weeks and found a full response in 80% for plane warts in a pilot trial and 86% in a double-blind trial without recurrence 2 to 6 months afterwards.[85] Common warts responded in only 11%. A similar randomized, double-blind controlled trial of 44 subjects with treatment of topical zinc oxide 20% ointment or salicylic acid 15% + lactic acid 15% ointment twice daily was conducted for 3 months or until cure occurred. In the zinc oxide-treated group, 50% of the subjects showed complete cure and 19% failed to respond, compared with 42% and 26%, respectively, in the salicylic acid-lactic acid-treated group.[86] Zinc is thought to have worked through an unspecified upregulation of immunologic events.

Old-world cutaneous leishmaniasis Several groups assessed the efficacy of zinc sulfate for the treatment of acute old-world cutaneous leishmaniasis by systemic preparations[87] and intralesional injections.[88–90] Iraji's double-blinded, case-controlled clinical study included 35 subjects receiving intralesional meglumine antimoniate (MA) and 31 subjects receiving intralesional zinc sulfate. A greater cure rate was reported for zinc sulfate (84%) than for MA (60%). After 2 and 4 weeks, treatment efficacy with zinc sulfate was higher than that with MA (P<.01), but after 6 weeks, there was no significant difference between the two groups (P>.05).[89] Oral zinc sulfate given at 10 mg/kg divided into three daily doses appeared to be effective in eradicating cutaneous leishmaniasis. This effect was associated with increments in serum zinc levels.[91] Studies where different doses of zinc sulfate are given show that subjects receiving 10 mg/kg versus 2.5 or 5 have higher response rates, although the difference was not statistically significant.[87,92] The efficacy of intralesional zinc sulfate in cutaneous leishmaniasis is reportedly high, though its advantage over meglumine antimoniate remains controversial.[89]

Miscellaneous conditions

Necrolytic acral erythema Necrolytic acral erythema (NAE) is a cutaneous marker of hepatitis C virus (HCV) infection classified within a group of diseases known as necrolytic erythemas. Necrolytic erythema is linked to nutrient deficiencies and includes necrolytic migratory erythema, acrodermatitis enteropathica, pellagra, and essential fatty acid deficiencies.[93] However, in most reported cases of NAE there is an absence of nutrient deficiency. Nofal observed five subjects with NAE, two of whom had low serum zinc and albumin levels.[93] All subjects responded to oral zinc sulfate, whereas mild or no improvement was seen with oral amino acid supplementation. In addition, DeCarvalho described a case of NAE with a zinc deficiency in Brazil, which responded to oral zinc sulfate 210 mg twice daily with complete resolution over 7 weeks.[94]

Case reports by Khanna and Abdallah both describe subjects with HCV and NAE with normal serum zinc treated successfully with oral zinc at 220 mg daily.[95,96] Khanna, however, also treated the subject with interferon alpha-2b injections in addition to zinc. Many explanations exist for zinc's role in cases where serum zinc levels are normal. Geria suggests that because albumin is the main carrier of zinc and essential fatty acids in plasma, decreased serum albumin levels may cause transitory deficiency in one or more of these nutrients, which could play a role in the development of NAE.[97] Furthermore, decreased serum zinc levels may be a late indicator of zinc deficiency. Thus, skin manifestations of zinc deficiency may occur despite having serum zinc levels within reference range.

Psoriasis Zinc was linked to psoriasis by a chain of case reports on the beneficial effects of locally applied zinc pyrithione-containing preparations on psoriatic plaques.[98] However, in a well-planned controlled study of 24 subjects, topical zinc pyrithione was ineffective when compared with topical clobetasol propionate in the treatment of psoriasis.[99] Furthermore, no additive effects were noted when combining zinc-pyrithione with clobetasol propionate. Systemic zinc sulfate supplementation was also ineffective as compared with placebo in the treatment of psoriasis.[100] The authors conclude that, based on currently available data, zinc has no apparent role in the treatment of psoriasis.

Chronic cutaneous ulcers Patients suffering from chronic skin ulcers have low skin and serum levels of zinc.[101] In addition, zinc deficiency may be caused by excessive wound drainage.[102] Ackerman and colleagues[103] noted an altered zinc distribution in the skin of subjects with varicose ulcers. Topical preparations containing zinc oxide were effective in the treatment of arterial and venous leg ulcers,[104,105] pressure ulcers,[106] and necrotic diabetic foot ulcers.[107] The therapeutic effects of zinc oxide or zinc sulfate on leg ulcers were most pronounced in subjects who were zinc-deficient.[108] Zinc oxide was superior to zinc sulfate because the latter was not as effective and caused local irritation at high concentrations (see the earlier discussion of acne vulgaris). The use of oral zinc (zinc sulfate) for chronic leg ulcers remains controversial and may be of benefit in patients who are zinc deficient.[109] Few studies have demonstrated a response to oral supplements including zinc; however, the exact cause of improvement is difficult to ascertain because many supplements are used at once.[110,111] The therapeutic effects of zinc in chronic cutaneous ulcers are thought to be derived from its ability to enhance reepithelialization, decrease inflammation, and inhibit bacterial growth.[108]

Local zinc deficiency A poorly understood concept is local zinc deficiency (ie, low levels of tissue zinc with normal serum levels). Michaelsson and colleagues[112] reported a lack of correlation between skin and serum zinc levels among healthy subjects. When zinc levels were surveyed in subjects with dermatitis herpetiformis, acne, psoriasis, and Darier disease, they were lower than normal.[113] However, there was no association between serum and skin zinc levels, because many subjects had normal serum zinc. This finding may indicate tissue zinc depletion as contributing to disease etiology. Another plausible explanation is that serum zinc levels do not reflect total zinc capacity. Amer and colleagues[25] reported a significantly lower serum zinc level in subjects with severe acne. Perhaps a more extensive examination of skin and serum levels corrected to the severity of the condition in question will yield a more significant correlation in the future.

Melasma This pigmentation deposition usually occurs in association with elevated levels of hormones during pregnancy or from oral contraceptives, and is treated with topical bleaching agents, chemical peels, lasers, and sun avoidance. Bolanca and colleagues[114] suggested sunscreens containing physical blockers, such as titanium dioxide and zinc oxide, are preferred over chemical blockers because of their broader protection. In addition to sunscreen containing zinc, Sharquie treated 28 subjects with 10% zinc sulfate solution twice daily for 2 months and found a statistically significant difference with its use.[115] Sharquie postulated that zinc aids in melasma by its peeling, antioxidant, and sun-screening effects.

DISCUSSION

In summary, from a review of the readily available peer-reviewed medical literature it appears that the relevance of zinc as a first-line treatment in dermatology is limited at present, with the exceptions presented by verifiable systemic zinc deficiencies. Several studies examining acne vulgaris, chronic verrucae, and chronic cutaneous ulcer sections support a role for zinc, at least as an adjunct modality, to existing first-line therapies. In several conditions, there is limited evidence of possible benefit. These conditions include various disorders, including rosacea, seborrheic dermatitis, hand eczema, and cutaneous ulcers. The main reservation is that most of these studies are either case reports or small subject series. Even the few randomized clinical trials that have been reviewed are often of limited sample size. It should be pointed out that in several conditions topical zinc is effective but systemic zinc is not, and in others, the opposite is true. In some conditions, different zinc compounds have different efficacy profiles. For example, zinc sulfate is more effective than zinc acetate for acne,[44,45] whereas zinc oxide is more effective than zinc sulfate for chronic ulcers.[108] Obviously, more evidence is needed where promising results are based on anecdotal data. In conditions for which zinc treatment is of benefit, further research is necessary to establish guidelines for its application, the efficacy of different zinc salts, and preparations and their therapeutic indexes.

REFERENCES

1. Raulin J. Etudes cliniques sur la vegetation. Ann Sci Nat Bot Biol Veg 1869;11:93.
2. Coleman J. Zinc proteins: enzymes, storage proteins, transcription factors, and replication proteins. Annu Rev Biochem 1992;61:897–946.
3. Prasad A. Zinc and enzymes. New York: Plenum Press; 1993.
4. Prasad A. Zinc and gene expression. New York: Plenum Press; 1993.
5. Hernick M, Fierke C. Zinc hydrolases: the mechanisms of zinc-dependent deacetylases. Arch Biochem Biophys 2005;433:71–84.
6. Vallee B, Falchuk K. The biochemical basis of zinc physiology. Physiol Rev 1993;73:79–118.
7. Prasad A. Zinc deficiency. BMJ 2003;326:409–10.
8. King J, Shames D, Woodhouse L. Zinc homeostasis in humans. J Nutr 2000;130(5S Suppl): 1360S–6S.
9. Murphy E, Willis B, Watt B. Provisional tables on the zinc content of foods. J Am Diet Assoc 1975;66: 345–55.
10. Hunt J. Bioavailability of iron, zinc, and other trace minerals from vegetarian diets. Am J Clin Nutr 2003;78(3 Suppl):633S–9S.
11. Krebs N. Overview of zinc absorption and excretion in the human gastrointestinal tract. J Nutr. 2000;130(5S Suppl):1374S–7S.
12. Bibi Nitzan Y, Cohen A. Zinc in skin pathology and care. J Dermatolog Treat 2006;17(4):205–10.
13. Prasad A, Halsted J, Nadimi M. Syndrome of iron deficiency anemia, hepatosplenomegaly, hypogonadism, dwarfism and geophagia. Am J Med 1961;31:532–46.
14. Prasad A. Zinc in growth and development and spectrum of human zinc deficiency. J Am Coll Nutr 1988;7:377–84.
15. Gibson R. Zinc nutrition in developing countries. Nutr Res Rev 1994;7:151–73.
16. Prasad A, Miale A Jr, Farid Z, et al. Zinc metabolism in patients with the syndrome of iron deficiency anemia, hepatosplenomegaly, dwarfism, and hypogonadism. J Lab Clin Med 1963;61:537–49.
17. Sandstead H, Prasad A, Schulert A, et al. Human zinc deficiency, endocrine manifestations and response to treatment. Am J Clin Nutr 1967;20: 422–42.
18. Danbolt N, Closs K. Acrodermatitis enteropathica. Acta Derm Venereol 1942;23:127–69.
19. Barnes P, Moynahan E. Zinc deficiency in acrodermatitis enteropathica: multiple dietary intolerance treated with synthetic diet. Proc R Soc Med 1973; 66:327–9.
20. Michaelsson G. Zinc therapy in acrodermatitis enteropathica. Acta Derm Venereol 1974;54:377–81.
21. Kury S, Dreno B, Bezieau S, et al. Identification of SLC39A4, a gene involved in acrodermatitis enteropathica. Nat Genet 2002;31:239–40.
22. Perafan-Riveros C, Franca L, Alves A, et al. Acrodermatitis enteropathica: case report and review of the literature. Pediatr Dermatol 2002;19:426–31.
23. Kay R, Tasman-Jones C, Pybus J, et al. A syndrome of acute zinc deficiency during total parenteral alimentation in man. Ann Surg 1976; 183:331–40.
24. Fitzherbert J. Zinc deficiency in acne vulgaris. Med J Aust 1977;2:685–6.
25. Amer M, Bahgat M, Tosson Z, et al. Serum zinc in acne vulgaris. Int J Dermatol 1982;21:481–4.
26. Michaelsson G, Vahlquist A, Juhlin L. Serum zinc and retinol-binding protein in acne. Br J Dermatol 1977;96:283–6.
27. Michaelsson G, Juhlin L, Vahlquist A. Effects of oral zinc and vitamin A in acne. Arch Dermatol 1977; 113:31–6.
28. Hillstrom L, Pettersson L, Hellbe L, et al. Comparison of oral treatment with zinc sulfate and placebo in acne vulgaris. Br J Dermatol 1977;97:681–4.
29. Göransson K, Liden S, Odsell L. Oral zinc in acne vulgaris: a clinical and methodological study. Acta Derm Venereol 1978;58:443–8.
30. Verma K, Saini A, Dhamija S. Oral zinc sulfate therapy in acne vulgaris: a double-blind trial. Acta Derm Venereol 1980;60:337–40.
31. Liden S, Goransson K, Odsell L. Clinical evaluation in acne. Acta Derm Venereol Suppl (Stockh) 1980; 89(Suppl):47–52.
32. Orris L, Shalita A, Sibulkin D, et al. Oral zinc therapy of acne. Absorption and clinical effect. Arch Dermatol 1978;114:1018–20.
33. Weimar V, Puhl S, Smith W, et al. Zinc sulfate in acne vulgaris. Arch Dermatol 1978;114:1776–8.
34. Cunliffe W. Unacceptable side-effects of oral zinc sulfate in the treatment of acne vulgaris. Br J Dermatol 1979;101:363.
35. Dreno B, Amblard P, Agache P, et al. Low doses of zinc gluconate for inflammatory acne. Acta Derm Venereol Suppl (Stockh) 1989;69:541–3.

36. Dreno B, Moyse D, Alirezai M, et al. Multicenter randomized comparative double blind controlled clinical trial of the safety and efficacy of zinc gluconate versus minocycline hydrochloride in the treatment of inflammatory acne vulgaris. Dermatology 2001;203:135–40.
37. Meynadier J. Efficacy and safety study of two zinc gluconate regimens in the treatment of inflammatory acne. Eur J Dermatol 2000;10:269–73.
38. Michaelsson G, Juhlin L, Ljunghall K. A double-blind study of the effect of zinc and oxytetracycline in acne vulgaris. Br J Dermatol 1977;97:561–6.
39. Sharquie KE, Noaimi AA, Al-Salih MM. Topical therapy of acne vulgaris using 2% tea lotion in comparison with 5% zinc sulphate solution. Saudi Med J 2008;29(12):1757–61.
40. Feucht C, Allen B, Chalker D, et al. Topical erythromycin with zinc in acne. A double-blind controlled study. J Am Acad Dermatol 1980;3:483–91.
41. Habbema L, Koopmans B, Menke H, et al. A 4% erythromycin and zinc combination (Zineryt) versus 2% erythromycin (Eryderm) in acne vulgaris: a randomized, double-blind comparative study. Br J Dermatol 1989;121:497–502.
42. Schachner L, Eaglstein W, Kittles C, et al. Topical erythromycin and zinc therapy for acne. J Am Acad Dermatol. 1990;22(2 Pt 1):253–60.
43. Schachner L, Pestana A, Kittles C. A clinical trial comparing the safety and efficacy of a topical erythromycin-zinc formulation with a topical clindamycin formulation. J Am Acad Dermatol 1990;22:489–95.
44. Langner A, Sheehan-Dare R, Layton A. A randomized, single-blind comparison of topical clindamycin + benzoyl peroxide (Duac) and erythromycin + zinc acetate (Zineryt) in the treatment of mild to moderate facial acne vulgaris. J Eur Acad Dermatol Venereol 2007;21:311–9.
45. Cochran R, Tucker S, Flannigan S. Topical zinc therapy for acne vulgaris. Int J Dermatol 1985;24:188–90.
46. Cunliffe WJ, Fernandez C, Bojar R, et al. Zindaclin Clinical Study Group. An observer-blind parallel-group, randomized, multicentre clinical and microbiological study of a topical clindamycin/zinc gel and a topical clindamycin lotion in patients with mild/moderate acne. J Dermatolog Treat 2005;16:213–8.
47. Dreno B, Foulc P, Reynaud A, et al. Effect of zinc gluconate on propionibacterium acnes resistance to erythromycin in patients with inflammatory acne: in vitro and in vivo study. Eur J Dermatol 2005;15:152–5.
48. Strauss J, Stranieri A. Acne treatment with topical erythromycin and zinc: effect of Propionibacterium acnes and free fatty acid composition. J Am Acad Dermatol 1984;11:86–9.
49. Toyoda M, Morohashi M. An overview of topical antibiotics for acne treatment. Dermatology 1998;196:130–4.
50. Bojar R, Eady E, Jones C, et al. Inhibition of erythromycin-resistant propionibacteria on the skin of acne patients by topical erythromycin with and without zinc. Br J Dermatol 1994;130:329–36.
51. Fluhr J, Bosch B, Gloor M, et al. In-vitro and in-vivo efficacy of zinc acetate against propionibacteria alone and in combination with erythromycin. Zentralbl Bakteriol 1999;289:445–56.
52. Rebello T, Atherton D, Holden C. The effect of oral zinc administration on sebum free fatty acids in acne vulgaris. Acta Derm Venereol. 1986;66:305–10.
53. Dreno B, Trossaert M, Boiteau H, et al. Zinc salts effects on granulocyte zinc concentration and chemotaxis in acne patients. Acta Derm Venereol Suppl (Stockh) 1992;72:250–2.
54. Pierard G, Pierard-Franchimont C. Effect of a topical erythromycin-zinc formulation on sebum delivery. Evaluation by combined photometric-multi-step samplings with Sebutape. Clin Exp Dermatol 1993;18:410–3.
55. Pierard-Franchimont C, Goffin V, Visser J, et al. A double-blind controlled evaluation of the sebosuppressive activity of topical erythromycin–zinc complex. Eur J Clin Pharmacol 1995;49:57–60.
56. Van Hoogdalem E, Terpstra I, Baven A. Evaluation of the effect of zinc acetate on the stratum corneum penetration kinetics of erythromycin in healthy male volunteers. Skin Pharmacol 1996;9:104–10.
57. Degitz K, Ochsendorf F. Pharmacotherapy of acne [review]. Expert Opin Pharmacother 2008;9:955–71.
58. Sharquie KE, Najim RA, Al-Salman HN. Oral zinc sulfate in the treatment of rosacea: a double-blind, placebo-controlled study. Int J Dermatol 2006;45:857–61.
59. Ead R. Oral zinc sulfate in alopecia areata – a double blind trial. Br J Dermatol 1981;104:483–4.
60. Brocard A, Knol AC, Khammari A, et al. Hidradenitis suppurativa and zinc: a new therapeutic approach. A pilot study. Dermatology 2007;214:325–7.
61. Abeck D, Korting HC, Braun-Falco O. Folliculitis decalvans. Long-lasting response to combined therapy with fusidic acid and zinc. Acta Derm Venereol 1992;72:143–5.
62. Najim RA, Sharquie KE, Abu-Raghif AR. Oxidative stress in patients with Behcet's disease: I correlation with severity and clinical parameters. J Dermatol 2007;34:308–14.
63. Sharquie KE, Najim RA, Al-Dori WS, et al. Oral zinc sulfate in the treatment of Behcet's disease: a double blind cross-over study. J Dermatol 2006;33:541–6.

64. Berger R, Fu J, Smiles K, et al. The effects of minoxidil, 1% pyrithione zinc and a combination of both on hair density: a randomized controlled trial. Br J Dermatol 2003;149:354–62.
65. Rushton D. Nutritional factors and hair loss. Clin Exp Dermatol 2002;27:396–404.
66. Warner R, Schwartz J, Boissy Y, et al. Dandruff has an zinc pyrithione shampoo. J Am Acad Dermatol 2001;45:897–903.
67. Imokawa G, Okamoto K. The inhibitory effect of zinc pyrithione on the epidermal proliferation of animal skins. Acta Derm Venereol 1982;62:471–5.
68. Gibson W, Hardy W, Groom M. The effect and mode of action of zinc pyrithione on cell growth. II. In vivo studies. Food Chem Toxicol 1985;23:103–10.
69. Gupte T, Gaikwad U, Naik S. Experimental studies (in vitro) on polyene macrolide antibiotics with special reference to hamycin against Malassezia ovale. Comp Immunol Microbiol Infect Dis 1999;22:93–102.
70. Schmidt A, Ruhl-Horster B. In vitro susceptibility of Malassezia furfur. Arzneimittelforschung 1996;46: 442–4.
71. Marks R, Pearse A, Walker A. The effects of a shampoo containing zinc pyrithione on the control of dandruff. Br J Dermatol 1985;112:415–22.
72. Rapaport M. A randomized, controlled clinical trial of four anti-dandruff shampoos. J Int Med Res 1981;9:152–6.
73. Pierard-Franchimont C, Goffin V, Decroix J, et al. A multicenter randomized trial of ketoconazole 2% and zinc pyrithione 1% shampoos in severe dandruff and seborrheic dermatitis. Skin Pharmacol Appl Skin Physiol 2002;15:434–41.
74. Shin H, Kwon OS, Won CH, et al. Clinical efficacies of topical agents for the treatment of seborrheic dermatitis of the scalp: a comparative study. J Dermatol 2009;36(3):131–7.
75. Van Coevorden AM, Coenraads PJ, Svensson A. Overview of studies of treatments for hand eczema the EDEN hand eczema survey. Br J Dermatol 2004;151:446.
76. Faghihi G, Iraji F, Shahingohar A, et al. The efficacy of 0.05% Clobetasol + 2.5% zinc sulfate' cream vs. 0.05% Clobetasol alone' cream in the treatment of the chronic hand eczema: a double-blind study. J Eur Acad Dermatol Venereol 2008;22:531–6.
77. Lansdown A. Zinc in the healing wound. Lancet 1996;347:706–7.
78. Baldwin S, Odio MR, Haines SL, et al. Skin benefits from continuous topical administration of a zinc oxide/petrolatum formulation by a novel disposable diaper. J Eur Acad Dermatol Venereol 2001; 15(Suppl 1):5–11.
79. Arad A, Ben-Amitai D, Zeharia A, et al. Efficacy of topical application of eosin compared with zinc oxide paste and corticosteroid cream for diaper dermatitis. Dermatology 1999;199:319–22.
80. Wananukul S, Limpongsanuruk W, Singalavanija S, et al. Comparison of dexpanthenol and zinc oxide ointment with ointment base in the treatment of irritant diaper dermatitis from diarrhea: a multicenter study. J Med Assoc Thai 2006;89:1654–8.
81. Al-Gurairi F, Al-Waiz M, Sharquie K. Oral zinc sulfate in the treatment of recalcitrant viral warts: randomized placebo-controlled clinical trial. Br J Dermatol 2002;146:423–31.
82. Gibbs S. Zinc sulfate for viral warts. Br J Dermatol 2003;148:1082–3.
83. Sadighha A. Oral zinc sulfate in recalcitrant multiple viral warts: a pilot study. J Eur Acad Dermatol Venereol 2009;23:715–6.
84. Yaghoobi R, Sadighha A, Baktash D. Evaluation of oral zinc sulfate effect on recalcitrant multiple viral warts: a randomized placebo-controlled clinical trial. J Am Acad Dermatol 2009;60:706–8.
85. Sharquie KE, Khorsheed AA, Al-Nuaimy AA. Topical zinc sulfate solution for treatment of viral warts. Saudi Med J 2007;28:1418–21.
86. Khattar JA, Musharrafieh UM, Tamim H, et al. Topical zinc oxide vs. salicylic acid-lactic acid combination in the treatment of warts. Int J Dermatol 2007;46:427–30.
87. Sharquie K, Najim R, Farjou I, et al. Oral zinc sulfate in the treatment of acute cutaneous leishmaniasis. Clin Exp Dermatol 2001;26:21–6.
88. Firooz A, Khatami A, Khamesipour A, et al. Intralesional injection of 2% zinc sulfate solution in the treatment of acute old world cutaneous leishmaniasis: a randomized, doubleblind, controlled clinical trial. J Drugs Dermatol 2005;4:73–9.
89. Iraji F, Vali A, Asilian A, et al. Comparison of intralesionally injected zinc sulfate with meglumine antimoniate in the treatment of acute cutaneous leishmaniasis. Dermatology 2004;209:46–9.
90. Sharquie K, Najim R, Farjou I. A comparative controlled trial of intralesionally-administered zinc sulfate, hypertonic sodium chloride and pentavalent antimony compound against acute cutaneous leishmaniasis. Clin Exp Dermatol 1997;22:169–73.
91. Sharquie KE, Najim RA. Disseminated cutaneous leishmaniasis. Saudi Med J 2004;25:951–4.
92. Minodier P, Parola P. Cutaneous leishmaniasis treatment [review]. Travel Med Infect Dis 2007;5: 150–8.
93. Nofal AA, Nofal E, Attwa E, et al. Necrolytic acral erythema: a variant of necrolytic migratory erythema or a distinct entity? Int J Dermatol 2005; 44(11):916–21.
94. de Carvalho Fantini B, Matsumoto FY, Arnone M, et al. Necrolytic acral erythema successfully treated with oral zinc. Int J Dermatol 2008;47(8): 872–3.
95. Khanna VJ, Shieh S, Benjamin J, et al. Necrolytic acral erythema associated with hepatitis C: effective

treatment with interferon alfa and zinc. Arch Dermatol 2000;136:755–7.
96. Abdallah MA, Hull C, Horn TD. Necrolytic acral erythema: a patient from the United States successfully treated with oral zinc. Arch Dermatol 2005;141:85–7.
97. Geria AN, Holcomb KZ, Scheinfeld NS. Necrolytic acral erythema: a review of the literature [review]. Cutis 2009;83:309–14.
98. Rowlands C, Danby F. Histopathology of psoriasis treated with zinc pyrithione. Am J Dermatopathol 2000;22:272–6.
99. Housman T, Keil K, Mellen B, et al. The use of 0.25% zinc pyrithione spray does not enhance the efficacy of clobetasol propionate 0.05% foam in the treatment of psoriasis. J Am Acad Dermatol 2003;49:79–82.
100. Burrows N, Turnbull A, Punchard N, et al. A trial of oral zinc supplementation in psoriasis. Cutis 1994; 54:117–8.
101. Rojas A, Phillips T. Patients with chronic leg ulcers show diminished levels of vitamins A and E, carotenes, and zinc. Dermatol Surg 1999;25:601–4.
102. Posthauer ME. Do patients with pressure ulcers benefit from oral zinc supplementation? [review]. Adv Wound Care 2005;18:471–2.
103. Ackerman Z, Loewenthal E, Seidenbaum M, et al. Skin zinc concentrations in patients with varicose ulcers. Int J Dermatol 1990;29:360–2.
104. Brandrup F, Menne T, Agren M, et al. A randomized trial of two occlusive dressings in the treatment of leg ulcers. Acta Derm Venereol Suppl (Stockh) 1990;70:231–5.
105. Stromberg H, Agren M. Topical zinc oxide treatment improves arterial and venous leg ulcers. Br J Dermatol 1984;111:461–8.
106. Agren M, Stromberg H. Topical treatment of pressure ulcers. A randomized comparative trial of Varidase and zinc oxide. Scand J Plast Reconstr Surg 1985;19:97–100.
107. Apelqvist J, Larsson J, Stenstrom A. Topical treatment of necrotic foot ulcers in diabetic patients: a comparative trial of DuoDerm and MeZinc. Br J Dermatol 1990;123:787–92.
108. Agren M. Studies on zinc in wound healing. Acta Derm Venereol Suppl (Stockh) 1990;154:1–36.
109. Wilkinson E, Hawke C. Oral zinc for arterial and venous leg ulcers. Cochrane Database Syst Rev 2000;(2):CD001273.
110. Cereda E, Gini A, Pedrolli C, et al. Disease-specific, versus standard, nutritional support for the treatment of pressure ulcers in institutionalized older adults: a randomized controlled trial. J Am Geriatr Soc 2009;57:1395–402.
111. Desneves KJ, Todorovic BE, Cassar A, et al. Treatment with supplementary arginine, vitamin C and zinc in patients with pressure ulcers: a randomized controlled trial. Clin Nutr 2005;24:979–87.
112. Michaelsson G, Ljunghall K, Danielson B. Zinc in epidermis and dermis in healthy subjects. Acta Derm Venereol 1980;60:295–9.
113. Michaelsson G, Ljunghall K. Patients with dermatitis herpetiformis, acne, psoriasis and Darier's disease have low epidermal zinc concentrations. Acta Derm Venereol 1990;70:304–8.
114. Bolanca I, Bolanca Z, Kuna K, et al. Chloasma–the mask of pregnancy [review]. Coll Antropol 2008; 32(Suppl 2):139–41.
115. Sharquie KE, Al-Mashhadani SA, Salman HA. Topical 10% zinc sulfate solution for treatment of melasma. Dermatol Surg 2008;34:1346–9.
116. Reinar LM, Forsetlund L, Bjørndal A, et al. Interventions for skin changes caused by nerve damage in leprosy. Cochrane Database Syst Rev 2008;3: CD004833.

Innovative Use of Dapsone

V.E. Gottfried Wozel, MD

KEYWORDS

• Dapsone • Dermatology • Sulfone

In the past, sulfones were used preferentially as antimicrobial/chemotherapeutic agents to treat infections caused by streptococcus, mycobacteriaceae, and other bacteria.[1] Currently, dapsone (4,4′ diaminodiphenylsulfone) is the only remaining sulfone congener used in human therapeutics. Because of its dual mechanism of action—antimicrobial and anti-inflammatory/immunomodulatory effects—dapsone alone or in conjunction with other drugs is used worldwide for preventing and treating pathogen-caused diseases (eg, leprosy, *Pneumocystis jiroveci* pneumonia in individuals with HIV infection) or chronic inflammatory diseases, especially in the field of dermatology (eg, autoimmune bullous eruptions).

Synthesis of dapsone was reported in 1908 by Emil Fromm (**Fig. 1**), professor of organic chemistry in Freiburg/Germany, and Jakob Wittmann during their experiments in dye chemistry.[2] When first synthesized, dapsone was not envisioned as a medical agent. In 1937, soon after the discovery of sulphonamides as antibiotics, two research groups (one in England and one in France) were the first to investigate dapsone. Both groups concurrently published the observed anti-inflammatory potency of dapsone in experimentally induced infections in mice.[3,4] In the narrowest sense, that marked the beginning of the sulfone story.

From a historical perspective, it is remarkable that other sulfones, and not the so-called "parent sulfone" (dapsone), were first used to treat gonorrhoea.[5,6] After extensive use of with promin and related sulfones in the treatment of Hansen's disease at the U.S. leprosarium in Carville, Louisiana early in the 1940s by Faget and coworkers,[7] sulfones ultimately developed from simple chemical compounds into valuable therapeutic agents.

In 1950, the Portuguese Esteves and Brandão[8] introduced sulfones (eg, Sulphetrone, Diasone) into dermatology through their reports of their successful use in treating dermatitis herpetiformis (Duhring's disease), which was subsequently confirmed by other groups.

Later, Sneddon and Wilkinson[9] in England reported a remission in subcorneal pustulosis after dapsone administration. Since that time, dapsone has been increasingly considered effective in treating neutrophil-mediated processes and autoimmune skin diseases, and retains its place in the therapeutic armamentarium as a unique and essential agent.

CHEMISTRY AND PHARMACOLOGY

Chemically, dapsone is an aniline derivative. All sulfones share the structure of a sulfur atom linking to two carbon atoms (**Fig. 2**). The solubility of dapsone varies over a large range depending on the solvent used (eg, water, 0.2 mg/mL, methanol, 52 mg/mL). Dapsone has been considered a difficult-to-handle compound for experimental investigations, especially using living cell assays.[10]

After oral administration, dapsone is almost completely absorbed from the gastrointestinal tract with bioavailability of more than 86%. Peak serum concentrations are generally attained within 2 to 8 hours. After ingestion of a single 50- to 300-mg dose of dapsone, maximal serum concentrations are reached between 0.63 and 4.82 mg/L.[10–12] Under steady-state conditions, the most frequently used dosage of 100 mg/d

Department of Dermatology, University Hospital Carl Gustav Carus, Technical University of Dresden, Fetscherstr. 74, D-01307 Dresden, Germany
E-mail address: Verena.Huebner@uniklinikum-dresden.de

Dermatol Clin 28 (2010) 599–610
doi:10.1016/j.det.2010.03.014
0733-8635/10/$ – see front matter © 2010 Elsevier Inc. All rights reserved.

derm.theclinics.com

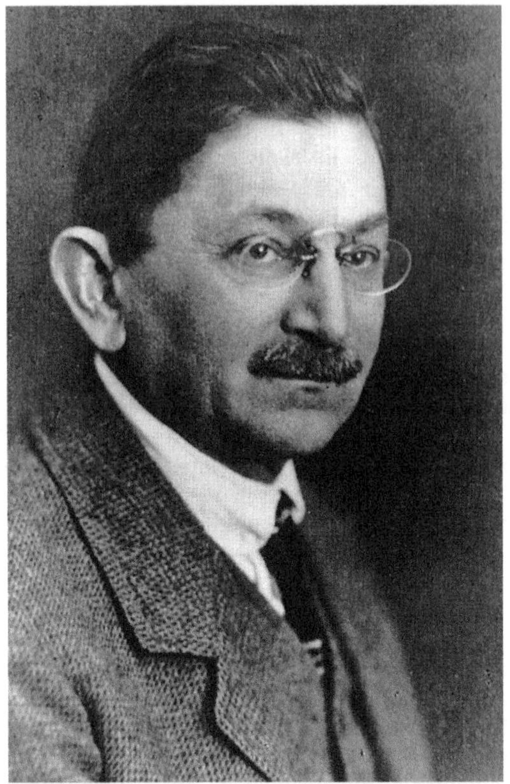

Fig. 1. Emil Fromm (1865–1928). (*Courtesy of* Institut für Geschichte der Medizin der Universität Wien; with permission.)

results in serum concentration of 3.26 (maximum) and 1.95 mg/L (after 24 hours).[13] These dapsone serum concentrations, attainable in vivo, must be strictly considered when interpreting the results of in vitro investigations.

After absorption, dapsone undergoes enterohepatic circulation. It is metabolized both by the liver and activated polymorphonuclear leucocytes (PMN) or mononuclear cells.[14] In the liver, dapsone is metabolized primarily through acetylation by *N*-acetyltransferase to monoacetyldapsone (MADDS), and through hydroxylation by cytochrome P-450 enzymes, resulting in generation of dapsone hydroxylamine (DDS-NOH) (**Fig. 3**). Acetylation is genetically determined, resulting in significant variability in acetylation (rapid or slow acetylator). In fact, dapsone can be administered to determine the acetylation phenotype.

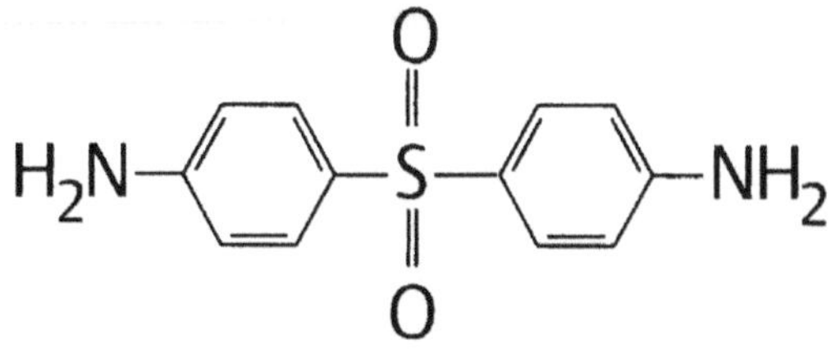

Fig. 2. Structural formula of dapsone (4,4′ diaminodiphenylsulfone).

In terms of both efficacy and induction of adverse effects, the most important factor is the generation of DDS-NOH; this occurs in lesional inflammatory processes in skin mediated by activated PMN.[14] Dapsone is distributed to all organs, crosses the blood–brain barrier and placenta, and is detectable in breast milk.[15,16] Approximately 20% of dapsone is excreted in urine as unchanged drug and 70% to 85% as water-soluble metabolites. Additionally, a small amount may be excreted in feces. The complex metabolic pathway of dapsone has been reviewed in detail several times.[10,12,14,17,18]

MECHANISM OF ACTION

The therapeutic efficacy most likely is based on differing drug activities when considering pathogen-caused diseases and noninfectious dermatologic disorders (**Fig. 4**). Antimicrobial activity is usually bacteriostatic in nature and seems to mimic that of sulfonamides (inhibition of folic acid synthesis in susceptible organisms), because antibacterial activity is inhibited by para-aminobenzoic acid.

When used as therapy for inflammatory disorders, however, alternate mechanisms are at work. Recent investigation shows that dapsone alone (and through its metabolites) has similarities to nonsteroidal anti-inflammatory drugs (NSAIDs).[10] However, these data were obtained through varying methods and under different experimental conditions. These discrepancies raise some important questions, such as which types of investigations render the most valid data for human use: in vitro versus in vivo investigation, animal versus human model, or single administration versus steady-state administration.

Additionally, several investigations have evaluated the capability of dapsone to ameliorate or block specific pathways using drug concentrations that are not achieved in humans. Therefore, despite many experimental investigations using dapsone, the relevance of observed effects remains unclear. This problem is even more obvious because the pathogenesis of dapsone-sensitive dermatoses has not been fully elucidated.

The ability of dapsone to inhibit reactive oxygen species (ROS) seems to contribute to the drug's anti-inflammatory effects.[19] ROS can be generated through two major pathways: the PMN-mediated

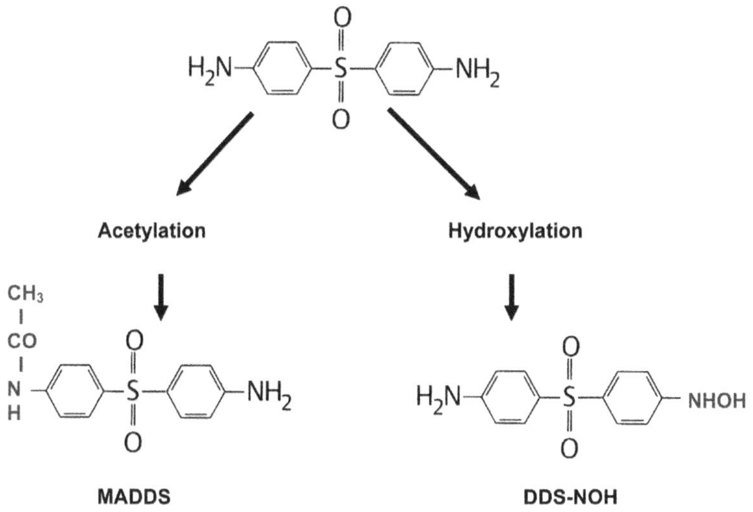

Acetylation

Hydroxylation

MADDS

DDS-NOH

Fig. 3. Main metabolic pathway of dapsone. MADDS, monacetyl dapsone; DDS-NOH, dapsone hydroxylamine.

intracellular system and an extracellular xanthine/xanthine–oxidase system. Both are affected by dapsone to the same extent.[20]

Niwa and colleagues[20] showed that dapsone has a scavenger-like effect; it quenches all ROS except the oxygen intermediate, O_2^-. Although Stendahl and colleagues[21] ascribed the depression of cytotoxic and cytopathic functions of PMNs to the ability of dapsone to directly inhibit the myeloperoxidase (MPO)–H_2O_2–halide system, it may also be caused by the marked decrease in hydrogen peroxide (H_2O_2), hydroxyl radical (OH), and oxygen (O_2) levels as a result of scavenger-like functions of dapsone. The cytotoxic potency in the MPO–H_2O_2–halide system may not be highly powerful, because patients with MPO deficiency are not unduly susceptible to infections.

Being one of the strongest scavengers known, dapsone decreases H_2O_2 as effectively as catalase and is as potent as colchicine, superoxide-dismutase, catalase, benzoate, and xanthine in lowering OH levels. Severe tissue injury observed in patients with disorders such as dermatitis herpetiformis, linear IgA bullous dermatosis, prurigo pigmentosa, leukocytoclastic vasculitis, Behçet's disease, and lupus erythematosus (LE) must be considered partly as a consequence of excessive PMN-generated oxygen intermediates.[20,22,23] The beneficial effects of dapsone on these dermatologic disorders are most likely a result of its quenching effects. Whether O_2^- and OH concentrations are linked by an iron-dependent mechanism is still unknown.

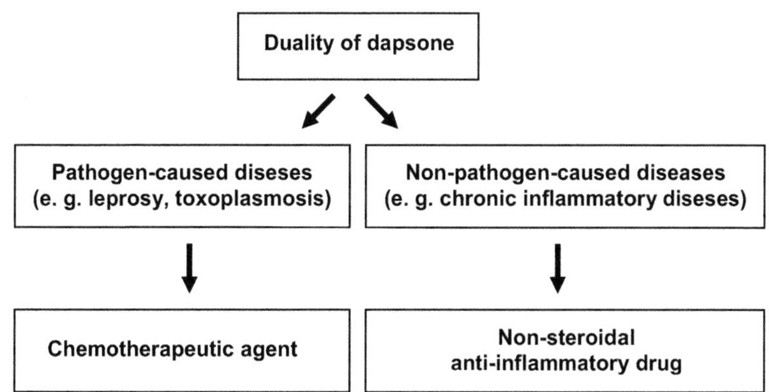

Fig. 4. Different dermatologic targets of dapsone.

Several reports indicate that dapsone may also affect additional inflammatory effector systems through

- Suppression of integrin-mediated neutrophilic adherence[24]
- Inhibition of generation of 5-lipoxygenase products (eg, leukotriene B_4 [LTB_4], 12-hydroxyeicosatetrenoate [HETE])[25]
- Inhibition of spontaneous or induced synthesis of prostaglandin E_2[26]
- Inhibition of cyclooxygenase I– and II–mediated generation of thromboxane B_2[27]
- Interference with activation or function of the G-protein, resulting in an inhibition of signal transduction[28]
- A protective effect on α1-protease inhibitor[29]
- Inhibition of cysteinyl leukotrienes (leukotriene C_4)[30]
- Inhibition of LTB_4 receptor binding of human PMN[31]
- Inhibition of interleukin (IL)-8 production/releasing of peripheral blood stimulated with lipopolysaccharide[32]
- Inhibition of mitogen-induced lymphocyte transformation.[33]

Moreover, it has been shown that dapsone has neuroprotective effects against quinolate- and kainate-induced striatal neurotoxicities in rats and attenuates kainic-induced seizures in rats.[34–36]

Summarizing these diverse mechanisms, growing evidence shows that dapsone is considered to be a pharmacodynamically active compound. The anti-inflammatory capacity of dapsone is generally attributed to the parent compound. The authors therefore addressed the question as to whether the two major dapsone metabolites (MADDS and DDS-NOH) possess anti-inflammatory properties of their own. High performance liquid chromatography analysis of 5-lipoxygenase products from calcium ionophore–stimulated isolated PMN showed that DDS-NOH is one magnitude more effective than dapsone and MADDS in suppressing the generation of LTB_4 and 5-HETE (eg, IC_{50} LTB_4: DDS-NOH, 0.490 μmol; dapsone, 15 μmol; MADDS, 40 μmol). Moreover, determination of lucigenin- and luminal-enhanced chemiluminescence of zymosan-stimulated human whole blood and isolated PMN showed that DDS-NOH (0.1–100 μmol) causes a significant and dose-dependent inhibition of oxidative burst, leading to almost complete suppression at the highest concentration tested.[37] Again, DDS-NOH was more effective than dapsone or MADDS.

After topical pretreatment with MADDS and DDS-NOH (both 1% dissolved in acetone) for 2 weeks, 10 ng LTB_4 were applied on the upper arm skin of eight healthy volunteers. Biopsies were taken after 24 hours and PMNs were quantified fluorometrically using elastase as a marker enzyme. MADDS did not show any inhibitory activity on PMN trafficking compared with the corresponding control and nontreated area (untreated: 790 ± 450 PMN per 10 μg skin; $P>.05$, acetone: 840 ± 578 PMN per 10 μg skin; MADDS: 1099 ± 556 PMN per 10 μg skin), whereas DDS-NOH caused a statistically significant inhibition of PMN accumulation, as did the reference clobetasol-17-propionate (CP) (DDS-NOH: 128 ± 143 PMN per 10 μg skin; CP: 86 ± 131 PMN per 10 μg skin; $P<.01$).[38] These results again indicate that only DDS-NOH can inhibit LTB_4-induced accumulation of PMN in healthy individuals.

In line with these in vivo experiments are results with dapsone, MADDS, and DDS-NOH to determine their effect on ultraviolet (UV)-induced erythema. Skin areas were irradiated with UVB (295 nm, two minimal erythema doses). Twenty-four hours later, UVB-induced erythema was quantified using the CR-200b handheld Chroma Meter (Minolta, Osaka, Japan) and cutaneous blood flow was measured using a Moor Laser Doppler Imager (Moor Instruments, Devon, England). In control skin, tissue blood flow was measured to be 227 units and was significantly ($P<0.05$) decreased by dapsone (186 units), DDS-NOH (154 units), and MADDS (195 units). UVB-induced erythema was also significantly reduced in DDS-NOH– or MADDS-treated skin when compared with controls. Thus, these explorations show that dapsone metabolites exert pharmacodynamic effects when applied topically to the skin and may at least be equal to dapsone in their anti-inflammatory properties.[39,40]

In general, the UVB-suppressing activity of dapsone was subsequently confirmed by Schumacher,[41] who observed significant inhibitory capability of both topically applied (0,1%, 0,5%, 1%, 5%, 10%) and systemically applied dapsone (100 mg/d) on UV-induced erythema in healthy volunteers having sun-reactive skin type II and III (**Fig. 5**, **Table 1**). A theoretical explanation for the observed erythema-suppressing effect of dapsone could be the drug's inhibitory action on prostaglandins. Against this background, it is noteworthy that dapsone unexpectedly showed no substantial effect on anthralin-induced erythema, sodium dodecylsulfate–induced erythema, LTB_4-induced chemotaxis of PMN, and in psoriasis plaque test.[41,42] However, the investigators did not consider dapsone metabolites like MADDS and

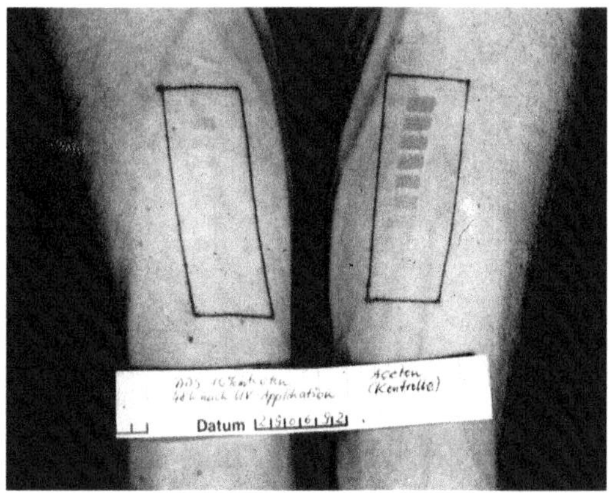

Fig. 5. Right forearm: suppression of ultraviolet (UV)-induced erythema with topically applied dapsone (1% solved in acetone, 48 hours after UV exposition). Left forearm: control.

DDS-NOH in the human models used. Regarding the effect of dapsone on chemotaxis, some controversial disparate results have been noted especially when comparing in vitro and in vivo studies. Some authors postulate even a selective inhibition of dapsone on specific chemotactic factors (eg, formyl-methionyl-leucyl-phenylalanine [fMLP]).[24,43]

Summarizing the mechanism of action of dapsone, a few theories have been postulated in an attempt to explain drug efficacy in chronic inflammatory disease states. However, little is known about the specific molecular effector systems targeted by dapsone or its metabolites, which leads to clinical efficacy. Further exploration of dapsone's mechanism of action in sulfone-sensitive dermatoses is needed.[44]

UNIQUE CHARACTERISTICS OF DAPSONE

Dapsone has unique pharmacologic properties among the spectra of available antiphlogistic agents. Currently, no other drug produces such a wide variety of beneficial activities:

1. Combination of antimicrobial and antiphlogistic effects (eg, treatment of opportunistic infections in patients with acquired immunodeficiency syndrome, use of dapsone in acne)
2. Safety of long-term treatment (eg, life-long use in leprosy, long-term ongoing or chronic intermittent approach in inflammatory dermatoses)
3. Disease-specific antiphlogistic activity (eg, prompt decrease of pruritus and control of skin lesions in dermatitis herpetiformis and amelioration of loxoscelism associated with brown recluse spider bites)
4. Steroid-sparing effect (eg, long-term treatment in autoimmune blistering diseases and as an adjuvant treatment in bronchial asthma)
5. UV protection (eg, suppression of UVB-induced erythema by dapsone and DDS-NOH)
6. Anticonvulsive effect (eg, in animal models)
7. Pharmacoeconomic benefits (eg, low cost of treatment).

CLINICAL USE OF DAPSONE

Dapsone, as a sulfone antibiotic, is used in rifampin-based multiple-drug regimens for treating multibacillary and paucibacillary leprosy.[10,13] Additionally, the sulfone alone or as part of drug combination with other antibiotic agents is used to treat prophylaxis of *P jiroveci* (*P carinii*) pneumonia and toxoplasmosis in individuals infected with HIV. The sulfone is designated an orphan

Table 1
Dapsone and erythema threshold

Application		Erythema Threshold Time (minimum)[a]		
Topical %	Systemic	Dapsone	Control	Difference
10	—	6.75 ± 1.27	4.14 ± 0.85	2.62 ± 0.74
5	—	5.79 ± 1.08	4.08 ± 0.74	1.72 ± 0.72
1	—	4.78 ± 0.82	3.38 ± 0.45	1.40 ± 0.55
0.5	—	4.97 ± 0.87	3.83 ± 0.51	1.14 ± 0.93
0.1	—	5.11 ± 1.07	4.22 ± 0.76	0.88 ± 0.46
—	100 mg/d	5.37 ± 1.19[b]	4.30 ± 1.06[b]	1.07 ± 0.34

[a] Dependent on the method of exposure in healthy volunteers (topical, n = 10; systemic, n = 8) with ultraviolet skin type II and III.
[b] Comparison between pre and posttreatment.
Data from Schumacher K. Humane in-vivo-Untersuchungen zur antientzündlichen Wirksamkeit von Diaminodiphenylsulfon (Dapson) [thesis]. Dresden, Germany: Department of Dermatology, University Hospital Carl Gustav Carus; 1996.

drug by US Food and Drug Administration for use in the latter condition.[10,13]

Extensive clinical experience in treating patients with dapsone shows that the sulfone can suppress disease activity in several chronic inflammatory dermatoses. Dapsone is considered the preferred drug for treating dermatitis herpetiformis, subcorneale pustulosis, erythema elevatum diutinum, acropustulosis infantilis, and prurigo pigmentosa. In these entities, dapsone is primarily indicated as monotherapy. In a second group of dermatoses, dapsone is used as an adjuvant treatment, especially in patients who experience insufficient therapeutic response to corticosteroids or other first-line agents, who have a need to reduce corticosteroid dosage, or in whom other first-line drugs are contraindicated or not tolerated. These entities are summarized in **Box 1**.[10,17,18,45–47]

In yet a third group of disorders, dapsone was reported anecdotally as being useful, but initial enthusiasm has been tempered with subsequent controversial or contradictory results or a total lack of properly controlled trials showing efficacy. Thus, use of dapsone in these latter entities is only justified in totally recalcitrant or refractory cases, such as those listed in **Box 2**.

Current perspective precludes using dapsone in psoriasis because of the lack of experimental evidence for its efficacy or inferential evidence derived from mechanism of action (eg, dapsone lacks T-cell targeting, tumor necrosis factor α antagonism, or IL-12/23 p40 blocking ability).[48] In line with this statement, topical 5% dapsone in a psoriasis plaque test showed no sulfone efficacy compared with inactive vehicle.[42] In all conditions in which dapsone is used, specific disease-related adjuvant treatment modalities should be considered when appropriate (eg, gluten-free diet in dermatitis herpetiformis, adequate UV protection in LE).

Because the potential for adverse hematologic effects associated with systemically administered dapsone, considerable work had gone into developing a safe topical formulation. Only one topical gel formulation of 5% dapsone is currently available on the market (Aczone, Allergan, Inc, Irvine, CA, USA) for treating acne vulgaris. Results of two large-scale studies (dapsone: n = 1506; vehicle: n = 1504) show an 8% reduction of noninflammatory lesions compared with placebo after a 12-week treatment period (mean change: 32% dapsone vs 24% vehicle). Inflammatory lesions improved nearly in the same low level (mean change: 48% dapsone vs 42% vehicle).[49] The authors highlight that a potential mechanism of action of dapsone in acne could be the direct

Box 1
Dapsone used in dermatologic entities as an adjunctive treatment modality (group II)

- Linear IgA dermatosis
- Bullous pemphigoid
- Pemphigus vulgaris
- Sweet's syndrome
- Recurrent neutrophilic dermatosis of the dorsal hands
- Pyoderma gangrenosum
- Relapsing polychondritis
- Leukocytoclastic vasculitis/urticaria vasculitis
- Brown recluse spider bite (loxoscelism)
- Eosinophilic folliculitis (Ofuji's disease)
- Cutaneous lupus erythematosus

Box 2
Miscellaneous dermatoses in which dapsone is used with uncertain benefit (group III)

- Alopecia areata
- Pressure urticaria
- Acute febrile neutrophilic dermatosis (Sweet's syndrome)
- Mycetoma
- Eosinophilic cellulitis (Well's syndrome)
- Behçet's syndrome
- Lupus miliaris disseminatus faciei
- Granuloma faciale
- Granuloma annulare
- Hypereosinophilic syndrome
- Lymphomatoid papulosis
- Nocardiosis
- Mucinosis follicularis/reticular erythematous mucinosis syndrome
- Transient acantholytic dermatosis (Grover's disease)
- Herpes gestationis
- Lymphocytic infiltrate (Jessner-Kanof syndrome)
- Acrodermatitis continua suppurativa (Hallopeau's disease)
- Pityriasis rosea
- Pemphigus benignus chronicus familiaris
- Kaposi sarcoma (AIDS)
- Psoriasis
- Erosive lichen planus/lichen planus pemphigoides
- Granulomatous rosacea

inhibition of PMN trafficking. However, early investigations clearly indicate that dapsone itself in vivo seems to exert only a minimal inhibitory effect in this regard,[50–55] whereas in healthy human volunteers, the dapsone metabolite DDS-NOH shows a strong inhibitory activity on LTB_4-induced accumulation of PMN into skin.[38] Therefore, an explanation for efficacy of topical dapsone in treating acne obviously could be the generation of DDS-NOH through activated PMN in the skin.

DOSAGE OF DAPSONE IN CHRONIC INFLAMMATORY DERMATOSES

The dosage of dapsone for nearly all sulfone-sensitive disorders must be individually titrated to determine the daily dosage that most effectively controls lesions. Dosage in adults is usually initiated at 50 to 100 mg/d. If the treatment goal is not achieved after some weeks, a higher dosage may be tried (150–300 mg/d); administration of higher doses depends on tolerability and laboratory monitoring. When a favorable response is attained, the dosage should then be reduced to the minimum that maintains a satisfactory clinical state.

Prophylactic administration of ascorbic acid, folate, iron, and vitamin E reportedly may prevent, to a small degree, the hematologic adverse effects associated with dapsone. In this regard, vitamin E (800 U/d) administration seems to be useful but still not in a substantial proportion of patients. Moreover, these therapeutic recommendations are not based on randomized, placebo-controlled, double-blinded trials.[10]

For administration to children, commercially available tablets of dapsone must be crushed and dissolved, for example, in strawberry syrup. Studies evaluating bioavailability of dapsone after administration of this preparation have not been published. For some indications in childhood, such as infantile acropustulosis or eosinophilic folliculitis, a daily dosage of 2 mg per kilogram of body weight is recommended.[56] Dosing of children with this dosage, or 4 mg/kg weekly, results in concentrations equivalent to these reached in adults receiving 100 mg/d.[57]

MONITORING GUIDELINES AND PITFALLS

Unfortunately, literature on dapsone often suggests a high degree of toxicity, although this toxicity is comparable to that of NSAIDs. If dapsone is used strictly according treatment recommendations, it is safe. Millions of patients tolerate the drug without serious problems.[58]

Before initiation of dapsone therapy, patients must undergo a careful clinical evaluation that includes a complete history and physical examination. Use must be avoided in patients with prior allergy to dapsone or sulfa antibiotics. In patients with severe cardiac or lung diseases, dapsone doses should be carefully adjusted because of the drug's inherent ability to cause some degree of hemolysis. Dapsone is contraindicated in patients with glucose-6-phosphate dehydrogenase (G6PD) deficiency and in those with severe hepatic abnormality. Dapsone should be avoided during pregnancy and nursing.

Laboratory evaluation before initiation of the medication includes complete blood cell (CBC) count with differential, white blood cell count, and reticulocyte count; liver and renal function tests and; G6PD determination. Consideration should also be given to determining methemoglobin (met-Hb) level and urinalysis.[18]

Follow-up visits should include a thorough history to determine adverse effects and periodic screening evaluation of neurologic functions. Laboratory tests include CBC with differential and reticulocytes count at least every 2 weeks for the first 3 to 6 months, and then every 2 months. Liver and renal function tests and urinalysis should be performed monthly in the first 3 to 6 months and then every 2 months. Special caution when treating patients with dapsone must be considered in those who are receiving or have been exposed to other drugs or agents that are capable of inducing met-Hb production or hemolysis. Unfortunately, this issue is not yet widely recognized. For example, some patients treated with dapsone have been reported who received aromatic amine drugs to accomplish local anesthesia, which resulted in a serious increase of met-Hb concentration.[59] After initiation of dapsone therapy, evaluation of met-Hb levels should be carefully addressed. Different time points generally are of relevance (**Fig. 6**):

1. The kinetics of met-Hb generation after a single dapsone dose is maximal after approximately 6 hours (**Fig. 7**A).
2. Approximately 14 days after initiation of treatment, determination of met-Hb will estimate the level under steady-state conditions and may also allow evaluation of patient's adherence to therapy.
3. Other met-Hb determinations can be considered at any time point if the patient's condition has changed (eg, occurrence of clinical complaints, comedication with other drugs, smoking, use of pump water in agricultural regions with potential content of nitrites/anilines, increased dapsone dosage).

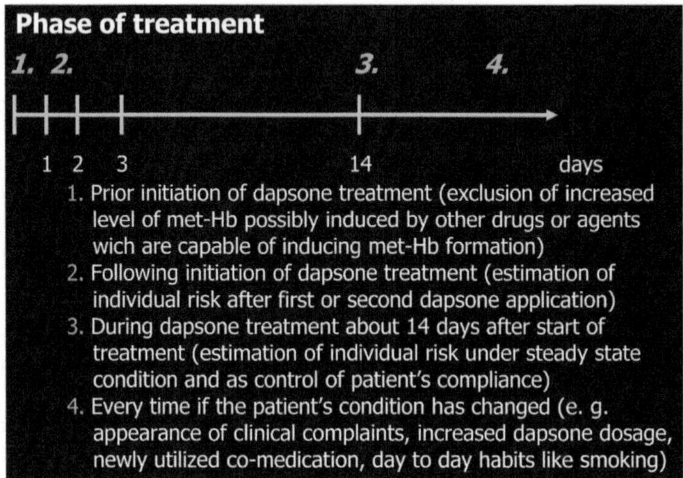

Fig. 6. Schedule for determining methemoglobin level in patients being treated with dapsone.

If clinical conditions of the patient remain stable, met-Hb levels should be checked only if clinically indicated.

ADVERSE EVENTS

In general, dapsone toxicity may be categorized as either dose-dependent or independent of dosage. Most adverse reactions are dose-related and uncommon at low doses of 50 to 100 mg/d. Classifying adverse events according to organ system manifestations is uselful[10,13,18,60]:

- Hematologic effects
- Dermatologic reactions
- Nervous system effects
- Gastrointestinal effects/hepatic effects
- Renal effects
- Hypersensitivity syndrome.

Hematologic Effects

The most frequent effects of dapsone are dose-related hemolytic anemia and production of met-Hb. Both effects are essentially unavoidable. However, some individuals experience only mild hematologic effects, whereas in others hemolysis and/or met-Hb production occur to a significant degree. Met-Hb caused by dapsone is normally well tolerated at a dosage of 100 mg/d. A few patients develop clinical cyanosis even at very low dosage. Met-Hb has a greater likelihood of becoming a serious problem at higher dapsone dosages (>200 mg/d) or in patients who are concomitantly exposed to other potentially met-Hb–producing agents (eg, anesthetics, nitrites, nitrates).

Methemoglobinemia may be poorly tolerated by patients with severe cardiopulmonary diseases. The dapsone hydroxylamine metabolites that react with hemoglobin cause met-Hb formation.[61,62] The generation of met-Hb undergoes a time-dependent process (**Fig. 7**B). In the early treatment phase, therefore, met-Hb should be determined 4 to 6 hours after ingestion of dapsone, because the maximum level of met-Hb in peripheral blood is indicative of real cardiopulmonary risk. For this reason, dapsone intake should be recommended in the evening in some patients.

Hemolysis is also dose-dependent. Therefore, nearly all patients treated with dapsone experience some degree of hemolysis. Unless it is severe, hemolysis does not generally require discontinuation of sulfone therapy. The manufacturer states that the hemoglobin level in patients treated with dapsone is generally decreased by 1 to 2 g/dL, the reticulocyte count is increased 2% to 12%, and erythrocyte life span is shortened. Heinz body formation also occurs frequently. Methemoglobinemia and hemolytic anemia are observed to a greater extent in patients with G6PD deficiency.

Agranulocytosis and aplastic anemia in patients treated with dapsone have been reported rarely.[13,60] Most cases of agranulocytosis developed within the first 8 to 12 weeks of therapy. This hematologic effect is usually reversible within 1 to 2 weeks, but it can also be fatal. Administration of hematopoietic growth factors is recommended for treatment of agranulocytosis.[63]

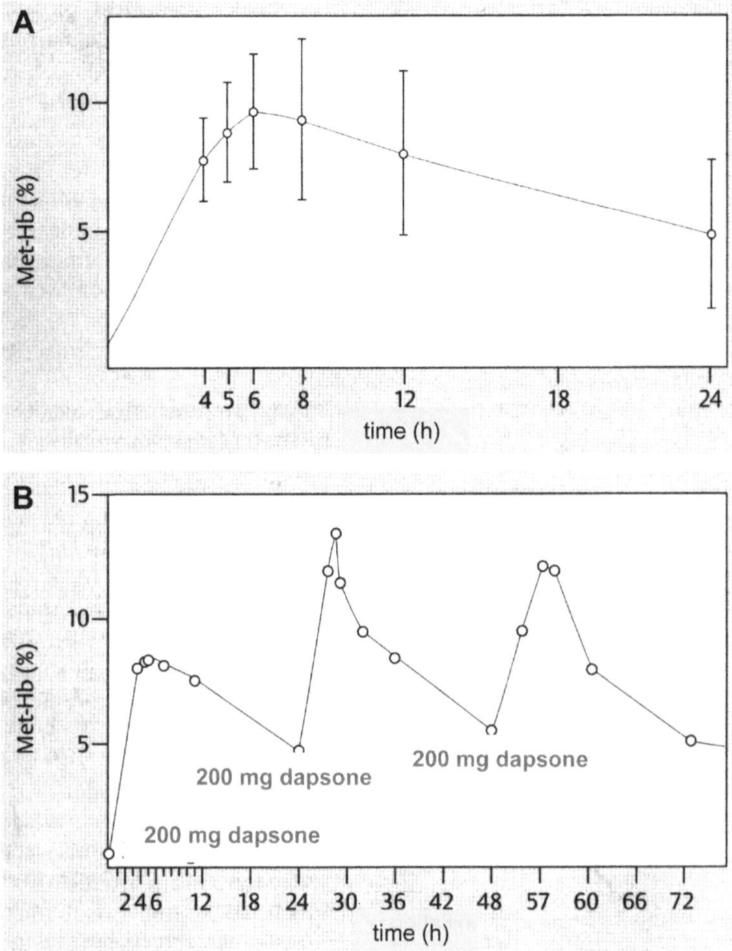

Fig. 7. Methemoglobin concentration (%) after single ingestion of dapsone, 200 mg, in dependence of time (*A*), methemoglobin concentration (%) after daily oral application of dapsone, 200 mg (*B*).

Dermatologic Reactions

Cutaneous reactions from dapsone include various skin eruptions: exfoliative dermatitis, erythema multiforme, urticaria, erythema nodosum, morbilliform and scarlatiniform exanthema, and toxic epidermal necrolysis. Dapsone-induced photosensitivity is not restricted to leprosy. Cutaneous reactions are rare, are not dose-dependent, and might be caused by not only the parent compound dapsone but also dapsone metabolites.[64]

Nervous System

Peripheral neuropathy with primarily motor loss has been reported rarely in patients receiving dapsone. If patients observe muscle weakness during dapsone treatment, the drug should be discontinued. Recovery may occur; however, this may take many months to several years. Tragic cases of patients ingesting dapsone on purpose to commit suicide confirm the ability of the drug to damage the peripheral nervous system, including the optic nerve (resulting in blindness).[65,66]

Gastrointestinal/Hepatic Reaction

Three different hepatic reactions must be considered:

1. Isolated abnormalities of liver function test (eg, increased bilirubin, aspartate aminotransferase, alanine aminotransferase, lactate dehydrogenase) without evidence of hepatitis or hepatosis. If any abnormality is detected, the dosage of dapsone should be decreased or the drug should be discontinued until the source is established.
2. Prehepatic jaundice induced by hemolytic anemia. Hyperbilirubinemia may occur more

often in patients with G6PD deficiency. All patients should be monitored periodically after reduction of dapsone dosage or discontinuation of treatment.
3. Toxic or cholestatic hepatitis in conjunction with a hypersensitivity syndrome. Hepatic coma is the most frequent cause of death.

Some other adverse effects of dapsone with unknown mechanisms have been recognized. Fortunately, most are rare (eg, albuminuria, insomnia, psychosis, impairment of electrolytes, atrioventricular block).[67] Some of these rarely reported adverse effects may be partially attributed to anemia and/or methaemoglobinemia.

Hypersensitivity Syndrome

A rare adverse reaction of dapsone is the hypersensitivity syndrome to dapsone, which is potentially life-threatening. The real frequency of hypersensitivity syndrome has been a continued subject of controversial speculation.[68] Until the end of October, 2009, only 343 patients with hypersensitivity syndrome, aged 5 to 83 years, were analyzed from the literature worldwide.[69] According to the results of this analysis, the most frequent dapsone dosage was 100 mg/d as monotherapy or in combination with additional drugs (eg, rifampin, clofazimine). No evidence was seen that concomitant therapy with corticosteroids avoided the risk for hypersensitivity syndrome. The median latency between dapsone initiation and first clinical complaint was 2 to 6 weeks (6 hours minimum, 20 weeks maximum).

In terms of clinical presentation of hypersensitivity syndrome to dapsone, nearly all patients had a various exanthem, fever, or lymphadenopathy. Most patients additionally showed hepatic dysfunction, varying in severity from abnormal liver function studies to overt hepato(spleno)megaly, jaundice, and finally hepatic coma. Hematologic changes were unexpectedly rare (leukocytosis, 23,6%; eosinophilia, 24,8%). After withdrawal of dapsone, and in some cases therapy with glucocorticosteroids, most patients recovered, whereas approximately 10.2% had a fatal outcome. Hepatic coma was the most frequent cause of death. Early discontinuation of dapsone therapy improves the prognosis of hypersensitivity syndrome. It seems likely that

1. The hypersensitivity syndrome to dapsone clearly is a dose-independent drug reaction.
2. Within the first 5 months of dapsone therapy, a relative risk for development of hypersensitivity syndrome is present. Consequently during this period, frequent clinical and laboratory evaluations are most important. Nonetheless, no reliable way exists to predict the risk for dapsone hypersensitivity.
3. If clinically suspected, a prompt discontinuation of dapsone therapy seems to be the best way to improve prognosis.

Considering the widespread use of dapsone and the paucity of reports, the hypersensitivity syndrome to dapsone must be considered an extremely rare side effect.

SUMMARY

Although the mechanism of action of dapsone and its metabolites is not precisely known, the sulfone is useful in two groups of entities: infections and chronic inflammatory diseases. Especially in dermatology, dapsone is considered the preferred drug for treating select inflammatory disorders. Moreover, dapsone is useful in several neutrophilic, eosinophilic, or autoimmune dermatoses. Dapsone retains its place in the therapeutic armamentarium as a unique and essential agent.

REFERENCES

1. Doull JA. Sulfone therapy of leprosy. Background, early history and present status. Int J Lepr 1963; 31:143–60.
2. Fromm E, Wittmann J. Derivate des p-nitrophenols. Berichte Deutsch Chem Ges 1908;41:2264–73.
3. Buttle GAH, Stephenson D, Smith S, et al. The treatment of streptococcal infections in mice with 4:4′diaminodiphenylsulfone. Lancet 1937;1:1331–4.
4. Fourneau E, Trèfouel J, Nitti F, et al. Action anti-streptococcique des derives sulfures organiques. C R Acad Sci 1937;204:1763–6.
5. Boyer H, Nitti F, Tréfouel J. Note preliminaire sur l' action de la paradiacetyl-aminodiphenyl sulfone (1399F) dans la blennorrhagic. Bull Soc Fr Dermatol Syphiligr 1889;1937:44.
6. Palazzoli M, Bovet D. Action de la di(paracetylaminophenyl)sulfone (1399F) dans les urétrites gonococciques aiguës et chroniques. Bull Soc Fr Dermatol Syphiligr 1900;1937:44.
7. Faget GH, Pogge RC, Johansen FA, et al. The promin treatment of leprosy. Public Health Rep 1943;58: 1729–41.
8. Esteves J, Brandão FN. Acerca da acção das sulfamidas e das sulfonas na doença de Duhring. Trab Soc Portuguesa Dermatol Venereol 1950;8:209–17.
9. Sneddon IB, Wilkinson DS. Subcorneal pustular dermatosis. Br J Dermatol 1956;68:385–94.
10. Wozel G, editor. Dapson—Pharmakologie, Wirkmechanismus und klinischer Einsatz. Stuttgart (Germany): Georg Thieme Verlag; 1996. New York.

11. Ahmad RA, Rogers HJ. Pharmacokinetics and protein-binding of dapsone and pyrimethamine. Br J Clin Pharmacol 1980;10:519–24.
12. Zuidema J, Hilbers-Modderman ESM, Merkus FWHM. Clinical pharmacokinetics of dapsone. Clin Pharmacokinet 1986;11:299–315.
13. Mc Evoy GK, editor. AHFS drug information. Bethesda (MD): American Society of Health-System Pharmacists; 2009. p. 605–9.
14. Uetrecht J, Zahid N, Shear NH, et al. Metabolism of dapsone to a hydroxylamine by human neutrophils and mononuclear cells. J Pharmacol Exp Ther 1988;245:274–9.
15. Branski D, Kerem E, Gross-Kieselstein E, et al. Bloody diarrhea—a possible complication of sulfasalazine transferred through human breast milk. J Pediatr Gastroenterol Nutr 1986;5:316–7.
16. Sanders SW, Zone JJ, Foltz RL, et al. Hemolytic anemia induced by dapsone transmitted through breast milk. Ann Intern Med 1982;96:465–6.
17. Wolf R, Tüzün B, Tüzün Y. Dapsone: unapproved uses or indications. Clin Dermatol 2000;18:37–53.
18. Zhu YI, Stiller MJ. Dapsone and sulfones in dermatology: overview and update. J Am Acad Dermatol 2001;45:420–34.
19. Wozel G, Barth J. Current aspects of modes of action of dapsone. Int J Dermatol 1988;27:547–52.
20. Niwa Y, Sakane T, Miyachi Y. Dissociation of the inhibitory effect of dapsone on the generation of oxygen intermediate—in comparison with that of colchicine and various scavengers. Biochem Pharmacol 1984;33:2344–60.
21. Stendahl O, Molin L, Dahlgren C. The inhibition of polymorphonuclear leukocyte cytotoxicity by dapsone. J Clin Invest 1978;62:214–40.
22. Niwa Y, Sakane T, Shingu M, et al. Neutrophil-generated active oxygens in linear IgA bullous dermatosis. Arch Dermatol 1985;121:73–8.
23. Miyachi Y, Niwa Y. Effects of potassium iodide, colchicine and dapsone on the generation of polymorphonuclear leukocyte-derived oxygen intermediates. Br J Dermatol 1982;107:209–14.
24. Booth SA, Moody CE, Dahl MV, et al. Dapsone suppresses integrin-mediated neutrophil adherence function. J Invest Dermatol 1992;98:135–40.
25. Wozel G, Lehmann B. Dapsone inhibits the generation of 5-lipoxygenase products in human polymorphonuclear leukocytes. Skin Pharmacol 1995;8:196–202.
26. Ruzicka TH, Wassermann SI, Soter NA, et al. Inhibition of rat mast cell arachidonic acid cyclooxygenase by dapsone. J Allergy Clin Immunol 1983;72:365–70.
27. Lehmann B, Wozel G. Inhibition of the prostaglandin endoperoxide H synthases-1 and -2 mediated by TBX2 production by dapsone in human whole blood stimulated ex vivo [abstract]. Presented at: 16th European Workshop on Inflammation. Leipzig, Germany, December 5–8, 1996.
28. Debol SM, Herron MJ, Nelson RD. Anti-inflammatory action of dapsone: inhibition of neutrophil adherence is associated with inhibition of chemoattractant-induced signal transduction. J Leukoc Biol 1997;62:827–36.
29. Theron A, Anderson R. Investigation of the protective effects of the antioxidants ascorbate, cysteine, and dapsone on the phagocyte-mediated oxidative inactivation of human alpha-1-protease inhibitor in vitro. Am Rev Respir Dis 1985;132:1049–54.
30. Bonney RJ, Wightman PD, Dahlgren ME, et al. Inhibition of the release of prostaglandins, leukotrienes and lysosomal acid hydrolases from macrophages by selective inhibitors of lecithin biosynthesis. Biochem Pharmacol 1983;32:361–6.
31. Maloff BL, Fox D, Bruin E, et al. Dapsone inhibits LTB_4 binding and bioresponse at the cellular and physiologic level. Eur J Pharmacol 1988;158:85–9.
32. Blasum CH. Untersuchungen zur Beeinflussung der Interleukin-8-Produnktion in LPS-stimuliertem Vollblut durch dermatlogisch relevante Radikalfänger [thesis]. Dresden, Germany: Department of Dermatology, University Hospital Carl Gustav Carus Dresden; 1996.
33. Beiguelman B, Pisani CB. Effect of DDS on phytohemagglutinin-induced lymphocyte transformation. Int J Lepr Other Mycobact Dis 1974;42:412–5.
34. Hamada K, Hiyoshi T, Kobayashi S, et al. Anticonvulsive effect of dapsone (4,4′-diaminodiphenyl sulfone) on amygdale-kindled seizures in rats and cats. Epilepsy Res 1991;10:93–102.
35. Ishida S, Hamada K, Yagi K. Comparing the anticonvulsive effects of dapsone on amygdale-kindled seizures and hippocampal-kindled seizures in rats. Acta Neurol Scand 1992;85:132–5.
36. Altagracia M, Monroy-Noyola A, Osorio-Rico L, et al. Dapsone attenuates kainic acid-induced seizures in rats. Neurosci Lett 1994;176:52–4.
37. Blasum CH, Lehmann B, Blümlein K, et al. The dapsone metabolite dapsone hydroxylamine is a highly effective anti-inflammatory agent in experimental models of inflammation. Arch Dermatol Res 1998;290:P34.
38. Wozel G, Blasum C, Winter C, et al. Dapsone hydroxylamine inhibits the LTB_4-induced chemotaxis of polymorphonuclear leukocytes into human skin: results of a pilot study. Inflamm Res 1997;46:420–2.
39. Aschoff R, Wozel G. In vivo modulation of UV-induced erythema by topical dapsone and dapsone metabolites. Skin Pharmacol Appl Skin Physiol 2000;13:219.
40. Wozel G, Blümlein K, Blasum C, et al. Comments to 'preventive effect of dapsone on renal scarring following mannose-sensitive piliated bacterial

infection' by Mochida, et al. (Chemotherapy 1998;44:36–41). Chemotherapy 1999;45:233–4.
41. Schumacher K. Humane in-vivo-Untersuchungen zur antientzündlichen Wirksamkeit von Diaminodiphenylsulfon (Dapson) [thesis]. Dresden, Germany: Department of Dermatology, University Hospital Carl Gustav Carus Dresden; 1996.
42. Wozel G, Köstler E, Barth J. Ergebnisse von Therapiestudien mit antientzündlichen Substanzen unter Okklusivbedingungen bei Psoriasis. Dermatol Monatsschr 1988;174:421–3.
43. Harvath L, Yancey KB, Katz St. I. Selective inhibition of human neutrophil chemotaxis to N-formylmethionyl-leucyl-phenylalanine by sulfones. J Immunol 1986;137:1305–11.
44. Pfeiffer CH, Wozel G. Comments to 'dapsone and sulfones in dermatology: overview and update'. J Am Acad Dermatol 2003;48:308–9.
45. Cohen DM, BenAmitai D, Feinmesser M, et al. Childhood lichen planus pemphigoides: a case report and review of the literature. Pediatr Dermatol 2009; 26:569–74.
46. Fredenberg MF, Malkinson FD. Sulfone therapy in the treatment of leukocytoclastic vasculitis. J Am Acad Dermatol 1987;16:772–8.
47. Kardos M, Levine D, Gürcan HM, et al. Pemphigus vulgaris in pregnancy: analysis of current data on the management and outcomes. Obstet Gynecol Surv 2009;64:739–49.
48. Nestle FO, Kaplan DH, Barker J. Mechanisms of disease: psoriasis. N Engl J Med 2009;361:496–509.
49. Draelos ZD, Carter E, Maloney JM, et al. Two randomized studies demonstrate the efficacy and safety of dapsone gel, 5% for the treatment of acne vulgaris. J Am Acad Dermatol 2007;56:439 e1–10.
50. Esterly NB, Furey NL, Flanagan LE. The effect of antimicrobial agents on leukocyte chemotaxis. J Invest Dermatol 1978;70:51–5.
51. Millar BW, Macdonald KJS, Macleod TM, et al. Dapsone and human polymorphonuclear leukocyte chemotaxis in dermatitis herpetiformis. Acta Derm Venereol 1984;64:433–6.
52. Esca SA, Pehamberger H, Silny W, et al. Polymorphonuclear leukocyte chemotaxis in dermatitis herpetiformis. Acta Derm Venereol 1981;61:61–3.
53. Anderson R, Gatner EMS, Van Rensburg CE, et al. In vitro and in vivo effects of dapsone on neutrophil and lymphocyte functions in normal individuals and patients with lepromatous leprosy. Antimicrob Agents Chemother 1981;19:495–503.
54. Jones RR. Effect of roaccutane and dapsone on leucotriene B4-induced microabscess formation in vivo. J Invest Dermatol 1985;84:446.
55. Ruzicka TH, Bauer A, Glück S, et al. Effect of dapsone on passive Arthus reaction and chemotaxis and phagocytosis of polymorphonuclear leukocytes. Arch Dermatol Forsch 1981;270:347–51.
56. Bundino S, Zina AM, Ubertalli S. Infantile acropustulosis. Dermatologica 1982;165:615–9.
57. Mirochnick M, Cooper E, McIntosh K, et al. Pharmacokinetics of dapsone administered daily and weekly in human immunodeficiency virus-infected children. Antimicrob Agents Chemother 1999;43: 2586–91.
58. Wozel G. The story of sulfones in tropical medicine and dermatology. Int J Dermatol 1989;28:17–21.
59. Frayling IM, Addison GM, Chattergee K, et al. Methaemoglobinaemia in children treated with prilocaine-lignocaine cream. Br Med J 1990;301:153–4.
60. Grunwald MH, Amichai B. Dapsone—the treatment of infectious and inflammatory diseases in dermatology. Int J Antimicrob Agents 1996;7: 187–92.
61. Coleman MD. Dapsone toxicity: some current perspectives. Gen Pharmacol 1995;26:1461–7.
62. Rhodes LE, Tingle MD, Park BK, et al. Cimetidine improves the therapeutic/toxic ratio of dapsone in patients on chronic dapsone therapy. Br J Dermatol 1995;132:257–62.
63. Miyagawa S, Shiomi Y, Fukumoto T, et al. Recombinant granulocyte colony-stimulating factor for dapsone-induced agranulocytosis in leukocytoclastic vasculitis. J Am Acad Dermatol 1993;28:659–61.
64. Stöckel S, Meurer M, Wozel G. Dapsone-induced photodermatitis in a patient with linear IgA dermatosis. Eur J Dermatol 2001;11:50–3.
65. Homeida M, Babikr A, Daneshmend TK. Dapsone-induced optic atrophy and motor neuropathy. Br Med J 1980;281:1180.
66. Kenner DJ, Holt K, Agnello R, et al. Permanent retinal damage following massive dapsone overdose. Br J Ophthalmol 1980;64:741–4.
67. Zhu KJ, Het FT, Jin N, et al. Complete atrioventricular block associated with dapsone therapy: a rare complication of dapsone-induced hypersensitivity syndrome. J Clin Pharm Ther 2009;34:489–92.
68. Wozel G, Göbel K. Hypersensitivity syndrome to dapsone—an epidemiological review. In: Ring J, Weidinger S, Darsow U, editors. Skin and environment—perception and protection. 10th EADV Congress, Munich, 2001. Bologna (Italy): Medimond Inc; 2001. p. 105–10.
69. Lorenz M, Wozel G. Hypersensitivity syndrome to dapsone: an epidemiological review and re-evaluation. Basic Clin Pharmacol Toxicol 2009;104: 508–9.

Innovative Use of Spironolactone as an Antiandrogen in the Treatment of Female Pattern Hair Loss

Deepani Rathnayake, MD[a], Rodney Sinclair, MBBS, MD[a,b,c,*]

KEYWORDS

• Female pattern hair loss • Androgenetic alopecia
• Antiandrogen therapy • Spironolactone

Female pattern hair loss (FPHL) is the most common cause of diffuse hair loss in women.[1–3] Ludwig described the hair loss pattern in 1977 and stated it to be the female equivalent of male baldness.[1] It also is referred to as female androgenetic alopecia. Although considerable histologic similarities exist between male pattern hair loss (MPHL) and FPHL, the age of onset, rate of progression, and response to therapy in females differ from that of males.[4]

A population survey performed in 2001 indicated that the age-adjusted prevalence of FPHL among Australian women of European descent aged 20 and over is 32.2% (95% confidence interval [CI], 28.8% to 35.6%). Among these women, 10.5% (95% CI, 8.2% to 12.7%) or approximately 800,000 Australian women were assessed as having moderate-to-severe FPHL as defined by stage 3, 4, or 5 on the clinical grading scale shown in **Fig. 1**. The prevalence of FPHL increases with advancing age, from approximately 12% among women aged between 20 and 29 years to over 50% of women over the age of 80.[5–7]

The impact of FPHL is predominately psychological. When compared with control women, FPHL has a significant detrimental effect on self-esteem, psychological well-being and body image[8] that is consistent across different cultures.[9–12] Affected women report a poorer health-related quality of life (QOL) than nonaffected women.[13]

Topical minoxidil is the only US Food and Drug Administration (FDA)-approved treatment for FPHL. Globally, the antiandrogens cyproterone acetate, spironolactone, and flutamide are widely used for treating FPHL. Prolonged continuous use is required for sustained effect. Poor donor hair density over the occipital scalp precludes many women from hair transplantation. Nonpharmacologic methods such as hair coloring, permanent waves, careful hair styling, and camouflage powders and creams also can provide temporary benefit.

ETIOLOGY OF FPHL

The hair loss progresses in a highly reproducible pattern. Exposure of genetically susceptible hair follicles to androgen leads to several changes including hair follicle miniaturization and changes

[a] Department of Dermatology, St Vincent's Hospital Melbourne, Post Office Box 2900, Fitzroy, Melbourne, Victoria 3065, Australia
[b] Department of Medicine, University of Melbourne, Victoria, Australia
[c] Skin and Cancer Foundation, Drummond Street Carlton, Victoria, Australia
* Corresponding author. Department of Dermatology, St Vincent's Hospital Melbourne, Post Office Box 2900, Fitzroy, Melbourne, Victoria 3065, Australia.
E-mail address: Rod.SINCLAIR@svhm.org.au

Dermatol Clin 28 (2010) 611–618
doi:10.1016/j.det.2010.03.011
0733-8635/10/$ – see front matter © 2010 Elsevier Inc. All rights reserved.

derm.theclinics.com

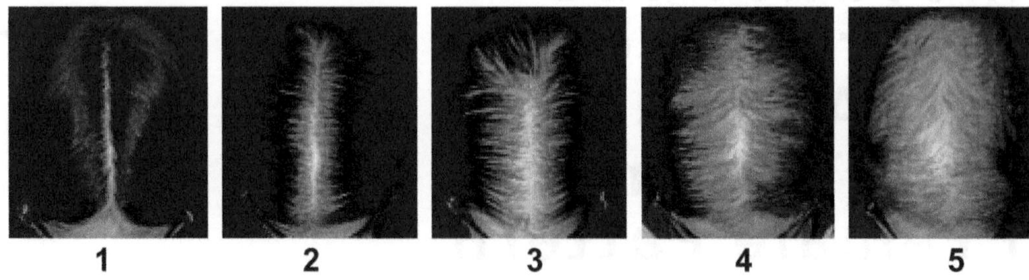

Fig. 1. Five-stage scale in FPHL.

in hair cycle dynamics with shortening of anagen duration and prolongation of telogen duration.

Genetics and Androgenetic Alopecia

Twin studies have confirmed the strong genetic predisposition to male pattern baldness.[14] Androgenetic alopecia (AGA) is complex polygenic condition. The first gene associated with AGA was the androgen receptor gene on the X chromosome[15]; however, this does not explain the high frequency of balding fathers among affected men.[16] Balding risk increases with the number of affected family members. There is racial variation in the age-related prevalence of balding, with Asian men having a lower prevalence than European men.

The cytochrome p 450 alpha aromatase enzyme also has been found to contribute to AGA in females.[17] Aromatase is a key enzyme in estrogen biosynthesis. Aromatase catalyzes the conversion of testosterone to estradiol, androstenedione to estrone, and 16- hydroxylated dehydroepiandrosterone to estriol. and thereby diminishes the amount of intrafollicular testosterone available for conversion to dihydrotestosterone (DHT). Young women have higher levels of aromatase compared with the male scalp and much higher levels in the frontal hair line.[18] This may explain the less severe baldness and relative sparing of the frontal hair line in FPHL.

Androgens and AGA

The role of androgen in MPHL was established by the anatomist James Hamilton, who observed that castrated males did not develop AGA unless treated with testosterone.[19] Testosterone is the main circulating androgen, and the tissue effects of androgens are mediated by biding to the intracellular androgen receptor.[20] In androgen insensitivity syndrome, caused by a mutation in the androgen receptor gene, there is neither baldness nor development of the beard, or axillary and pubic hair, despite the presence of normal circulating androgens.[21]

In most body sites, secondary sexual hair growth is mediated by DHT. The androgen receptor has a several fold higher sensitivity to DHT than its precursor testosterone. Conversion of testosterone to DHT is catalyzed by the enzyme 5 alpha reductase. There are two isoforms of the enzyme (types 1 and 2). Although both are capable of producing DHT from testosterone, they have distinct tissue-specific expression patterns.[22] High concentrations of 5 alpha reductase type 2 are observed in the dermal papillae and androgen dependant sites. Low levels of 5 alpha reductase are seen in the occipital hair, which shows little or no response to androgen.[18] This may explain in part the site-specific behavior within the hair follicle in different body sites.[23,24]

Itami proposed that the second messenger system determines whether androgen-sensitive follicles will respond to androgens by miniaturization rather than enhancement. Androgen stimulation of cultured beard dermal papilla cells (DPC) lead to increased transcription of insulin-like growth factor-1 and enhanced growth of cocultured keratinocytes. Androgen stimulation of DPC derived from a balding scalp leads to suppression of growth of cocultured keratinocytes. This growth suppression of keratinocytes was mediated by transforming growth factor-beta1 (TGF-beta1) derived from DPC of AGA, suggesting that TGF-beta1 is a paracrine mediator for AGA expressed.[25]

The important role of 5 alpha reductase activity in AGA is supported by absent temporal regression and baldness in men with 5 alpha reductase deficiency caused by mutation in 5 alpha reductase gene,[26] and the proven role of the 5 alpha reductase inhibitors finasteride and dutasteride in treating men with AGA.[27]

Although patterned hair loss and hirsutism are seen in women with hyperandrogenism, most women with FPHL have androgen levels within the normal range.[28] Sawaya and Price[18] reported that the concentration of androgen receptors in women is 40% less compared with men, and also women have low concentrations of 5 alpha reductase levels. A single case report of clinically and histologically proven FPHL in a woman with hypopituitarism and undetectable androgens raises the possibility that this pattern of hair loss also can be induced by events independent of androgens.[29]

Pathophysiology of FPHL

In a normal individual, the hair follicle undergoes a repetitive sequence of growth and rest known as the hair cycle (shown in **Fig. 2**). The period of active hair growth (anagen) determines the final length of hair. At the end of anagen, the hair follicle involutes during the course of a 2-week phase known as catagen. Catagen is followed by telogen, during which time the proximal part of the hair shaft is keratinized to form a club-shaped structure. Telogen lasts approximately 3 months, during which time the club hair lies just below the insertion of arrector pili muscle. Club hair is shed actively in the exogen phase, which usually occurs before the commencement of the next hair cycle with the onset of anagen phase growth.[30]

In FPHL, the duration of anagen decreases with each successive cycle, while the duration of telogen remains constant. This leads to progressive shortening of the terminal hairs. Concurrently, the entire size of the hair follicles decreases, leading to a progressive reduction in fiber diameter. Both processes combine to replace long terminal hairs with short fine vellus hairs (**Fig. 3**). The histologic hallmark of the AGA in both men and women is an increase in the ratio of miniaturized hair follicles; this is appreciated best on horizontally sectioned scalp biopsy.

The histologic decline in mean total follicle count, the reduction in terminal follicle counts, the increase in absolute number of vellus follicles, and terminal/vellus ratio all correlate with clinical severity of FPHL as graded using a five-point scale.[31]

Scalp follicles exist as compound follicles, with a single arrector pili muscle with two or three terminal hairs exiting from a single pore. Histologically this correlates with follicular units (FUs). In FPHL, mean numbers of FUs remain constant, but the mean number of terminal hairs per FU decreases while there is a corresponding increase in the mean number of vellus hairs per FU. This suggests a hierarchy of susceptibility within FUs to AGA. Complete miniaturization of all hairs within the FU is uncommon in women[32] explaining why, unlike men, women rarely progress to complete baldness.

Clinical Features and Diagnosis

The main clinical feature in both men and women is the patterned hair loss over the crown. Women can present early with recurring episodes of increased hair shedding and reduction in the volume of the pony tail, or later with thinning of hair over the crown.[4] Widening of the central part is used to assess the severity of the hair loss.[33] Ludwig first introduced clinical grading of FPHL.[1] He described three stages of severity that range from rarefaction of the hair on the crown (stage 1) to near total baldness (stage 3). One of the authors (RDS) later described a scale with five stages, which the authors have found to be more helpful in assessing the progression of the disease and the treatment response[34] (see **Fig. 1**). Although most women maintain their frontal hair line, about 13% of premenopausal women and

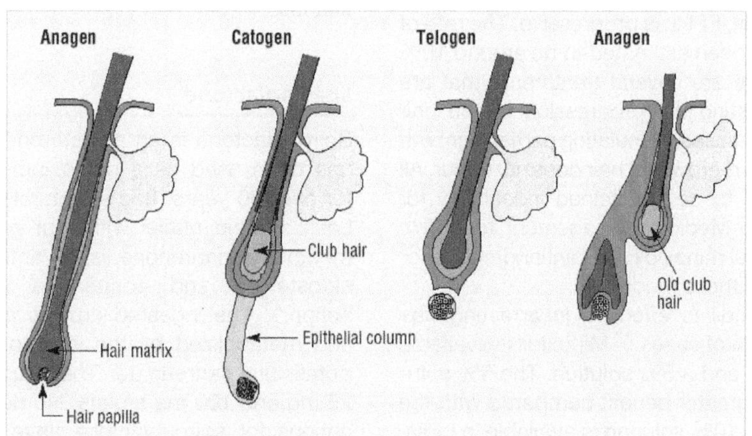

Fig. 2. Normal hair cycle. Each telogen hair is replaced by a new anagen hair.

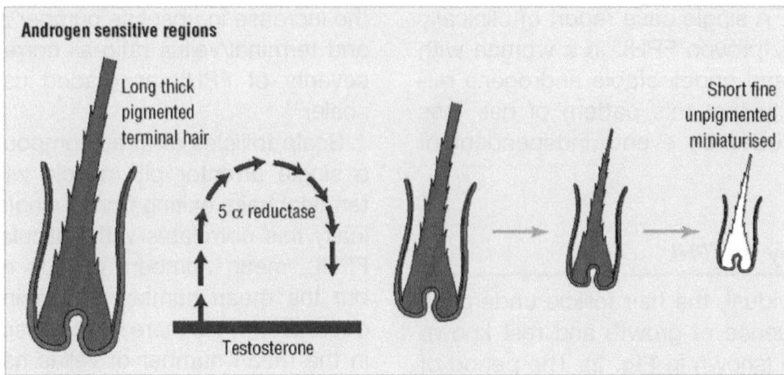

Fig. 3. Stepwise miniaturization of the hair follicle and shortening of the anagen growth phase, mediated by dihydrotestosterone.

37% of postmenopausal women show bitemporal recession.[35]

The diagnosis of FPHL is largely clinical. Reduction in hair density over the crown and widening of the central part enable a confidant clinical diagnosis. Scalp biopsy is helpful for women who present early with increased hair shedding, reduction in the ponytail volume but no obvious widening of the central part line. Horizontal sectioning is more informative and allows calculation of the vellus hairs to terminal hair ratio. Women with associated hirsutism, acne, menstrual irregularities, or other evidence of virilization should be evaluated for polycystic ovary syndrome or other causes of hyperandrogenism.

Chronic telogen effluvium is an important differential diagnosis for women who present with increased hair shedding, reduction in the ponytail volume but no obvious widening of the central part-line. Miniaturization is not seen on scalp biopsy. This condition tends not to progress to baldness nor respond to oral antiandrogens.

Treatment

Without treatment, FPHL is progressive. The rate of progression has been estimated to be around 10% per year.[36] There are several treatments that are effective in arresting the progression of the hair loss and, in some cases, stimulating partial regrowth of hair. Complete regrowth of hair does not occur. All treatments need to be maintained indefinitely for sustained effect. Medical management for FPHL consists of topical minoxidil, oral antiandrogens, or a combination of these modalities.

Topical minoxidil is effective in arresting hair loss in about 60% of cases.[37] Minoxidil is available in a 2% solution and a 5% solution. The 5% solution has shown greater benefit compared with the 2% solution.[38] A 10% solution is available in India. Minoxidil is a piperidinopyrimidine derivative and a vasodilator and has been used as an oral antihypertensive agent. Minoxidil is thought to act by initiating telogen-to-anagen transition and prolonging anagen duration.[39] Minoxidil is thought to act directly on potassium channel K (ATP) in the follicular dermal papilla.

Oral antiandrogens such as cyproterone acetate (CPA), flutamide, and spironolactone have been available for many years. All are FDA category D drugs, and thus contraindicated in pregnancy. CPA is used in Europe, South America, Asia, Australia, and Canada but is not FDA-approved for use in the United States. Use of Flutamide is limited by its potential severe liver toxicity. The 5 alpha reductase inhibitor finasteride is contraindicated in premenopausal women because of the risk of teratogenesis. A 12-month, randomized, double-blinded placebo-controlled study of postmenopausal women with FPHL failed to demonstrate superiority of finasteride over placebo.[40] Dutasteride, a combined 5 alpha reductase types 1 and 2 inhibitor, has not been systematically tested in women with FPHL, even though beneficial effects have been reported in isolated case studies.[41]

Spironolactone

Spironolactone is an aldosterone antagonist and has been used as a potassium-sparing diuretic for over 50 years. It is structurally a steroid, with basic steroid nuclei with four rings. Its primary metabolite, canrenone, is the active antagonist of aldosterone and contributes to the diuretic action.[42] The ingested drug is absorbed rapidly and metabolized by the liver to canrenone and potassium canrenoate. The drug is available in 25 mg and 100 mg tablets. No dermatologic indications for spironolactone have been approved by the FDA.

Mechanism of Action of Spironolactone in Treatment of FPHL

Spironolactone is an antiandrogen. It acts by decreasing the production and blocking the effect of androgens in the target tissue.[43] Spironolactone decreases testosterone production in the adrenal gland by depleting microsomal cytochrome p450 and by affecting the cytochrome p450-dependant enzyme 17a-hydroxylase and desmolase. The action of spironolactone is limited to tissues with a high microsomal 17a-hydroxylase activity and thereby decreasing steroid 17–hydroxylation. Spironolactone also is a competitive inhibitor of the androgen receptor and thereby blocks the androgen action on the target tissues.

Uses of Spironolactone in Dermatology

Antiandrogenic properties of spironolactone have been exploited for over 30 years in treating hirsutism, acne, and seborrhea. The benefit of spironolactone in hirsutism was discovered when a female with polycystic ovary syndrome was being treated for concurrent hypertension. The patient had noticed improvement in her hirsutism after 3 months of spironolactone therapy.[44] Several studies have shown the clinical efficacy of spironolactone in hirsutism associated with polycystic ovary syndrome (PCOS).[45,46] When compared, the efficacy of CPA 50 mg/d and ethynylestradiol 35 μg/d with spironolactone 200 mg for idiopathic hirsutism and PCOS, idiopathic hirsutism responded equally while the latter showed better results with CPA-ethynylestradiol combination. Spironolactone has shown superior efficacy when compared with finasteride in treating hirsutism.[47]

Spironolactone also has shown efficacy and long-term safety in treating acne,[48,49] and it is effective in treating seborrhea. Conflicting results were recorded after using topical spironolactone for seborrhea. Topical 5% spironolactone solution is reported to inhibit dihydrotestosterone receptors in human sebaceous glands. On the other hand, small case studies have failed to demonstrate the effect of topical spironolactone in reducing sebum excretion.[50] Further studies are necessary to determine the antiandrogenic properties of topical spironolactone and the possibility of using it for FPHL.

Spironolactone is the most widely used, albeit off-label, antiandrogen for FPHL in the United States. In Australia, spironolactone has been used for FPHL for more than 20 years, especially in premenopausal women. The standard dose used is 100 to 200 mg daily.[51,52] Lower doses of 50 to 75 mg also have been shown to stabilize hair loss in some women; however, daily doses in excess of 150 mg have been shown to work better.[53]

Sinclair and colleagues investigated 80 women with biopsy-proven FPHL. Forty women received spironolactone 200 mg daily, and 40 received cyproterone acetate. Premenopausal women received cyproterone acetate 100 mg daily for the first 10 days of each menstrual cycle for 12 months in combination with an oral contraceptive pill. Postmenopausal women received 50 mg daily of cyproterone acetate continuously. Women were followed with serial scalp global photography under standardized conditions. At the end of 12 months, thirty-five (44%) women had clearly visible hair regrowth; 35 (44%) had no change in hair density, and 10 (12%) had reduced hair density at the end of the study, indicating continuing hair loss during the treatment period. There was no significant difference between the two drugs.[52] Most of the women in this study did not have clinical or biochemical evidence of hyperandrogenism. Several other small case studies have shown the beneficial effect of spironolactone in AGA.[54] Additive effects of combination of spironolactone and 5% minoxidil have been noted.[55]

Adverse effects of spironolactone are dose-dependant. Hyperkalemia, although rare in the presence of normal renal function, is a potential adverse effect. Regular monitoring of serum potassium and blood pressure is recommended. Concurrent use of drugs that increase serum potassium should be avoided. Menstrual irregularity, tiredness, and breast tenderness are common, albeit usually mild and rarely necessitating cessation of the medication. As it can feminize the male fetus, spironolactone should be avoided in pregnancy. Chemical hepatitis has been reported,[56] as has chloasma.[57]

Monitoring of Treatment Response

Monitoring clinical response is important for the physician and patient. The response to treatment is slow, and accurate monitoring is facilitated by good-quality photographs (**Fig. 4**). In the absence of photographs, periodic midscalp clinical grading is the most reliable measure to assess the treatment response. The midscalp clinical grading scale was developed from midscalp photographs and used to assess the severity of hair loss among women undergoing treatment for hair loss. The five-point visual analog grading scale has good interobserver reproducibility[34] and can be used for patient self-assessment.[58] Seasonal fluctuations in hair shedding make counting the

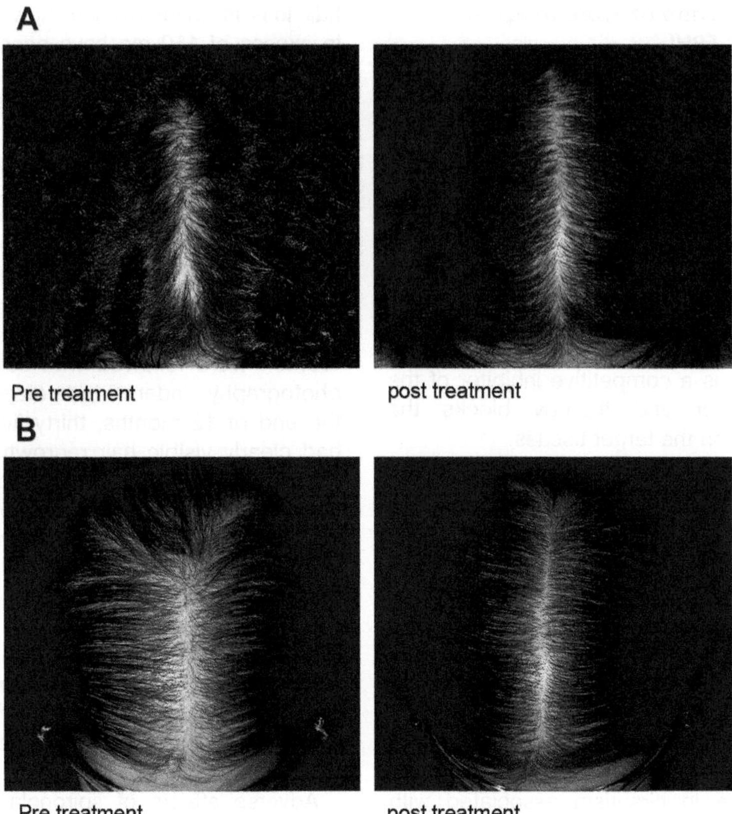

Fig. 4. Photographic evaluation of treatment response to spironolactone. (*A*) In a 34-year-old woman. (*B*) In a 15-year-old girl.

number of falling hairs an unreliable method of evaluation.

SUMMARY

Women find patterned hair loss distressing. The inconvenience of topical therapy and the slow response and the potential for adverse effects with systemic therapy deter many women from pursuing treatment, as does the need for life-long therapy. Nevertheless, most women who do embark on treatment tolerate the medications well and satisfactorily arrest further hair loss. Many also achieve a moderate degree of hair regrowth that is sustained for the duration of the treatment. Women with FPHL who present early often achieve the best regrowth.

For women with very early hair loss and no noticeable baldness, where the goal of therapy is to prevent future hair loss, spironolactone should be used a monotherapy. For women with more advanced balding where the goal of treatment is to stimulate maximal regrowth, spironolactone can and likely should be combined with topical minoxidil.

In the absence of prospective double-blind placebo-controlled trials, further work is required to establish the precise utility of spironolactone in FPHL and to determine the optimal dose.

REFERENCES

1. Ludwig E. Classification of the types of androgenetic alopecia (common baldness) occurring in the female sex. Br J Dermatol 1977;97:247–54.
2. Norwood OT. Male pattern baldness. Classification and incidence. South Med J 1975;68:1359–70.
3. Olsen EA. Female pattern hair loss. J Am Acad Dermatol 2001;45:S70–80.
4. Sinclair RD, Dawber RP. Androgenetic alopecia in men and women. Clin Dermatol 2001;19:167–78.
5. Gan DC, Sinclair RD. Prevalence of male and female pattern hair loss in Maryborough. J Investig Dermatol Symp Proc 2005;10:184–9.

6. Birch MP, Messenger JF, Messenger AG. Hair density, hair diameter and the prevalence of female pattern hair loss. Br J Dermatol 2001;144:297–304.
7. Norwood OT. Incidence of female androgenetic alopecia (female pattern alopecia). Dermatol Surg 2001;27:53–4.
8. Van der Donk J, Passschier J, Knegt-Junk C, et al. Psychological characteristics of women with androgenetic alopecia: a controlled study. Br J Dermatol 1991;125:248–52.
9. Cash TF. The psychology of hair loss and its implications for patient care. Clin Dermatol 2002;19:161–6.
10. Budd D, Himmelberger D, Rhodes T, et al. The effect of hair loss in European men: a survey of four countries. Eur J Dermatol 2000;10:122–7.
11. Lee HJ, Ha SJ, Kim D, et al. Perception of men with androgenetic alopecia by women and non bolding men. Int J Dermatol 2002;41(12):867–9.
12. Cash TF, Price VH, Savin RC. Psychological effects of androgenetic alopecia on women: comparisons with balding men and with female control subjects. J Am Acad Dermatol 1993;29(4):568–75.
13. Williamson D, Gonzalez M, Finlay AY. The effect of hair loss on quality of life. J Eur Acad Dermatol Venereol 2001;15(2):137–9.
14. Nyholt DR, Gillespie NA, Heath AC, et al. Genetic basis of male pattern baldness. J Invest Dermatol 2003;121:1561–4.
15. Ellis JA, Stebbing M, Harrap SB. Polymorphism of the androgen receptor gene is associated with male pattern baldness. J Invest Dermatol 2001; 116:452–5.
16. Kuster W, Happle R. The inheritance of common baldness. Two B or not two B? J Am Acad Dermatol 1984;11:921–6.
17. Yip L, Zaloumis S, Irwin D, et al. Gene-wide association study of the aromatase gene (CYP19A1) with female pattern hair loss. Br J Dermatol 2009; 161(2):289–94.
18. Sawaya ME, Price VH. Different levels of 5 alpha reductase type I and II, aromatase, and androgen receptor in hair follicles of women and men with androgenetic alopecia. J Invest Dermatol 1997; 109:296–300.
19. Hamilton JB. Male hormone stimulation is prerequisite and an insitant in common baldness. Am J Anat 1942;71:451–80.
20. Williams GR, Franklyn JA. Physiology of the steroid-thyroid hormone nuclear receptor superfamily. Baillieres Clin Endocrinol Metab 1974;38:811–9.
21. Patterson MN, McPhaul MJ, Hughes IA. Androgen insensitivity syndrome. Baillieres Clin Endocrinol Metab 1994;8:379–404.
22. Jenkins EP, Andersson S, Imperato McGinley J, et al. Genetic and pharmacological evidence for more than one human steroid 5-alpha-reductase. J Clin Invest 1992;89:293–300.
23. Orentreich N. Autografts in alopecias and other selected dermatological conditions. Ann N Y Acad Aci 1959;83:463–79.
24. Nordstrom RE. Synchronous balding of scalp and hair bearing grafts of scalp transplanted to the skin of the arm in male pattern baldness. Acta Derm Venereol (Stockh) 1979;59:266–8.
25. Itami S, Inui S. Role of androgen in mesenchymal epithelial interactions in human hair follicle. J Investig Dermatol Symp Proc 2005;10(3):209–11.
26. Imperato MJ. 5 alpha-reductase-2 deficiency and complete androgen insensitivity: lessons from nature. Adv Exp Med Biol 2002;511:121–31.
27. Kaufman KD, Olsen EA, Whiting D, et al. Finasteride in the treatment of men with androgenetic alopecia. J Am Acad Dermatol 1998;39:578–89.
28. Schmidt JB, Lindmaier A, Trenz A, et al. Hormone studies in females with androgenetic hair loss. Gynecol Obstet Invest 1991;31:235–9.
29. Orme S, Cullen DR, Messenger AG. Diffuse female hair loss: are androgens necessary? Br J Dermatol 1999;141(3):521–3.
30. de Berker DA, Messenger AG, Sinclair RD. Disorders of hair In: Burns T, Breathnach S, Cox N, et al, editors. Rook's textbook of dermatology, vol. 4. 7th edition. Oxford (UK): Blackwell Publishing; 2004. p. 63.8–63.10.
31. Messenger AG, Sinclair R. Follicular miniaturization in female pattern hair loss: clinicopathological correlations. Br J Dermatol 2006;155: 926–30.
32. Yazdabadi A, Magee J, Harrison S, et al. The Ludwig pattern of androgenetic alopecia is due to a hierarchy of androgen sensitivity within follicular units that leads to selective miniaturization and a reduction in the number of terminal hairs per follicular unit. Br J Dermatol 2008;159:1300–2.
33. Oslen EA. The midline part: an important physical clue to the clinical diagnosis of androgenetic alopecia in women. J Am Acad Dermatol 1999;40: 106–9.
34. Sinclair R, Jolly D, mallari R, et al. The reliability of horizontally sectioned scalp biopsies in the diagnosis of chronic diffuse telegen hair loss in women. J Am Acad Dermatol 2004;51:189–99.
35. Venning VA, Dawber RP. Patterned andrgenetic alopecia in women. J Am Acad Dermatol 1988;18: 1073–7.
36. Rushton DH, Ramsay ID, Norris MJ, et al. Natural progression of male pattern baldness in young men. Clin Exp Dermatol 1991;16:188–92.
37. De Villez RL, Jacobs JP, Szpunar CA, et al. Androgenetic alopecia in the female. Treatment with 2% topical minoxidil solusions. Arch Dermatol 1994; 130:303–7.
38. Lucky AW, Piacquadio DJ, Ditre CM, et al. A randomised placebo controlled trial of 2% and 5%

topical minoxidil solutions in the treatment of female pattern hail loss. J Am Acad Dermatol 2004;50:541–53.
39. Messenger AG, Rundegen J. Minoxidil:mechanisms of action on hair growth. Br J Dermatol 2004;150: 186–94.
40. Price VH, Roberts JL, Hordinsky M, et al. Lack of efficacy of finasteride in postmenopausal women with androgenetic alopecia. J Am Acad Dermatol 2000;43:768–76.
41. Olszewska M, Rudnicka L. Effective treatment of female androgenetic alopecia with dutasteride. J Drugs Dermatol 2005;4(5):637–40.
42. Gómez R, Núñez L, Caballero R, et al. Spironolactone and its main metabolite canrenoic acid block hKv1.5, Kv4.3 and Kv7.1+minK channels. Br J Pharmacol 2005;146(1):146–61.
43. Shaw JC. Antiandrogen therapy in dermatology. Int J Dermatol 1996;35:770–6.
44. Ober KP, Hennessy JF. Spironolactone therapy for hirsutism in a hyperandrogenetic woman. Ann Intern Med 1978;89:643–4.
45. Evans DJ, Burke CW. Spironolactone in the treatment of idiopathic hirsutism and the polycystic ovary syndrome. J R Soc Med 1986;79(8):451–3.
46. Christy NA, Franks AS, Cross LB. Spironolactone for hirsutism in polycystic ovary syndrome. Ann Pharmacother 2005;39(9):1517–21.
47. Lumachi F, Rondinone R. Use of cyproterone acetate, finesteride and spironolactone to treat idiopathic hirsutism. Fertil Steril 2003;79:942–6.
48. Shaw JC, White LE. Long term safety of spironolactone in acne: results of an 8-year follow-up study. J Cutan Med Surg 2002;6:541–5.
49. Yemisci A, Gorgulu A, Piskin S. Effects and side effects of spironolactone therapy in women with acne. J Eur Acad Dermatol Venereol 2005;19(2):163–6.
50. Waltron S, Cunliffe WJ, Lookingbill P, et al. Lack of effect of topical spironolactone on sebum excretion. Br J Dermatol 1986;114(2):261–9.
51. Shapiro J. Hair loss in women. N Engl J Med 2007; 357(16):1620–30.
52. Sinclair R, Wewerinke M, Jolley D. Treatment of female pattern hair loss with oral antiandrogens. Br J Dermatol 2005;152:466–73.
53. Rushton DH, Futterweit W, Kingsley D, et al. Quantitative assessment of spironolactone treatment in women with diffuse androgen dependant alopecia. J Soc Cosmet Chem 1991;42:317–25.
54. Yazdabadi A, Green J, Sinclair R. Successful treatment of female-pattern hair loss with spironolactone in a 9-year-old girl. Australas J Dermatol 2009;50(2):113–4.
55. Carlijn H, Sylvia AE, Sinclair R. Treatment of female pattern hair loss with a combination of spironolactone and minoxdil. Australas J Dermatol 2007;48:43–5.
56. Thai KE, Sinclair RD. Spironolactone indused hepatitis. Australas J Dermatol 2001;42:180–2.
57. Hughes BR, Cunliffe WJ. Tolerance of spironolactone. Br J Dermatol 1988;118(5):687–91.
58. Biondo S, Goble D, Sinclair R. Women who present with female pattern hair loss tend to underestimate the severity of their hair loss. Br J Dermatol 2004;150:750–2.

Innovative Therapeutics in Pediatric Dermatology

Carlo Gelmetti, MD[a,b,*], Adina Frasin, MD[c], Lucia Restano, MD[b]

KEYWORDS

- Pediatric dermatology • Infantile hemangiomas
- Propranolol • Atopic dermatitis • 5-Finger socks
- UV-A1 • Gene targeting

Despite a plethora of new drugs for sundry dermatologic disorders, the armamentarium for pediatric patients remains limited because clinical trials often exclude this age group. Nevertheless, advances in understanding the physiology and molecular biology of infantile skin are improving the therapy for some pediatric and adolescent skin conditions. Advances have been observed in the following areas: infantile hemangiomas (IHs), atopic dermatitis (AD), cutaneous infections, and autoimmune dermatoses. Present and future approaches to some genetic skin diseases are also forthcoming.

ANGIOMAS

IHs, among the most common tumors affecting children, most often arise in the first days or weeks after birth. Most IHs are benign vascular neoplasms with a self-limited course and transient cosmetic disfigurement. However, a significant minority of such lesions may cover an extensive surface (segmental hemangiomas) or may occur in sensitive and important areas (periorificial) and thus may cause major problems and require appropriate treatment.[1–5] Complex cases include broad facial IH (including PHACE [*p*osterior fossa malformations, *h*emangiomas, *a*rterial anomalies, *c*oarctation of the aorta and other cardiac defects, and *e*ye abnormalities] syndrome), periorbital and retrobulbar IH (associated with a risk of amblyopia), mandibular and central neck IH (with a potential for concomitant airway hemangiomas), and lumbosacral/perineal IH (including SACRAL [*s*pinal dysraphism, *a*nogenital, *c*utaneous, *r*enal and urologic anomalies, associated with an *a*ngioma of *l*umbosacral localization]/PELVIS [*p*erineal hemangioma, *e*xternal genitalia malformations, *l*ipomyelomeningocele, *v*esicorenal abnormalities, *i*mperforate anus, and *s*kin tag] syndrome, with potential risk for tethered spinal cord and/or genitourinary anomalies). All these should be managed in a multidisciplinary manner.

For uncomplicated IH, compression alone or in combination with other treatments (eg, glucocorticoids, laser ablation) is a well-established treatment regimen.[6] However, this plan may be limited by the ease with which the treatment is applied, especially in neonates. In fact, the traditionally used pressure garments provide adequate compression, but they need to be custom-made and are usually expensive. Moreover, they are characterized by compliance difficulties with regards to comfort, restricted movement, and unsightly appearance; use of these garments can sometimes burden parents with psychosocial distress. Thus, pressure garments are generally used for lesions likely to cause important disfigurement. Another limitation of pressure garments is that they cannot be used to treat lesions in the periorificial area and must be avoided on lesions

[a] Department of Anesthesia, Intensive Care and Dermatologic Sciences, Università degli Studi di Milano, Milan, Italy
[b] Unit of Pediatric Dermatology, Fondazione IRCCS Ca' Granda "Ospedale Maggiore Policlinico", Mangiagalli eRegina Elena, Milan, Italy
[c] Unit of Dermatology, Ospedale A. Manzoni, Lecco, Italy
* Corresponding author. Clinica Dermatologica, Via Pace 9, 20122 Milan, Italy.
E-mail address: carlo.gelmetti@unimi.it

Dermatol Clin 28 (2010) 619–629
doi:10.1016/j.det.2010.03.005
0733-8635/10/$ – see front matter © 2010 Elsevier Inc. All rights reserved.

of the head until the fontanelles have closed because of the risk of bone deformity.[7] Elastic bandages and Coban wraps (3M, St Paul, MN, USA)[6] are more practical and have been used successfully but are suitable only for lesions located on the limbs.

Self-adhesive polyurethane strips designed for the treatment of hypertrophic scars can also be used to achieve mild yet effective compression of small (<5 cm), superficial, nonulcerated IHs. These strips (Hansaplast Scar Reducer, Beiersdorf, Germany) are elastic, self-adhesive, and almost transparent and can be cut to precisely fit the lesion. The method of use consists of stretching the strip sufficiently beyond the limits of the lesion before application so as to provide adequate compression. Flattening and blanching of the IH will indicate the correct application of the strip (**Figs. 1** and **2**). After use, the strip is usually removed with ease without leaving adhesive residue. The strip can be used on almost all body parts and easily adapted to fit areas difficult to compress with elastic garments, such as the periorbital and zygomatic regions. The treatment is well tolerated except for rare, mild local irritation. Moreover, parents are often pleased to "do something" for the angioma in the child that does not involve the use of drugs. In the treatment of IH, the strip should be applied for 12 hours daily throughout the expansive phase of the lesion. Despite some obvious restrictions (IH located in diaper area, lips, eyelid, and areas without an underlying bony structure; large or deeply located lesions), in the authors' experience, the compression obtained with this technique can be useful in selected cases (Restano and Gelmetti, personal observation, 2009). Although the efficacy of this method has clear limits, its safety and ease of use make it a useful tool in the broad spectrum of treatment of IH.

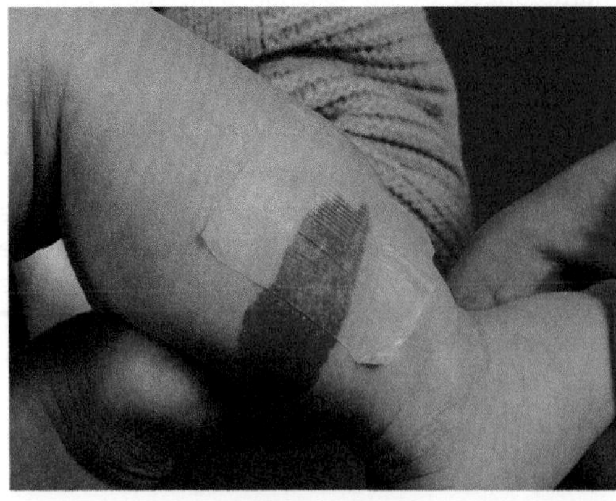

Fig. 1. An infant with IH growing on her leg. The parents did not accept a steroid treatment. Thus, a self-adhesive polyurethane strip was applied to half the lesion.

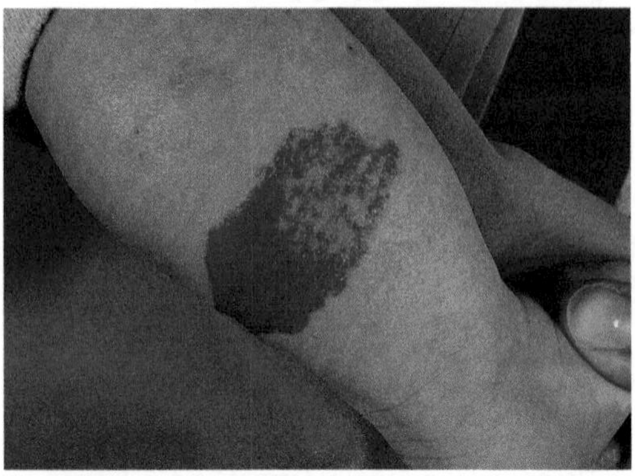

Fig. 2. The part of IH that was compressed with the polyurethane strip during nighttime appeared clear and flattened in the infant 1 month later.

IHs that develop in perioral and perineal areas have an increased potential of ulceration, which can lead to pain and scarring. According to the classic "Guidelines of care for hemangiomas of infancy" published in the *Journal of the American Academy of Dermatology*,[8] preventing or treating ulceration to reduce scarring, infection, and pain is the major goal of hemangioma management. In the last decade, laser treatment has been adopted for ulcerated IH. Pulsed dye laser (PDL) was used initially. In a review of 78 patients treated with PDL for ulcerated IH, 71 patients (91%) responded after 2 treatments with only PDL, whereas 6 patients needed concomitant oral corticosteroid.[9] Today, long-pulsed dye laser seems safer and more efficient. Currently, there are no optimal laser systems for IH treatment.[10] The benefits of vascular laser treatment are limited by the depth of light penetration because PDL can only penetrate to a depth of around 1.2 mm. For this reason, it is not effective in treating deeper components of IH, which may continue to grow even as the superficial component recedes. PDL treatment is an accepted therapy for ulcerating IH despite potential complications. In addition, PDL therapy almost always decreases pain related to ulceration and therefore remains an important element in the global management of IH.[11] Other lasers, such as Nd:YAG or KTP, can reach the deeper parts of the lesion but carry significantly greater risks of posttherapy scarring, dyspigmentation, or textural abnormalities.

With the exception of small, isolated IHs located in nonproblematic anatomic sites for which a benign neglect is considered an appropriate treatment, all the other IHs require some specific therapeutic intervention. Management is individualized, and oral corticosteroids have been considered the mainstay of therapy,[1] at least for the last 3 decades. Other treatment modalities include laser ablation,[2] surgery,[3] and administration of oral interferon[4] and vincristine.[5] All these interventions have significant risk. Recently, Leauté-Labreze and colleagues[12] described a case series of 11 infants in which IH demonstrated dramatic improvement after treatment with oral propranolol. This response was observed serendipitously during the treatment of obstructive hypertrophic myocardiopathy that followed high-dose systemic corticosteroids treatment in an infant with a large segmental IH.

Propranolol, a nonselective β-blocker, has been used for several decades to treat hypertension, ischemic heart disease, arrhythmias, endocrine and neurologic disorders, and eye disorders. At normal doses (0.5–4 mg/d), it has good tolerance and rare side effects. The latter may include bradycardia, hypotension, and hypoglycemia (especially in infants younger than 3 months). IHs are composed of a complex mixture of clonal endothelial cells associated with pericytes, dendritic cells, and mast cells. Regulators of IH growth and involution are poorly understood. During the expansion stage, when the endothelial and interstitial cells divide actively, the basic fibroblast growth factor (bFGF) and the vascular endothelial growth factor (VEGF) are involved; in contrast, during the regression stage, apoptosis is observed. Potential explanations for the therapeutic effect of propranolol on IH include vasoconstriction (which is immediately visible as a change in color and temperature associated with a palpable softening of the hemangioma in 1–3 days), decreased expression of VEGF and bFGF genes through the downregulation of the ras derived from RAt Sarcoma (RAF)–mitogen-activated protein kinase pathway (which explains progressive improvement of the hemangioma), and triggering of capillary endothelial cell apoptosis. Perhaps propranolol could also induce apoptosis by antagonizing Glut-1 receptors or act through other unknown pathways to inhibit growth of the IH.[13] Recommendations for instituting treatment with propranolol in infants differ among academic centers. The authors' protocol includes a clinical evaluation with photographs and, when possible, an ultrasonographic and thermographic examination; a routine blood panel; and a preliminary cardiology visit including electrocardiographic and echocardiographic evaluations to rule out treatment contraindications. The drug is given at a starting dose of 2 mg/kg/d, in 2 doses, for 3 to 9 months depending on the severity of the clinical condition. If the optimal dose exceeds 3 mg/kg/d, gradual tapering of propranolol for 4 weeks will be considered as soon as clinically indicated.

Although Food and Drug Administration (FDA) labeling indicates that safety and effectiveness in pediatric patients have not been established, more than 40 years of clinical experience with infants and young children does not document death or serious cardiovascular morbidity resulting directly from adrenergic receptor blockade. However, the well-known possible side effects, including bradycardia, hypotension, bronchospasm, and hypoglycemia, justify a careful monitoring, especially at the onset of treatment. In accordance with a recent article that states that side effects were limited and mild,[14] no case with significant side effect has been observed among the more than 30 patients followed up for the past several years (personal observation, 2010).

Recently, Bonifazi and colleagues[15] proved the efficacy of 1% topical propranolol in a lipid-based cream on the red, superficial component of rapidly growing IHs in 6 children. The cream was applied twice daily with a good control of the superficial component in 4 of 6 cases; the deep components of treated hemangiomas did not improve.

In conclusion, although propranolol is a "new" agent for the treatment of IH, its long-standing good reputation and its robust advantages compared with steroids (**Table 1**) are evident. The rapidity of action and the dramatic change, together with optimal tolerability, make propranolol the drug of choice (**Figs. 3** and **4**).

ATOPIC DERMATITIS

AD is a chronic inflammatory skin disease affecting up to 20% of children. The skin lesions of AD affect the facial and extensor areas of the extremities in young infants, whereas in older children and adults there is a predilection for the flexural areas of the neck, elbows, and knees. The pathogenesis of AD includes complex interaction among the genetic background, skin barrier defects, abnormalities of innate and adaptive immune functions, and environmental influences. AD acute skin lesions exhibit increased expression of interleukin (IL) 4 and IL-13, whereas chronic lesions are characterized by overexpression of interferon-γ. Recent studies have reported significantly reduced filaggrin gene expression of keratinocytes differentiated in the presence of IL-4 and IL-13, suggesting improvement of skin barrier integrity by neutralization of these cytokines.[16] Disease management implications of these observations are directed in restoring the barrier and finding a long term anti-inflammatory treatment to control exacerbations.

Table 1
Differences between corticosteroids and propranolol in IH management

	Corticosteroids	Propranolol
Activity (% of Patients)	Approximately 70%	Approximately 100%
Activity (Stage of Evolution)	Growing phase	Growing, resting, and late phase
Onset of Action	Rapid (days)	Rapid (days)
HPA Axis Inhibition	Yes	No
Growth Impairment	Yes	No
Arterial Blood Pressure	Rising	Decreasing
Blood Glucose	Rising	Decreasing?
Gastric Hyperacidity	Yes	No
Irritability	Yes	No
Insomnia	Yes	Yes
Immunodepression	Yes	No
Increased Infection	Likely	Unlikely
Precipitation of Asthma	Unlikely	Likely
Bronchospasm	?	?
Nightmares	?	?
Course	Months (intermittent)	Months (continuous)
Compliance (Caregivers)	Low	High
Cost	Low	Low

Abbreviation: HPA, hypothalamic pituitary adrenal; ?, insufficient data.

Various active cosmeceutical ingredients, such as hydroxydecine, *N*-palmitoylethanolamine, and sunflower oil oleodistillate, have been tested to restore skin barrier function and alleviate the lack of epidermal lipid synthesis. Hydroxydecine (Ictyane HD), a fatty acid derivative from royal jelly, induces the production of filaggrin and involucrine and promotes lipoprotein cohesion of the horny layer. This regenerative action is combined with an antioxidant power to protect against noxious effects of free radicals. *N*-palmitoylethanolamine (Physiogel AI and Mimyx) is a cannabinoid that works by restoring the natural components of the stratum corneum (SC) and reestablishing barrier function of the outer layers of the epidermis.[17] Sunflower oil oleodistillate (Stelatopia) contains a concentrated extract of β-sitosterol and α-tocopherol well-known for antioxidant and anti-inflammatory properties. The 2% sunflower oil oleodistillate in cream has a restorative effect by inducing epidermal lipid neosynthesis.[18] The correction of skin barrier defects can prevent flares induced by external triggers of inflammation, including allergens or infections, especially *Staphylococcus aureus*. Staphylococcal superantigens interact with the cutaneous immune system to cause inflammation with increased production of IL-4 or IL-13. In this field, the use of special silk fabrics (DermaSilk) coated with an antimicrobial substance, AEM 5772/5, has been shown to be effective in improving the severity of AD in various trials. In a randomized, double-blind study designed to compare the efficacy of AEM 5772/5–treated silk with that of a similar but nonengineered fabric, long-term improvement of eczema

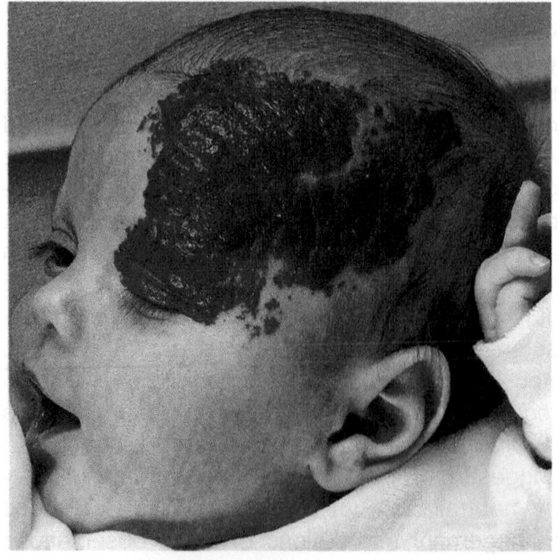

Fig. 3. An alarming, segmental IH growing on the face of a young girl despite a 1-month course on oral steroids.

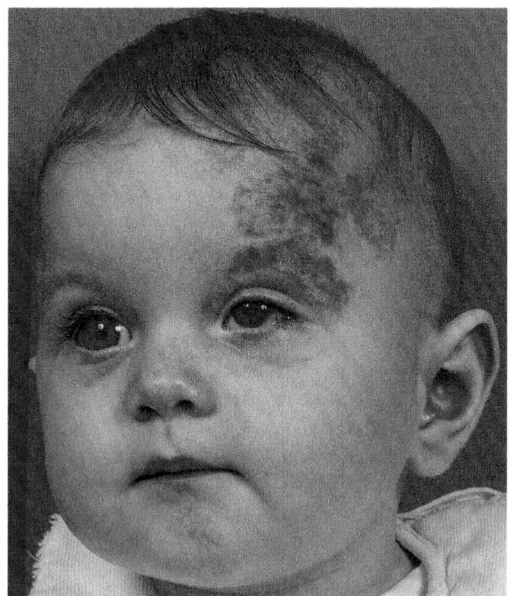

Fig. 4. The same lesion after a 6-month course of oral propranolol. The IH is completely flattened; only residual telangiectases are visible.

symptoms was greater for the AEM 5772/5–treated silk group after 28 days.[19] Moreover, a study of 15 children comparing the efficacy of the same antimicrobial silk fabric with that of a topical corticosteroid in the treatment of AD revealed no significant difference.[20] This result, if confirmed, would be of enormous importance.

Because normal-appearing skin in AD is associated with subclinical inflammation, long-term antiinflammatory therapy is essential to prevent acute flares. A proactive antiinflammatory approach was proposed as an alternative to the reactive strategy used in the traditional long-term management of AD. A randomized, multicenter study of 12 months investigated the low-dose, long-term intermittent use of 0.03% tacrolimus ointment (proactive strategy) to previously affected skin areas to prevent disease exacerbation. Tacrolimus is a topical calcineurin inhibitor (TCI) introduced to treat adult patients with moderate-to-severe AD (0.1%) and children older than 2 years (0.03%). This study demonstrated clearly that, regardless of the baseline severity of the patient's AD, twice-weekly 0.03% tacrolimus ointment application was effective in preventing, delaying, and reducing the occurrence of AD flares. The low incidence of application site pruritus and skin infection in this study was similar to those found in other clinical studies.[21]

A major concern among pediatricians is the risk of lymphoma in AD patients who receive treatment with TCIs. In a British case-control study involving a population of 3,500,194 individuals, Arellano and colleagues[22] identified an increased lymphoma risk (odds ratio, 1.83; 95% confidence interval, 1.41–2.36) in patients with AD but did not find any cases of lymphoma in TCI users. However, the study results did suggest an association between lymphoma (especially skin lymphoma) and the use of topical corticosteroids; the risk increased with duration of exposure and potency of topical corticosteroids.

Current evidence suggests that the epithelial cell–derived cytokine thymic stromal lymphopoietin (TSLP) may initiate asthma or AD through a dendritic cell–mediated T helper (T_H2) response in the absence of T lymphocytes and IgE antibodies through the innate immune system. Because TSLP can be released by skin cells in response to various stimuli (including microbes, physical injury, or inflammatory molecules), it may play a central role in "intrinsic" forms of AD and explain the vicious circle of infection and scratching in this disorder.[23] Therefore, systemic or topical application of anti-TSLP agents could inhibit the skin inflammation.[24]

It is well-known that neutralization of the physiologic acidic pH of SC can interfere with key epidermal functions, including barrier homeostasis and SC integrity. Most inflammatory dermatoses, including AD, exhibit an increased epidermal pH. Thus, it seems logical to hypothesize that acidification could influence positively the course of AD. A recent article focusing on murine AD showed that this modification induced an improvement in barrier function and a consequent antiinflammatory activity, which could be further attributed to normalization of lamellar body secretion and lamellar bilayer formation.[25]

At the same time, an important recent publication noted the benefits of a basic compound (sodium hypochlorite) in the management of AD. The group of Amy Paller investigated whether suppression of *S aureus* colonization with bleach baths and intranasal mupirocin could improve AD. The investigators concluded that the continuous use of dilute bleach baths with intermittent intranasal application of mupirocin ointment decreased the clinical severity of AD in patients with clinical signs of secondary bacterial infections.[26] Although bleach has a tendency to increase the pH, the improvement demonstrated with this regimen is undeniable. In this case, however, the concentration of bleach (0.005%) was probably too low to impair the skin barrier and further stimulate epidermal proteases; so the positive antiseptic effect superseded any negative effect of a higher pH in the skin.

Because it has been shown that defects in the innate immune system are present in AD, a possible strategy of treatment could be to increase the production of antimicrobial peptides. The discovery that active vitamin D (1,25-dihydroxyvitamin D) can induce the production of cathelicidin has led some investigators to pursue this option. A recent controlled study of 14 normal controls and 14 subjects with moderate-to-severe AD, in which oral vitamin D3 at 4000 IU/d was administered for 3 weeks, has suggested that supplementation with oral vitamin D can dramatically induce cathelicidin production in AD lesional skin and may also induce production in normal skin.[27] This is particularly interesting because a published report noted that topical application of active vitamin D3 can trigger a mouse AD-like syndrome, characterized by a red, scaly, and deteriorated skin, accompanied by an epidermal hyperplasia and a dermal infiltration of $CD4^+$ lymphocytes, eosinophils, dendritic cells, and mast cells and an increase of T_H2 cytokine level in skin along with an elevated level of serum IgE and blood eosinophilia.[28] Therefore, larger studies examining the benefits and risks of vitamin D supplementation will be necessary in future to see if this increase in cathelicidin is adequate for the prevention of infections and outweighs the potential side effects of this substance.

PSORIASIS

Psoriasis is a complex systemic immune inflammatory disease, most frequently diagnosed between ages 15 and 25 years; it can, however, appear at any time and may affect children of all ages, including infants. Although a host of newer biologic drugs are now available, some of them may be inappropriate for children because of possible long-term or delayed adverse effects. Although systemic medications for children and teenagers are not usually prescribed, in the face of severe psoriasis, systemic treatment may be indicated. Methotrexate, acitretin, and cyclosporine are some drugs that may be prescribed. Advances in understanding the immunopathogenesis of psoriasis have been recently translated into highly effective biologic therapies.

Etanercept (Enbrel), a tumor necrosis factor (TNF) receptor fusion protein approved for the treatment of juvenile rheumatoid arthritis, demonstrated safety and efficacy in children and adolescents with moderate-to-severe plaque psoriasis.[29] Recently, 211 patients with psoriasis (4–17 years of age) were initially randomly assigned in a double-blind trial of 12 once-weekly subcutaneous injections of placebo or 0.8 mg/kg of etanercept (to a maximum of 50 mg), followed by 24 weeks of once-weekly open-label etanercept. This multicenter, phase 3, randomized study demonstrated statistically significant and clinically meaningful reductions in disease severity as early as week 2 in the etanercept-treated group. After withdrawal of etanercept therapy, more than half of the patients maintained a Psoriasis Area and Severity Index of 75 until the end of the study (48 weeks). Patients who received weight-based dosing had a better response than did patients who received the maximum dose. A delayed side effect of its use is the associated immunogenicity to the drug. The development of antietanercept antibodies was associated in 0% to 18% of patients, without apparent effect on effectiveness or adverse events.[30] Use of etanercept for pediatric psoriasis remains unapproved by the FDA.

INFECTIOUS DISEASES

Molluscum contagiosum (MC) is a viral infection caused by a DNA poxvirus, more common in children aged 1 to 10 years. Usually MC affects the trunk, legs, and arms, and the virus can spread from one part of the body to another by autoinoculation or to other people through close skin-to-skin contact. MC can persist for several months or, rarely, years. There is no general agreement regarding treatment because no single approach has been convincingly effective. The different approaches for MC attempt to minimize side effects and depend on the location and number of lesions. Recently, cantharidin, an old blistering agent, has been evaluated.[31] In this survey, 92% of respondents reported satisfaction with cantharidin efficacy, but 79% reported side effects, with discomfort or pain and blistering being most common. Treatment options of MC should always be individualized to specific patients, but cantharidin cannot be excluded.

Athlete's foot (tinea pedis) is an infection of the skin that causes scaling, flaking, and itching between the toes, with the space between the fourth and fifth digits most commonly afflicted. This disease is commonly caused by fungi (*Trichophyton rubrum* and *Trichophyton mentagrophytes* most commonly; rarely caused by *Candida* spp) living on moist surfaces. Tinea pedis can be complicated by bacterial superinfections (eg, *Pseudomonas* spp) that transform a trivial disturbance into a quite severe disease with painful blisters and fissures. A recent prospective cross-sectional study performed in 1305 children between the ages 3 and 15 years has evaluated the prevalence of tinea capitis, tinea pedis, and tinea unguium in children from several schools in

Barcelona (Spain) during 2003–2004.[32] The results of this study demonstrated a low prevalence of tinea capitis and tinea unguium but a high prevalence of dermatophyte carriage. In addition, the high prevalence of healthy carriers of dermatophytes in feet was observed. Another study[33] performed in Latin America on 1387 adolescents in 2006 confirmed the high prevalence of tinea pedis (62.6% of the infected subjects), although 38.5% of confirmed cases were asymptomatic. This observation suggests that an infection may develop without symptoms in the interdigital region of the foot. To prevent more severe disease in later life, perhaps earlier identification and treatment are indicated.

Superficial fungal infection is a common ailment directing teenagers to seek medical attention from dermatologists. The presence of these lesions may negatively affect the development of teenagers' personalities and self-esteem.[34] Because fungi thrive in moist environments, feet and footwear should be kept as dry as possible. Hygiene, therefore, plays an important role in managing an athlete's foot infection. Prevention is more important than treatment because the causative organisms are essentially ubiquitous. Schoolchildren and adolescents may be at lower risk because they often walk barefoot, by contrast. These same groups wear sports shoes mostly made with occlusive and near impermeable synthetic rubber. Enclosing feet in such shoes generates a moisture-rich environment that stimulates overgrowth of aerobic bacteria and infectious fungi. The natural remedy to suppress microbial growth would be to expose the feet to air to enhance evaporation, when possible, or to change the type of shoe to a leather, perspirant, well-ventilated model. But this obvious behavior, together with the doctor's advice (eg, use a separate towel for drying infected skin areas; dry feet well after showering, paying particular attention to the web space between the toes), is almost always ignored by adolescents. Young patients are advised to wear lightweight, absorbent socks. Among these socks, cotton fabric is usually advised, although it has been shown that dermatophytes were also isolated from the sole after taking off cotton socks. In contrast, few dermatophytes were isolated from the sole after taking off wool socks or "tabi" (traditional Japanese socks with a separation between the big toe and other toes).[35] Recently, engineered tissues (silver-coated fabrics) have been used to produce antimicrobial underwear and socks. Another "trick" that can help reduce moisture and friction is the use of the so-called 5-finger socks (**Figs. 5** and **6**). This type of footwear is stylish, easily accepted by youngsters, and keeps traditional foot powder (zinc oxide, kaolin, and talcum) or other innovative substances[36] closer to the skin surface.

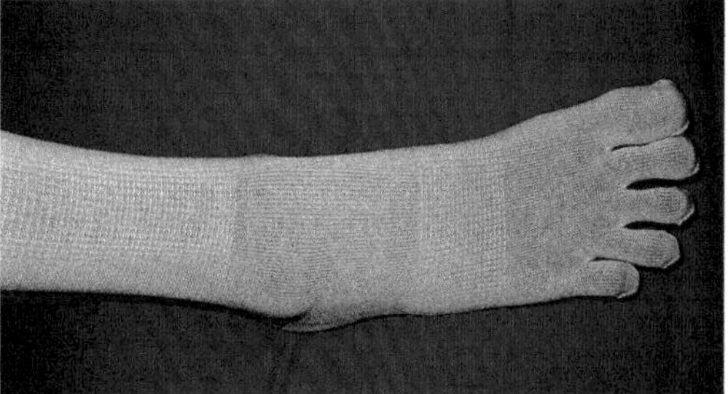

Fig. 5. A 5-finger sock. With this type of socks, the toes are always separated with 2 layers of tissue.

IMMUNE DISEASES

Alopecia Areata

The most common form of nonscarring hair loss in childhood is alopecia areata (AA); it may be patchy or involve any hair-bearing surface. Most children recover spontaneously, but sometimes the disorder demonstrates recurrent relapses or persistent hair loss. AA can cause great psychological distress, and the most important aspect of management is counseling the caregivers about the unpredictable nature and course of the disease. Although different modalities of treatment have been proposed to induce hair regrowth, there are only limited data on long-term efficacy and impact on quality of life. The most commonly used treatments are corticosteroids (topical, intralesional, and systemic), topical sensitizers, psoralen and UV-A phototherapy, topical minoxidil, and topical dithranol. A recent survey suggested that dermatologists recommend treatment less frequently for children than for adults and that offering no treatment for AA is relatively common.

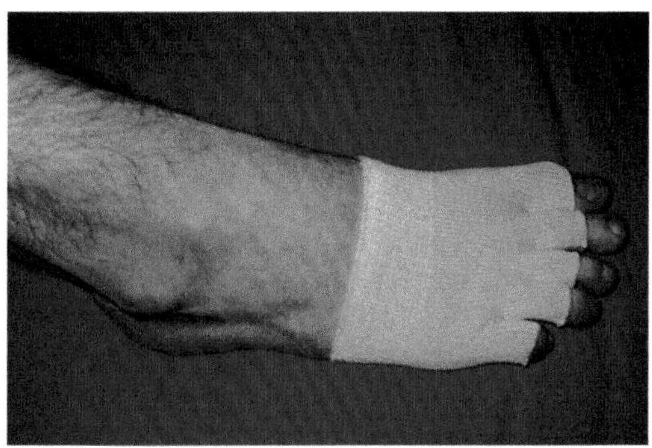

Fig. 6. A 5-finger sock. This model can be adopted by people who do not want to be seen wearing socks.

Thus, the article concludes that dermatologists' treatment of AA is inconsistent.[37]

Recently, photodynamic treatment (PDT) has been considered a new therapeutic option for extensive forms of AA. Although the precise pathophysiology of AA is not well understood, T lymphocytes are known to be involved in the pathogenesis of the disease. PDT could theoretically improve AA by inducing apoptosis in T lymphocytes clustered around hair follicles. However, many studies have been deceptive, including a recent one in which a special microneedle treatment system was used to enhance drug delivery.[38]

Because the inflammatory cytokine TNF-α has been hypothesized to be in connection with the development of AA, the TNF-α inhibitors have been cited as possible therapy. Nevertheless, some patients treated with TNF-α inhibitor for underlying diseases paradoxically developed AA. As a consequence, it is possible that TNF-α may not be involved in the pathogenesis of AA as in vitro studies have suggested.[39] Another study that aimed to assess the efficacy of alefacept for the treatment of severe AA failed to demonstrate a statistically significant improvement in AA when compared with a well-matched group receiving placebo.[40] In short, at present biologic drugs do not appear indicated for treating AA.

As no definitive treatment of AA has yet been introduced, it is understandable that many people use unconventional therapies for severe AA. This is especially true when AA affects children and parents fear aggressive or dangerous treatments and prefer homeopathic remedies (such as topical use of garlic and onions, both popular in many countries). For that reason, dermatologists should be aware of this tendency to use unconventional therapies and should guide patients toward the use of harmless treatments.

A few years ago, the effectiveness of topical crude onion juice in the treatment of patchy AA was reported. In a controlled study of 38 patients, divided into 2 groups (23 treated with onion juice and 15 treated with tap water), hair regrowth at 8 weeks of treatment was significantly higher among onion juice–treated group.[41] On the same premise, a combination of topical garlic gel and betamethasone valerate cream in the treatment of localized AA was studied more recently. In this study,[42] 40 patients were randomly divided into 2 groups, garlic gel treated and placebo. The 2 groups were advised to follow the treatment twice daily, for 3 months. Both groups received topical application of corticosteroid (betamethasone cream 0.1% in isopropyl alcohol) twice daily. The first group (garlic gel treated) consisted of 20 patients (12 men [60%] and 8 women [40%]), and the second group (control) consisted of 20 patients (10 men [50%] and 10 women [50%]). At the end of the treatment, good and moderate responses were observed in 19 (95%) and 1 (5%) patient of the garlic gel–treated group, respectively, that which was significantly better than the control group ($P = .001$).

As far as it concerns garlic and onion (which are botanically related), both are claimed to have hair growth–promoting properties, but the scientific basis for this claim is lacking.[43] Onion and garlic contain diallyl disulfide, which may provide their therapeutic effects through an irritative and/or immune mechanism. The high spontaneous remission rate of AA makes it difficult to clearly assess the true efficacy of any given therapy. Given the innocuous nature of this treatment, the authors have recently treated a 7-year-old boy with an inherited, recalcitrant form of AA with crude onion juice during summer twice daily for 2 months with moderate benefit (**Figs. 7** and **8**). Whether this regrowth is because of sun exposure, onion juice, or a combination of the two or simply because of coincidence will always be questionable.

Vitiligo

Vitiligo, a frequent depigmenting skin disease, affects adults and children, but in about half of patients the onset of disorder is before 20 years of age. The most common clinical variant is nonsegmental vitiligo; however, the prevalence of segmental vitiligo has been found to be higher in

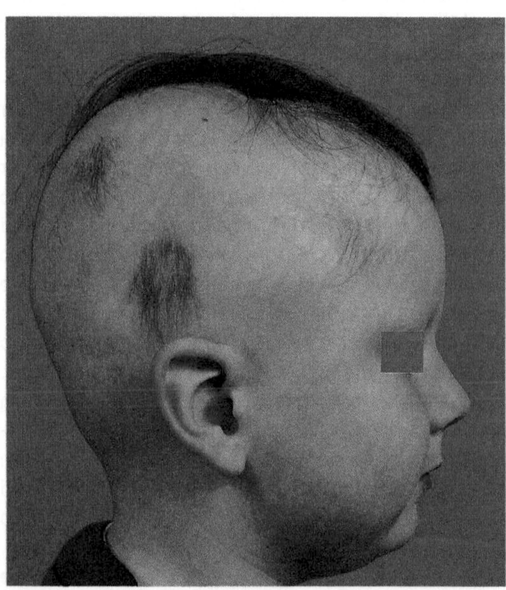

Fig. 7. A boy with severe AA that was resistant to topical steroids. Intralesional steroids gave limited results only at the site of injection.

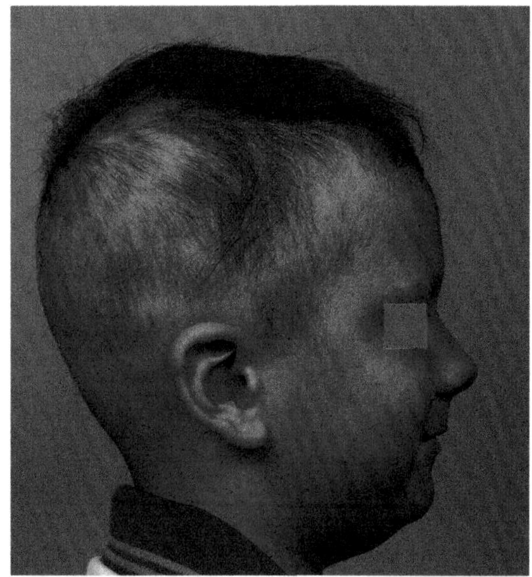

Fig. 8. The same patient after 3 months of treatment with topical crude onion juice (and after the summer season).

children compared with that in adults. At present, there is no cure for the disease, but new data on combined regimens are available. Topical therapy seemed to improve with the advent of TCI use, but the response is slow and limited to the thinnest skin areas. Narrow-band UV-B and UV-B are the most common treatments administered in children, but with variable response. Recently some studies reported that a 308-nm monochromatic excimer light is more effective than narrow-band UV-B in treating vitiligo lesions, inducing repigmentation more rapidly.[44]

Narrow-band UV-B radiation has proved to be effective in the treatment of widespread disease, and the authors recommend it as first-line therapy. In the case of localized disease, treatment should be started with a potent topical corticosteroid or TCI; on the face, TCIs, especially tacrolimus, are currently preferred because of the potential side effects of prolonged application of corticosteroids. The long-term safety of these molecules requires further study.[45] Surgical techniques, such as minigrafting and transplantation of autologous epidermal cell suspensions, are not recommended for children. The skin barrier is not altered in vitiligo compared with AD; hence, tacrolimus should be used at the highest available concentration (ie, 0.1%) also in children.

Scleroderma

Progressive facial hemiatrophy is a rare condition, usually occurring within the first 2 decades of life and characterized by slowly progressive atrophy of one side of the face involving the subcutaneous tissue and fat. Localized scleroderma (LS) and Parry-Romberg syndrome can cause facial hemiatrophy, sometimes associated with neurologic complications. It remains unclear whether these 2 conditions represent different clinical entities or belong to the same spectrum of disease. The patients are often treated with potent immunosuppressive agents, such as corticosteroids, cyclosporine, and methotrexate. In some patients, thermography and Doppler ultrasonography show active inflammation despite the systemic therapeutic strategy. Phototherapy, in particular use of UV-A1, seems to be an effective therapeutic option in patients with progressive facial hemiatrophy. UV-A1 phototherapy is an antiinflammatory treatment modality that influences fibroblast functions. An open, nonblinded, uncontrolled study was conducted on 30 adult patients with LS to evaluate sclerotic skin plaques before and after medium-dose UV-A1 therapy.[46] This study showed a positive short- and long-term efficacy of UV-A1 phototherapy in patients with LS, with a reduction in sclerotic plaques, an increase in skin elasticity, and a reduction of lesional skin thickness.

At present there are no reported results for UV-A1 phototherapy in pediatric population, but in selected cases a good control of the disease has been observed (Altomare GF and Gelmetti C, unpublished data, 2010). Further controlled studies investigating the efficacy of UV-A irradiation in connective tissue diseases are needed. The restoration of contour and symmetry of face of the patients has been achieved by autologous fat transplantation. However, this technique has not been used primarily in treating patients with hemifacial atrophy, and its efficacy and long-term outcome remain unknown.[47]

GENODERMATOSES

For all inherited skin diseases, the classical treatment has always been symptomatic in nature and to avoid triggering factors, such as mechanical trauma in epidermolysis bullosa (EB) and UV irradiation in xeroderma pigmentosum. Gene therapy, cell therapy, protein therapy, and gene silencing therapy are the new treatment horizons for genodermatoses.

Gene therapy with retroviral vectors corrected the underlying defect in a 36-year-old man affected by nonlethal junctional EB.[48] This study, with a follow-up of 4 years, showed that transplantation of autologous cultured epidermis derived from genetically corrected epidermal stem cells is feasible, is well tolerated, and leads to long-term cure. Other studies have highlighted the possibility of using allogeneic cells as a way of delivering type VII collagen to the dermal-epidermal junction and therefore as a treatment for dystrophic EB. These include local injection of fibroblasts obtained from healthy donors and expanded in culture and transplantation of bone marrow–derived hematopoietic stem cells.[49]

Gene silencing can be obtained through various oligonucleotides (ONs), which are synthetic fragments of nucleic acid designed to modulate the expression of target proteins. DNA-based ONs (antisense, antigene, aptamer, or decoy) and, more recently, a new class of RNA-based ONs, the small interfering RNAs, could be used in different diseases, including genodermatoses.[50] The ethical and practical problems connected with the treatment of genodermatoses remain to be thoroughly discussed, but the development of skin stem cells may also offer a chance at tremendous progress.

REFERENCES

1. Bennett ML, Fleischer AB, Chamlin SL, et al. Oral corticosteroid use is effective for cutaneous hemangiomas. Arch Dermatol 2001;137:1208–13.
2. Batta K, Goodyear HM, Moss C, et al. Randomised controlled study of early pulsed dye laser treatment of uncomplicated childhood haemangiomas: results of a 1-year analysis. Lancet 2002;360:521–7.
3. Mulliken JB, Fishman SJ, Burrows PE. Vascular anomalies. Curr Probl Surg 2000;37:517–84.
4. Bruckner AL, Frieden IJ. Hemangiomas of infancy. J Am Acad Dermatol 2003;48:477–93.
5. Perez J, Pardo J, Gomez C. Vincristine: an effective treatment of corticoid-resistant life-threatening infantile hemangiomas. Acta Oncol 2002;41:197–9.
6. Kaplan M, Paller A. Clinical pearl: use of self-adhesive, compressive wraps in the treatment of limb hemangiomas. J Am Acad Dermatol 1995;32:117–8.
7. Tanner JL, Dechert MP, Frieden IJ. Growing up with a facial haemangioma: parent and child coping and adaptation. Pediatrics 1998;101:446–52.
8. Frieden IJ, Eichenfield LF, Esterly NB, et al. Guidelines of care for hemangiomas of infancy. American Academy of Dermatology Guidelines/Outcomes Committee. J Am Acad Dermatol 1997;37:631–7.
9. David LR, Malek MM, Argenta LC. Efficacy of pulse dye laser therapy for the treatment of ulcerated hemangiomas: a review of 78 patients. Br J Plast Surg 2003;56:317–27.
10. Stier MF, Glick SA, Hirsch RJ. Laser treatment of pediatric vascular lesions: port wine stains and hemangiomas. J Am Acad Dermatol 2008;58(2):261–85.
11. Cordisco MR. An update on lasers in children. Curr Opin Pediatr 2009;21(4):499–504.
12. Leauté-Labreze C, Dumas de la Roque E, Hubiche F, et al. Propranolol for severe hemangiomas of infancy. N Engl J Med 2008;358:2649–51.
13. Lawley LP, Siegfried E, Todd JL. Propranolol treatment for hemangioma of infancy: risks and recommendations. Pediatr Dermatol 2009;26(5):610–4.
14. Sans V, Dumas de la Roque E, Berge J, et al. Propranolol for severe infantile hemangiomas: follow-up report. Pediatrics 2009;124:e423–31.
15. Bonifazi E, Colonna V, Mazzotta F, et al. Propranolol in rapidly growing hemangiomas. Eur J Pediatr Dermatol 2008;18:185–92.
16. Howell MD, Kim BE, Gao P, et al. Cytokine modulation of atopic dermatitis filaggrin skin expression. J Allergy Clin Immunol 2009;124(3 Suppl 2):R7–12.
17. Eberlein B, Eicke C, Reinhardt HW, et al. Adjuvant treatment of atopic eczema: assessment of an emollient containing N-palmitoylethanolamine (ATOPA study). J Eur Acad Dermatol Venereol 2008;22(1):73–82.
18. Msika P, De Belilovsky C, Piccardi N, et al. New emollient with topical corticosteroid-sparing effect in treatment of childhood atopic dermatitis: SCORAD and quality of life improvement. Pediatr Dermatol 2008;25(6):606–12.
19. Stinco G, Piccirillo F, Valent F. A randomized double-blind study to investigate the clinical efficacy of adding a non-migrating antimicrobial to a special silk fabric in the treatment of atopic dermatitis. Dermatology 2008;217:191–5.
20. Senti G, Steinmann LS, Fischer B, et al. Antimicrobial silk clothing in the treatment of atopic dermatitis proves comparable to topical corticosteroid treatment. Dermatology 2006;213(3):228–33.
21. Thaçi D, Reitamo S, Gonzalez Ensenat MA, et al. Proactive disease management with 0.03% tacrolimus ointment for children with atopic dermatitis: results of a randomized, multicentre, comparative study. Br J Dermatol 2008;159(6):1348–56.
22. Arellano FM, Arana A, Wentworth CE, et al. Lymphoma among patients with atopic dermatitis and/or treated with topical immunosuppressants in the United Kingdom. J Allergy Clin Immunol 2009;123(5):1111–6.
23. Allakhverdi Z, Comeau MR, Jessup HK, et al. Thymic stromal lymphopoietin is released by human epithelial cells in response to microbes, trauma, or inflammation and potently activates mast cells. J Exp Med 2007;204(2):253–8.
24. He R, Oyoshi MK, Garibyan L, et al. TSLP acts on infiltrating effector T cells to drive allergic skin inflammation. Proc Natl Acad Sci U S A 2008;105(33):11875.
25. Hatano Y, Man MQ, Uchida Y, et al. Maintenance of an acidic stratum corneum prevents emergence of

murine atopic dermatitis. J Invest Dermatol 2009;129(7):1824–35.
26. Huang JT, Abrams M, Tlougan B, et al. Treatment of Staphylococcus aureus colonization in atopic dermatitis decreases disease severity. Pediatrics 2009;123(5):e808–14.
27. Hata TR, Kotol P, Jackson M, et al. Administration of oral vitamin D induces cathelicidin production in atopic individuals. J Allergy Clin Immunol 2008;122(4):829–31.
28. Li M, Hener P, Zhang Z, et al. Induction of thymic stromal lymphopoietin expression in keratinocytes is necessary for generating an atopic dermatitis upon application of the active vitamin D3 analogue MC903 on mouse skin. J Invest Dermatol 2009;129(2):498–502.
29. Paller AS, Siegfried EC, Langley RG, et al. Etanercept treatment for children and adolescents with plaque psoriasis. N Engl J Med 2008;358(3):241–51.
30. Emi Aikawa N, de Carvalho JF, Artur Almeida Silva C, et al. Immunogenicity of anti-TNF-alpha agents in autoimmune diseases. Clin Rev Allergy Immunol 2010;38(2–3):82–9.
31. Coloe J, Morrell DS. Cantharidin use among pediatric dermatologists in the treatment of molluscum contagiosum. Pediatr Dermatol 2009;26:405–8.
32. Pérez-González M, Torres-Rodríguez JM, Martínez-Roig A, et al. Prevalence of tinea pedis, tinea unguium of toenails and tinea capitis in school children from Barcelona. Rev Iberoam Micol 2009;26(4):228–32.
33. Flores JM, Castillo VB, Franco FC, et al. Superficial fungal infections: clinical and epidemiological study in adolescents from marginal districts of Lima and Callao, Peru. J Infect Dev Ctries 2009;3(4):313–7.
34. Welsh O, Welsh E, Ocampo-Candiani J, et al. Dermatophytoses in Monterrey, México. Mycoses 2006;49:119–23.
35. Watanabe K, Taniguchi H, Nishioka K, et al. [Preventive effects of various socks against adhesion of dermatophytes to healthy feet]. Nippon Ishinkin Gakkai Zasshi 2000;41(3):183–6 [in Japanese].
36. Misner BD. A novel aromatic oil compound inhibits microbial overgrowth on feet: a case study. J Int Soc Sports Nutr 2007;4:3.
37. Mukherjee N, Morrell DS, Duvic M, et al. Attitudes of dermatologists in the southeastern United States regarding treatment of alopecia areata: a cross-sectional survey study. BMC Dermatol 2009;9(1):11.
38. Lee JW, Yoo KH, Kim BJ, et al. Photodynamic therapy with methyl 5-aminolevulinate acid combined with microneedle treatment in patients with extensive alopecia areata. Clin Exp Dermatol November 3, 2009 [online].
39. Kirshen C, Kanigsberg N. Alopecia areata following adalimumab. J Cutan Med Surg 2009;13(1):48–50.
40. Strober BE, Menon K, McMichael A, et al. Alefacept for severe alopecia areata: a randomized, double-blind, placebo-controlled study. Arch Dermatol 2009;145(11):1262–6.
41. Sharquie KE, Al-Obaidi HK. Onion juice (Allium cepa L.), a new topical treatment for alopecia areata. J Dermatol 2002;29(6):343–6.
42. Hajheydari Z, Jamshidi M, Akbari J, et al. Combination of topical garlic gel and betamethasone valerate cream in the treatment of localized alopecia areata: a double-blind randomized controlled study. Indian J Dermatol Venereol Leprol 2007;73(1):29–32.
43. Gönül M, Gül U, Cakmak SK, et al. Unconventional medicine in dermatology outpatients in Turkey. Int J Dermatol 2009;48(6):639–44.
44. Casacci M, Thomas P, Pacifico A, et al. Comparison between 308-nm monochromatic excimer light and narrowband UVB phototherapy (311–313 nm) in the treatment of vitiligo—a multicentre controlled study. J Eur Acad Dermatol Venereol 2007;21(7):956–63.
45. Taïeb A, Picardo M. Clinical practice. Vitiligo. N Engl J Med 2009;360(2):160–9.
46. Andres C, Kollmar A, Mempel M, et al. Successful ultraviolet A1 phototherapy in the treatment of localized scleroderma: a retrospective and prospective study. Br J Dermatol 2010;162:445–7.
47. Xie Y, Li Q, Zheng D, et al. Correction of hemifacial atrophy with autologous fat transplantation. Ann Plast Surg 2007;59(6):645–53.
48. De Luca M, Pellegrini G, Mavilio F. Gene therapy of inherited skin adhesion disorders: a critical overview. Br J Dermatol 2009;161(1):19–24.
49. Long HA, McMillan JR, Qiao H, et al. Current advances in gene therapy for the treatment of genodermatoses. Curr Gene Ther 2009;9(6):487–94.
50. Heo I, Kim VN. Regulating the regulators: posttranslational modifications of RNA silencing factors. Cell 2009;139(1):28–31.

Index

Note: Page numbers of article titles are in **boldface** type.

Dermatol Clin 28 (2010) 631–637
doi:10.1016/S0733-8635(10)00107-5
0733-8635/10/$ – see front matter © 2010 Elsevier Inc. All rights reserved.

derm.theclinics.com

U

V

W

Z

Moving?

Make sure your subscription moves with you!

To notify us of your new address, find your **Clinics Account Number** (located on your mailing label above your name), and contact customer service at:

Email: journalscustomerservice-usa@elsevier.com

800-654-2452 **(subscribers in the U.S. & Canada)**
314-447-8871 **(subscribers outside of the U.S. & Canada)**

Fax number: 314-447-8029

Elsevier Health Sciences Division
Subscription Customer Service
3251 Riverport Lane
Maryland Heights, MO 63043

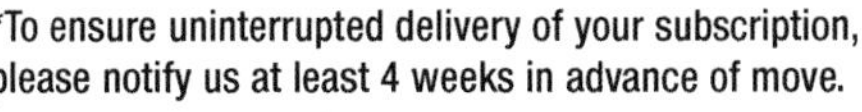
*To ensure uninterrupted delivery of your subscription, please notify us at least 4 weeks in advance of move.

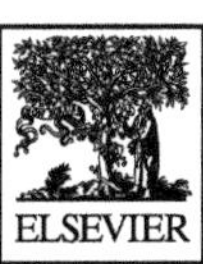